FLOORED

A Woman's Guide to Pelvic Floor Health at Every Age and Stage

Dr. Sara Reardon, PT, DPT, WCS

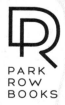

PARK
ROW
BOOKS

PARK
ROW
BOOKS™

Recycling programs
for this product may
not exist in your area.

ISBN-13: 978-0-7783-1053-2

Floored: A Woman's Guide to Pelvic Floor Health at Every Age and Stage

Medical Illustrations by Anna Bessmertnaia

TM is a trademark of Harlequin Enterprises ULC.

Park Row Books
22 Adelaide St. West, 41st Floor
Toronto, Ontario M5H 4E3, Canada
ParkRowBooks.com

Printed in U.S.A.

To all my people and their pelvic floors.

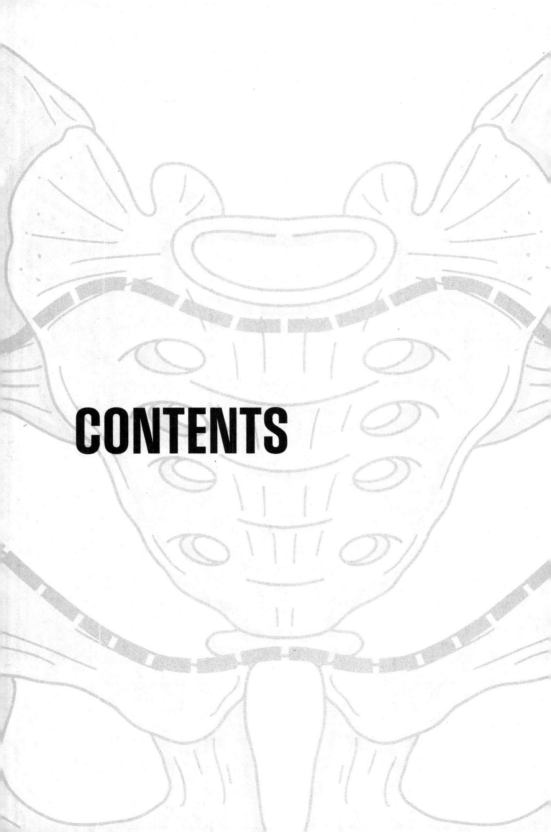

CONTENTS

The Current State of Down-There Care

If you fall, I'll be there.
—FLOOR

It starts when we are young—when we get our periods. When we first see blood, we feel scared. When the adults around us talk about it in hushed tones, we grow ashamed, as if discussions about our bodies should be hidden. As we get older, we slip tampons up our shirtsleeves when walking into bathrooms and roll used panty liners into toilet paper to hide them in trash cans. If we have a baby or menopause looms, we start wearing black pants instead of colorful ones in case we leak a little urine. We avoid intimacy with our partners because of pain, or perhaps worse, we silently endure sexual discomfort for fear of letting our partners down. When it comes to "down there," hushed conversations have become too much of the norm.

Women suffer in silence because our pelvic floors are not the priority in our healthcare system. In fact, we might not even know what a pelvic floor is. And when a pelvic floor issue arises, we are presented with three options:

1. Treat your symptoms by spending money on an array of medications and elaborate devices.
2. Have surgery or procedures to "rejuvenate" your vagina.
3. Deal with it.

If you are a woman, the culture of silence around matters relating to your vagina began when you were a teen, or even younger. And since then, pelvic health problems are either dismissed or you are presented with an extreme fix.

My patient Beth is just one example of many. When she first came to see me, her eyes were full of worry. Forty-five years old, a mom of two, and a surgical nurse at a hospital, she spent her days lifting patients in and out of bed and her evenings hoisting strollers, groceries, and kids into her SUV. Her children were growing like weeds, some of her patients were two times her size, and she felt like she could handle all of it . . . until one evening.

She was in the shower after a long day, rinsing her lower body, when she felt a lump at the opening of her vagina. She panicked, as one does when they feel a lump anywhere near down there. Concerned about cancer or an abnormal growth, she immediately made an appointment with her gynecologist. After a visual inspection lasting not even a minute, her doctor had an answer. "It's nothing unusual!" her doctor proclaimed. "Your bladder is falling out of your vagina. It's called prolapse and happens to a lot of women. Just don't lift anything too heavy."

That's it. Just don't lift anything too heavy.

As relieved as one would be to hear, "It's not cancer," a bladder falling out of your body still isn't good news. Beth's care that day was grossly insufficient, but it's also all too common. She is just one of many women who have left her doctor's appointment feeling dismissed, frustrated, and scared.

Over the past two decades in my pelvic floor therapy practice, I've treated thousands of women like Beth who, before seeing me, were denied open conversations and real tools to manage their pelvic floor problems. In every direction, we hear narratives that undermine the intimate issues women experience:

- Commercials advertising incontinence liners send the message to consumers that leaking is just part of being a lady (when physical therapy can improve or prevent this).
- Trusted medical professionals view pelvic organ prolapse as a normal part of motherhood (so countless women make do with unrelenting pelvic pain).
- Medications for an overactive bladder promise a better quality of life (but don't mind the laundry list of side effects).
- Scented vaginal washes declare a fresher, cleaner vagina (when vaginas aren't dirty and only water is needed to rinse them).

Nearly one in three women suffers from a pelvic floor disorder—from painful sex to prolapse, back pain to constipation, and urinary leakage to lack of orgasms. Although pelvic floor issues are common, they are *not* normal. But most of us aren't taught what the pelvic floor actually is, let alone how to care for it. So if problems begin to develop, we aren't equipped to identify them, and we are left completely unaware there are a number of noninvasive treatments available to us. Then we are blindsided when those problems become full-blown.

These conditions compromise our self-esteem, mental health, intimate relationships, ability to exercise, and even our pocketbooks. Over *20 billion dollars* a year is spent on treating urinary leakage in women in the United States alone. Some of these treatments are effective, mostly temporarily, and most of them just treat the symptoms without addressing the underlying pelvic floor dysfunction. This is the equivalent of putting a Band-Aid over the problem and why 30% of women who have surgery to fix a pelvic floor problem will require a repeat surgery for the same condition.

Too often we are met with responses that perpetuate a culture of defeat rather than empowerment. As a result, we start to accept that leakage, pain, and prolapse *are* just a normal part of life for people with vaginas. (*They are not.*) We feel embarrassed or broken. (*You aren't.*) We no longer trust our bodies. (*You will again.*) And we believe there is no other way. (*There is.*)

The Business of Our Business

With the rise of social media use and increased focus on self-care in the post-#MeToo era, there is a surge of products, procedures, and even formalwear bringing vaginas and vulvas into the spotlight and raising awareness that women are simply not getting the care we deserve. In 2018, the Vagina Museum opened in London as the world's first brick-and-mortar museum dedicated to the female reproductive system. In 2020, women's wellness company Goop launched a vagina-scented candle for $75 a pop . . . and it sold out! In 2024, actress Gillian Anderson wore a dress covered in images of vulvas to an awards show, and it went viral.

With every passing year, I see more and more consumer brands offering gadgets and creams promising your best vagina yet. The female intimate wellness industry in the United States is estimated to be roughly $5 billion dollars—and it will continue to grow. Vaginas have become big business, and you'd think that the more coverage vaginas and vulvas get, the better, right?

My answer is, theoretically, yes. Increased awareness pushes our society and medical system forward to recognize the deficits in women's healthcare and start taking steps to improve it. Yet this awareness simultaneously spawned a vulvovaginal and pelvic wellness industry focused on making one's vagina feel better, smell better, taste better, or look better but not necessarily *function* better. The emphasis sometimes seems to be how to make your vagina trendier rather than healthier. The real issues, the real problems, are still hush-hush. We moved from using medications, procedures, or total dismissal of vaginal and pelvic health issues to using vibrating chairs, scented washes, and libido gummies as alternative options for healthcare.

Some women's health and pelvic health brands perpetuate the narrative that vaginas are dirty, smelly, or unattractive by constantly bombarding women with products and procedures that are aimed to *improve* their vaginas when, in fact, there may be nothing wrong with their vaginas in the first place. Many of these trending products can actually diminish your pelvic health versus improve it, leading to a disruption of the vulvo-vaginal microbiome, increased risk of infection, onset of pelvic floor tension, or zero effect at all. And they can be a waste of money . . . and hope. Not to mention, many of the trends focus almost entirely on our vaginas—when the attention for true health down there needs to include the entire pelvic floor.

Women may be growing more comfortable talking about their vaginas, but we have a long way to go. Many women still carry so much shame and do not get meaningful advice for treatment or prevention of problems. While more attention on the vulva and vagina is great, we need to clarify which practices are actual *health*care. Health refers to a state where the body is free from disease. Wellness is a bit like putting fancy light fixtures in a house when it may not even have walls yet. As a culture, our attention needs to turn toward true healthcare for women. So let me put on my pelvic floor therapist hat to give you real advice for your vagina and pelvic floor.

The Vagina Whisperer

In 2017, I started making videos for social media dressed in a stuffed vulva costume to call attention to the extreme lack of quality down-there care. I named this account what my friends had been calling me for years: The Vagina Whisperer. Pregnant with my second child at the time, I shared all kinds of information from simple tips like "squeeze when you sneeze" to stretches that can ease painful sex to more advanced protocols to prepare for childbirth. I wanted to educate women about their pelvic floor, give them the tools to support their pelvic health, and offer them ideas for how to advocate for themselves with their healthcare providers. There is *so much* women can do daily to manage and improve pelvic floor issues, and even more, to prevent pelvic floor problems from arising. The instant and significant social media following was a testament that women wanted—no, *needed*—this information so badly that they were turning to a dancing vulva on social media to learn about their bodies.

When I started "vagina whispering," I'd already been a pelvic floor physical therapist for over a decade, having chosen pelvic floor health as my specialty immediately after graduate school. One of my professors was a pioneer in the field and offered a handful of lectures about the pelvic floor muscles that made my jaw drop.

> Tense muscles can cause constipation? *Mind blown!*
> Pushing your pee out is bad? *Who knew!?*
> Orgasms are pelvic floor muscle contractions? *Really?!!*
> Pelvic floor tightness can impact both sexual pleasure
> and our ability to give birth? *Wait, wait, wait, whhhhhhat?*

I loved learning how *my* body worked. Once I started working with patients, I loved teaching them about how *their* bodies worked. Whether they were experiencing prolapse, leakage, hemorrhoids, painful sex, or even tailbone pain, there were muscles in their pelvic floor that were responsible. Simply that . . . muscles! Nothing freaky. Nothing weird. Nothing scary. Just muscles. As a pelvic floor physical therapist (PT) for decades now, I myself remain "floored" over the number of women who are still suffering from pelvic floor dysfunction when there is so much that can be done to help them.

Forty-five percent of new mothers will experience birth trauma, like my patient Claire who wanted to have a second baby but was terrified after her first birth entailed hours of pushing and an emergency C-section.

One in four women will have pain with sex at some point in her lifetime, like my patient Deidre, who could not consummate her marriage because sex was so painful. Once she finally worked up the courage to tell her gynecologist, she was told to "just relax and use more lube."

Over 70% of menopausal women wake frequently at nighttime to pee, like my patient Marsha, who was waking eight to ten times at night to pee and experienced a fall when rushing to the bathroom in the dark.

All three of these women found their way to pelvic floor therapy. They were taught exercises and simple habitual adjustments to improve their discomfort, pelvic floor function, and quality of life. All of them finally felt seen, understood, and hopeful during their treatment. But each and every one asked the same question: *Why didn't anyone tell me about pelvic floor therapy sooner?*

In the pages that follow, I will tell you about all things pelvic floor. Contrary to popular belief, pelvic floor problems don't just affect aging or birthing women. They can affect anyone with a pelvic floor, *which is everyone.* In my practice, and in letters I've received from patients and followers, I have seen and heard countless success stories—about how learning to pee and poop properly helped manage prolapse, how stretches and working with vaginal dilators led to enjoyable sex after years of pain, how they were confident traveling again and no longer feared not being close to a restroom, and how they could now pick up their toddlers without back pain and they no longer spent their evenings with a heating pad and ibuprofen. I've written *Floored* because I want this, and more, for you.

I've titled this book *Floored* because it captures the awe that I feel over one of my favorite (and arguably one of the most important) parts of our body: the pelvic floor. I know that while reading this, you too will be surprised, and sometimes astonished, by what you will learn.

Some of you may have *heard* of the pelvic floor, but for many it's still a mystical part of the body. What does it actually do? And how do you know if there's a problem? Or even more, that it needs therapy? In Chapter 1, I get the party started by diving deep into both the anatomy and the function of the pelvic floor and show how it's connected to almost every part of our daily lives as women (breathing, peeing, pooping, sex, menstruation, pregnancy, birth, and menopause). In Chapter 2, I teach you the basics of how to care for it. And from Chapter 3 onward, we will look at each "system" and "passageway" of the pelvic floor, how it changes, and what it needs through the different seasons of a woman's life. In each chapter, I get real about the pelvic floor problems that can arise and offer techniques and exercises to relieve them. At the end of this book, my hope is that you:

1. Understand how the pelvic floor muscles play a role in your day-to-day function.
2. Tune in to your own body to identify if there is a pelvic floor issue that warrants addressing.
3. Implement strategies *right now* to help prevent or address pelvic floor problems.
4. Feel empowered to speak with your healthcare provider.
5. Share this information with your friends, daughters, sisters, mothers, grandmothers, and all people in your life with vaginas so others don't suffer silently.

Whether you're here for general pelvic health knowledge or for a solution to a specific problem, this book will provide information, tips, exercises, and other resources you need throughout your life.

I also can't write this book without addressing three very important topics. First, in an effort to simplify language, I use the words *woman, women, mom,* etc. throughout. I recognize that some people with vaginas don't identify as women, and some people who birth babies don't identify as moms. This book is, however, for everyone with a pelvic floor.

Second, this book is not one-size-fits-all. It's one-size-fits-*most*. In the coming chapters, my goal is to educate, support, and empower you, but the exercises and practices are not a replacement for individualized medical care. If you feel you would benefit from one-on-one support, I encourage you to see a licensed medical provider and pelvic health specialist.

Third, and most importantly, the challenges I mention in this book can affect all women and all races, but it is clear from research, statistics, and my own personal experience that women of color experience medical gaslighting, trauma, and inadequate medical care to a much greater extent. As much as I encourage advocating for oneself and offer guidance on approaching medical providers, systemic racism will continue to play a role in how women of color are treated in our society and throughout our healthcare systems. At the end of this book, I have included a list of organizations actively working to improve women's and maternal healthcare, particularly for people of color.

The New Normal

Remember my patient Beth from earlier who was told that the solution to her prolapse was to not lift anything heavy? After her disappointing doctor's visit, she went down a rabbit hole on Google and found my clinic. She proceeded to drive two hours each way to see me for pelvic floor therapy. After six one-hour sessions, Beth reported feeling 80% better. Her bladder prolapse was not completely gone, but she had the tools to improve her symptoms and prevent it from getting worse. She felt empowered. She understood her body. She no longer felt broken. This is what's possible.

I can't promise that I will cure your pelvic floor problem, you'll never leak again, sex will *always* be pleasurable, or your back will be pain-free. But I can promise that you will better understand your body and that you can find relief. You will feel less broken and alone, and more hopeful and empowered.

I told a friend that after I finished writing this book, I was going to create an event called "Running of the Vulvas" in New Orleans, where I live. A bunch of folks dressed as vulvas running down the streets would not be *that* odd as this city annually hosts a Naked Bike Ride, a Red Dress Run, and a Zombie Run. "But what are you trying to achieve?" he asked. "Wouldn't it be weird if there were a bunch of people dressed as penises running down the street?"

Fair question, and here's my response: women are screaming at the medical system and the world to pay attention to us. Medical gaslighting is more likely to happen to women than to men. More moms are dying in the first year after childbirth in the United States than any other developed country in the world. Currently twenty states in the US still have a tampon tax, which taxes menstrual products as nonessential "luxury goods" while Viagra, a well-known prescription erectile dysfunction drug for men, is not taxed in any state except for one. We as women are literally penalized, taxed, and often dismissed for having vaginas. My idea for Running of the Vulvas, and for writing *Floored*, is to say, "Pay attention to women. Pay attention to our vulvas, our vaginas, and of course, our pelvic floors." Let's get started. The pelvic floor revolution starts now.

PART 1
GETTING THE PELVIC FLOOR PARTY STARTED

CHAPTER 1

Pulling Back the Curtains

When I started PT school as a bright-eyed twenty-two-year-old, I planned to become a sports physical therapist. I was an avid runner and loved learning about the human body. The idea of spending my career helping people move better and feel better excited me. In high school, I ran track and loved the way exercise, and particularly running, made me feel. It required minimal equipment (just socks, shoes, and a good sports bra) and gave me the opportunity to be outside, breathe in fresh air, and feel free. I ran through my first heartbreak—crying as I rounded the corners in my neighborhood. I ran through college, five hundred miles away from home for the first time and often lonely in my dorm room. And I ran through the devastation of losing my family's home in Hurricane Katrina in 2005. Running was how I cleared my mind, healed my heart, battled depression, and settled my nerves. I wanted everyone to be able to exercise and move to feel that same release that running gave me.

In my second year of PT school, I was taking a class on specialty areas of physical therapy. The professor, Dr. Spitznagle (or Spitz, as we called her), spent two weeks lecturing on pelvic floor physical therapy. She introduced us to the pelvic floor muscles, which help us day in and day out with countless bodily functions like peeing, pooping, having sex, having a period, and even . . . exercising. All of a sudden, I understood that movement and function weren't just a matter of having a strong core and solid running legs; they also depended on having a healthy, well-functioning pelvic floor. I realized that problems related to the pelvic floor muscles could prevent people from doing almost everything they love—including running. If a woman has a pelvic floor problem, for example, she might leak urine when running or need to pee every fifteen minutes, both of which may force her to stop. During pregnancy, if a woman experiences hip pain that isn't treated, she might not be able to complete the recommended thirty minutes of daily exercise. A healthy pelvic floor, it turned out, was integral to healthy movement and exercise.

Learning how these complex and sophisticated muscles (that no one was openly talking about) work during our everyday activities not only fascinated me but also helped me understand my own body as a woman. When I took a bathroom break between those lectures, I found myself rethinking how I performed basic functions: *Wait, I should sit down to pee and not hover. Okay, don't push when you pee; just breathe and let your muscles relax.*

Out of the sixty-seven students in my graduating class, I was the only one who jumped right into practicing as a pelvic floor physical therapist. My early patients included a college-aged woman struggling with constipation, a fifty-year-old woman experiencing painful sex after breast cancer treatment, and an elderly woman with urinary leakage who stopped playing cards at the senior center because she was worried about the odor of her incontinence pads. These women were distraught and unable to enjoy basic activities—from gardening and walking to biking and carrying young children—that many of us take for granted. They also felt like their bodies were failing them.

Pelvic floor issues can limit us in countless ways. And I want all women to be able to pick up their toddlers, to enjoy their sex lives well into old age, to travel and socialize with friends, and to run or dance or hike or do any of the amazing activities that having a human body allows us to do.

A Bowl of Goodness

Before PT school, I had never heard the term "pelvic floor." This term has recently become more widely known with the help of social media and news articles that are slowly turning their focus onto this critical part of our body. But back then, when I told folks what I did as my specialty, I often heard: "*Why is it called a floor?*" We call it your pelvic floor because:

1. It literally acts as the floor supporting your pelvic organs.
2. Along with your abdominal and back muscles, it provides core stability for your entire body.
3. Like any floor or structure in a house, if you don't maintain and care for this foundation, things can start to crumble.

Your pelvic floor is a body part, just like your knee or shoulder, and can suffer an injury. But because our culture teaches that we should be hush-hush about anything happening in the region from our belly buttons to our thighs, we end up far more in the dark about what can go wrong in this arena. Every vagina owner deserves to know how these parts of her body work, so when something is off, we have an understanding of what could be the culprit. With that, let's dive into the anatomy of your floor.

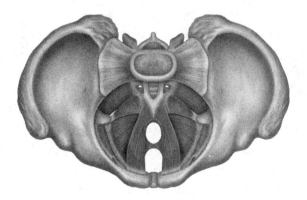

Pelvis and pelvic floor muscles: a view from above

YOUR PELVIS

Envision the white bones on the black skeleton jammies you see during Halloween or the skeleton model you've seen hanging in your doctor's office. Most likely, those two elephant-ear–shaped bones at the bottom of the spine stand out. You've seen images of the pelvis throughout your life, and unknowingly, you feel and touch your pelvic bones dozens of times throughout the day. Follow along with me to identify these bones, your iliac crests, ischial tuberosities, and pubic bones, which are all connected and create your pelvis.

1. Place your hand on your hips and squeeze in. The bones you feel are the top part of your pelvis. They are the elephant ears you see in most images and are called your iliac crests.
2. Sit down. The bones you can feel deep in your tush, supporting your weight, are the bottom part of your pelvis. These are your ischial tuberosities.
3. Place your hand on your belly and walk it down until you feel that hard bone. Often referred to as a vagina bone, these are your pubic bones at the front of your pelvis.

The word *pelvis* is Latin for "basin" because these bones form a bowl or basin at the bottom of your spine. Your pelvis is there for you, quietly supporting you when you sit, stand, and move. Your pelvis serves as the attachment site for all of your pelvic floor muscles. It acts as a funnel for the nerves at the bottom of your spinal cord that control bladder and bowel function, sensation to your genitals, and the movements of your hips all the way down to your toes. Located within this bony basin are your pelvic organs, supported by your pelvic floor muscles. In female bodies, those organs include your uterus, ovaries, bladder, and bowels. In male bodies, those organs include the prostate, bladder, and bowels. I like to think of the pelvis as a bowl of goodness because it holds essential anatomy for some important and joyful functions—from walking and running to having sex and making babies.

How is a woman's pelvis different from a dude's?

The female pelvis has a wider opening at the top (pelvic inlet) and bottom (pelvic outlet) compared to a male pelvis to accommodate the passage of a baby. Females also have their sit bones (ischial tuberosities) wider apart, which means birthing hips are a real thing. A male pelvis is taller and narrower with a smaller opening at the top and bottom and sit bones closer together.

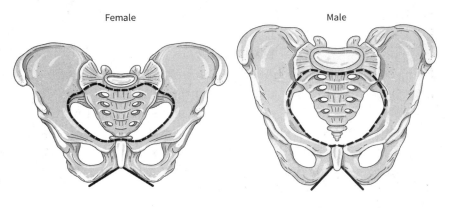

Shape of female pelvis compared to male pelvis

The pelvic floor sits at the lowest portion of this "basin" and has muscular attachments from the pubic bone in front to the tailbone in the back and from side to side between your sit bones. Everyone has a pelvic floor, even male bodies, which differ from female bodies in that male pelvic floors have two openings (for the urethra and anus) compared to three openings in female bodies (for the urethra, anus, and vagina).

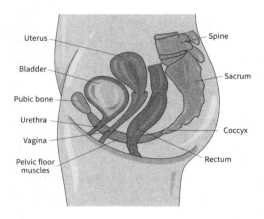

Female pelvic anatomy: side view of bladder, uterus, and rectum traversing through the pelvic floor muscles

Before we dive deeper to get to the muscles, let's start with the basics of female anatomy. Here we go from the outside in.

YOUR VULVA

Skin covers your entire genital region from your pubic bone and labia back toward your anus (aka butthole) and tailbone. This region is referred to as your external genitalia, also known as your vulva. The word *vulva* is derived from the Latin term *volva*, which means "wrapper" or "to roll." Your vulva includes the labia majora—your outer lips, which have hair—and the labia minora—your inner lips, which are hairless.

Pubic hair typically surrounds your genital area; it grows on the labia majora and region above the pubic bone, called the mons pubis, and serves as a barrier to protect your genitalia from foreign bodies, bacteria, and viruses. Pubic hair also protects the skin of your labia and mons pubis from friction during sexual activity, which can lead to dryness, irritation, and abrasions.

The labia minora, which surround the opening of the vagina and urethra, also form a protective barrier from irritation, dryness, and infection. The merger of the labia minora at the top of your vulva forms the clitoris, which is a *very* important sex organ, arguably the most important. This bulb of tissue is filled with over 10,000 nerves that enable arousal, pleasure, and, when we're lucky, an orgasm. (Yup, that's all it is for—pure pleasure, just for you.)

Does the size of my labia matter?

Labia come in different colors, shapes, and sizes, and these differences are not necessarily problematic. Labia are rarely symmetrical and won't look the same or be the same size in any two individuals, in the case that you see someone else's labia and think, "Wow, mine look different!" The size of your labia does not matter unless they rub against your underwear or pants, causing chafing, irritation, and discomfort. A surgical procedure called a labiaplasty removes excess labia tissue, but please proceed with caution as a lot of nerves are located in those tissues that can affect your sensation. There are also autoimmune conditions that cause problematic thinning of the labia and need additional medical attention. We'll get to that in Chapter 11, on pelvic pain.

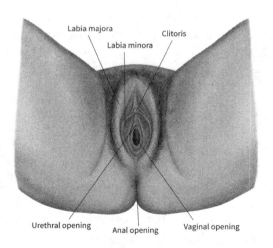

Female vulva with external genitalia labeled

YOUR VAGINA

Coochie, cookie, cha-cha, hoo-ha, vajayjay, and many more terms are used to refer to the vulva and vagina from the time we are little kids and even into adulthood. To set the record straight, I always recommend using the proper anatomical terms when teaching children and referring to these body parts. When I use the term "down there," I am being tongue-in-cheek, as a nod to how hush-hush we can be when it comes to conversations about our pelvic floor. But using the proper terminology gives children, our friends, and ourselves a shared understanding of our bodies, provides language to ask questions, and helps create healthier body images. Using a nickname for genitals can connote something shameful or bad that's inappropriate to discuss.

The terms vulva and vagina are often used interchangeably, but they are different and separate parts of your body. Your vulva is the gateway to your vagina. Your vagina is the muscular canal that leads from the vaginal opening in the vulva to your cervix, the opening to the uterus. The Latin origin of *vagina* means "sheath" or "scabbard for a sword." The vagina measures anywhere from two to four inches long, about the length of your middle finger. It serves multiple functions—for elimination (it's the pathway for menstrual blood to leave the body), for sexual pleasure and reproduction (through insertion of a penis, dildo, or sex toy), and for support (its muscular walls provide support for your pelvic organs). When you consider the fact that it also serves as the birth canal for a baby delivered vaginally, you get a sense of the tremendous strength and flexibility of your vaginal walls. All this to say, your vagina is pretty much a powerhouse.

YOUR PELVIC FLOOR MUSCLES

Your pelvic floor is the group of muscles, tissues, ligaments, vessels, and nerves that work together to perform a number of physical and biological activities for you. These pelvic floor muscles are organized into a superficial layer and a deeper layer, which you can think about like layers of an onion. The superficial muscles are four separate muscles that mainly act to close the urinary and anal sphincters and tighten your vaginal opening. The deeper layer is divided into four individual sections of muscles that join together to sit like a hammock at the base of the pelvis to support your pelvic organs. I'm going to nerd out for a bit and go into detail about what these muscles do, because if you understand *what* these muscles do, then you can better understand *how* to keep them healthy and exercise them if they aren't working optimally. Let's go.

SUPERFICIAL MUSCLES

While your labia and clitoris are visible externally, the superficial layer of pelvic floor muscles lies just underneath them. These thin slips of muscle are each smaller than your pinky finger, but their importance and impact are huge. These superficial muscles include the Ischiocavernosus, Bulbocavernosus, Deep transverse perineal muscle, and Superficial transverse perineal muscle, and lie in the shape of a triangle with a line down the middle, serving as the entryway into the pelvic floor.

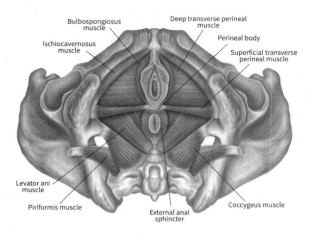

Superficial pelvic floor muscles: a view from below

The perineum, the area of tissue between the vaginal opening and anal opening, functions to support the pelvic floor and is also an erogenous zone for sexual pleasure. Underneath the skin of the perineum is the perineal body, which is the Grand Central Station of your pelvic muscles. At the perineal body, every single muscle of your pelvic floor has an attachment, and its integrity is critical for maintaining pelvic floor strength and support in women. It's also highly sensitive with a lot of nerve endings, which can make it a source of pleasure with rubbing or stimulation but also a source of pain after prolonged sitting or injury during vaginal birth.

Is a perineum the same as a "taint"?

Yes! The perineum, similar to the vulva and vagina, has a laundry list of slang terms like "taint" in female bodies, or "gooch" or "grundel" in male bodies. These terms make me chuckle. I have never heard a slang term for an elbow, yet we have one for the perineum, reflecting the challenge we have talking about intimate parts of our bodies in an appropriately anatomical way, especially when that body part relates to sex or sexual function. The slang term taint comes from the area being between the vagina and the anus, so it ain't (t'ain't) your vagina, and it ain't your anus. It's your taint.

During a vaginal birth, the perineal body stretches significantly; it can also tear or get cut by the physician (called an episiotomy) to aid in delivering the baby. Trauma to this area is a contributing factor to why so many women experience pelvic floor dysfunction after childbirth. But all is not lost; there's a ton of research that supports practices like perineal massage and alternative birth positions that can minimize the risk of a more severe perineal tear. Stay tuned for that in Chapter 8, when we discuss childbirth.

This superficial layer of the female pelvic floor muscles also has three openings. At the top is the urethral sphincter, where pee exits. In the middle is the vaginal opening for vaginal intercourse, vaginal birth, and menstruation. Below the vaginal opening is the anal sphincter, where poop and gas exit the body.

Just beneath the first layer of muscles is an area called the urogenital diaphragm. This layer is shaped like a flat triangle sandwiched between two other layers of tissues and muscles, like a piece of cheese between two slices of bread. The main function of the urogenital diaphragm is to help support the urethra (the tube that carries urine from your bladder out of your body) and to keep urine in the bladder until you're ready to empty. Before moving on, let's do a little pelvic floor activity, shall we? Sit up tall with your feet flat on the floor.

1. Cough.
2. Now lift your arm overhead and lower it back down.
3. Now tighten your vagina as if you are trying to stop your urine stream or hold in pee.

Great! Your superficial pelvic floor muscles just contracted with each of those activities.

AND EVEN DEEPER MUSCLES

Peeling back the outer, superficial layer, we get to the deepest and largest group of the pelvic floor muscles. The deeper muscles form a basket closing the bottom of the pelvis and do a lot of the heavy lifting for the pelvic floor. This layer forms a network of muscles known as the levator ani, whose major function is to support your pelvic organs. In addition, it assists with sexual functioning, peeing, pooping, breathing, and core support.

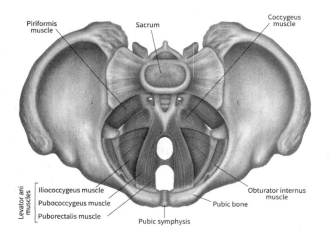

Piriformis muscle

Sacrum

Coccygeus muscle

Levator ani muscles
Iliococcygeus muscle
Pubococcygeus muscle
Puborectalis muscle

Obturator internus muscle

Pubic bone

Pubic symphysis

Deep pelvic floor muscles: a view from above

When it comes to muscles, you may have heard of "range of motion." For instance, when your arm is completely straight, your biceps muscle is at its full length, and then when you bend your elbow, your biceps muscle is contracted to its most shortened state. This is your biceps muscle's full range of motion. Your pelvic floor muscles also have a full range of motion. Most of the time they are resting in the middle of their range. They contract to their shortened state when you are holding in pee with a full bladder and racing down the hallway to make it to the restroom in time. They then relax to their lengthened state to have a bowel movement or to accommodate a baby coming down the birth canal.

Even though you can't see all of your pelvic floor muscles doing their work, try to tune in and feel them. Next time you go to the bathroom, make an effort to stop your urine stream (just once), and that's your pelvic floor contracting. Next time you are feeling stressed, take a deep breath and exhale, and that's your pelvic floor relaxing. The first step is learning that these muscles exist. Now let's look at what they do.

Your Pelvic Floor Is Always Doing Its Thing

When I was pregnant with my first son, I saw a pelvic floor physical therapist. That's right, I, Sara Reardon, aka The Vagina Whisperer, needed my own vagina whisperer. This was a no-brainer as I had worked with thousands of women over the years who reaped the benefits of therapy. And because it was my first pregnancy, I wanted to do everything I could to prepare my body and pelvic floor for birth. I had some heavy lifting to do.

My pelvic floor PT guided me through exercises to help strengthen my pelvic joints that had become stretched and misaligned during the course of my pregnancy. She helped relieve sciatica symptoms that were radiating into my left butt cheek, making it painful to bend over while I was working with patients. She also performed internal pelvic floor massage and prescribed a menu of stretches to prepare my pelvic floor for the required relaxation needed during birth. With the help of my husband during labor, I went on to have an unmedicated vaginal birth with no perineal tearing. Many women think this is due to luck. But a lot of it was the advanced preparation I had done. And it's preparation we can all do.

The muscles of your pelvic floor are working all throughout the day, every day, and even when you sleep, which most of us don't realize, perhaps because we don't see these muscles contracting and relaxing like we see our biceps muscles. When I am lounging on my couch, binge-watching crime documentaries, my pelvic floor is still at the gym. When I breathe, my pelvic floor is working. When I cough, my pelvic floor is working. When I stand up, yup, it's working again. Let's walk through all of the ways the pelvic floor works hard for us day in and day out.

IT SUPPORTS YOUR PELVIC ORGANS

As a basket for your pelvic organs, the pelvic floor can hold quite a bit of weight. In females, this includes your bladder that holds urine, your rectum that holds poop, and your uterus that holds a growing baby during pregnancy. A uterus weighs just one sixth of a pound in a nonpregnant state, but at forty weeks pregnant, your uterus and its contents (baby, placenta, and amniotic fluid) can weigh between thirteen and fifteen pounds. Have you ever lifted a fifteen-pound weight at the gym? It's hard work!

IT HOLDS IN PEE AND POOP

Your pelvic floor has openings for the urethra, which carries urine from the bladder out of your body, and your anus, which carries poop from your colon and rectum out of your body. When your bladder or rectum fills with pee or poop, respectively, urinary and anal sphincters contract to hold the contents in and then relax to allow them to empty the body . . . ideally at a convenient time. And when your bladder gets super full because perhaps you delay the urge to pee or you get constipated from too many carbs or not wanting to poop in public, your pelvic floor muscles are working overtime.

IT ENGAGES DURING SEX AND ORGASMS

In order to have vaginal sex, your pelvic floor muscles need to relax for the insertion of a finger, penis, or sex toy. During arousal, your superficial muscles engorge as they fill with blood. Upon climax, these muscles contract and relax in a rhythmic and pleasurable wave in what we know as an orgasm. Your pelvic floor muscles can contract anywhere from three to thirty-two times during an orgasm. And yes, the stronger your pelvic floor, the stronger your orgasms can be.

IT HELPS YOU BREATHE

Yup, that's how important the pelvic floor is. The muscles of your floor are literally working with every breath you take. Your diaphragm sits at the top of your abdomen like a dome-shaped muscle under your rib cage. Your pelvic floor sits like a bowl at the bottom of your abdomen. When you breathe in and out, your diaphragm and pelvic floor muscles lower and rise together like a piston. Taking some deep breaths into your rib cage can help your pelvic floor chill out and relax.

IT SUPPORTS THE BIRTHING OF BABIES

During vaginal birth, the pelvic floor muscles lengthen, relax, and can stretch anywhere from 25% up to 245%! Your pelvic floor muscles are not only strong enough to support a growing baby but also have the incredible ability to lengthen and stretch to accommodate a baby coming down the vaginal canal during birth.

IT SUPPORTS YOUR CORE

We talk all the time about working out our core, but we rarely realize that our core includes our pelvic floor. Your pelvic floor is the floor of your core. Other core muscles include your back muscles and abdominals, which attach to your pelvis and, along with the pelvic floor, support your trunk and spine. These pelvic core muscles stabilize your body every time you move a limb. When you reach for something overhead, your pelvic floor muscles activate. When you stand up, your pelvic floor muscles activate. When you lift a bag of groceries from your trunk, your pelvic floor muscles activate. During every movement you make, your core and pelvic floor are recruited to help.

IT HELPS YOU MAINTAIN YOUR POSTURE

Our pelvic floor engages to support our organs, but it also supports our spines. To sit or stand in an upright position, your core needs activation, and your pelvic floor, being a part of your core muscles, works to maintain that posture for you. So when you are sitting upright in your desk chair with a straight spine, your pelvic floor is making that possible.

WE OFTEN DON'T REALIZE THE LOAD OUR PELVIC FLOOR IS CARRYING— and how much its health contributes to our well-being. A case in point: In 2021 on my thirty-ninth birthday, my husband picked up my giant birthday cake (double-layer vanilla with rainbow sprinkles) at a local bakery as images of bright red and orange swirled across the television screen playing the local news behind the checkout counter. Hurricane Ida was heading toward New Orleans, exactly sixteen years to the day after Hurricane Katrina, which flooded and destroyed my childhood home in 2005. After he drove home with the cake, the news reported Hurricane Ida was predicted to be a major hurricane when it hit land, like Hurricane Katrina, which practically wiped out the entire city of New Orleans. Needless to say, my birthday plan was derailed. We hurriedly packed the car with our important documents, a few days' worth of clothes, and my son's baseball trophies to head west to Houston, Texas.

Typically just five hours, the drive took at least double the time due to the mass exodus out of town. We arrived at 4:00 a.m. at a random hotel room we booked while on the road, as so many were already at full capacity with other evacuees. After the storm passed, we drove back to New Orleans to check on our house and empty our refrigerator full of spoiled food, including my untouched birthday cake, which sadly did not make the evacuation packing list. The entire city of New Orleans was without power indefinitely, which meant no air conditioning or refrigeration, no ability to charge phones for communication, and school closures until power was restored. So we drove back to Texas and bounced to the homes of family and friends for three weeks until the power to our city and home were restored. From the time we evacuated to returning home for good, we drove over 1,600 miles. I was a ball of stress sitting in the passenger seat, tossing endless snacks back to my kids, for most of that. And you know what else was stressed? My pelvic floor!

I was constipated from all of the traveling. My tailbone hurt from sitting so much. And my whole body was in knots. My pelvic floor had been supporting me while lifting suitcases in and out of my car and while sitting and driving for hours. Sitting for long periods of time without changes in our posture can tighten our pelvic floors, as can stress. Mine had been working overtime as I experienced the stress of trying to hold it all together as a mom, homeowner, and business owner navigating uncertainty and hurricane devastation.

A question I get often, and perhaps what brings you to this book, is, *How do I even know if I have a pelvic floor issue?* Because your pelvic floor is intimately related to peeing, pooping, sex, menstruation, posture and core support, hip mobility, breathing, pregnancy, birth, and menopause, if you have a problem with any of these functions, you (and your medical provider) need to consider your pelvic floor as a potential source of the problem. For example, we often think of only urinary leakage being a pelvic floor problem, but difficulty starting your urine stream, feeling like you don't empty all the way, waking frequently at night to pee, and burning during urination can all also be caused by a pelvic floor muscle problem. Low back pain, often chalked up to weak abdominal muscles or terrible posture, can actually be a symptom of a pelvic floor problem too. Many women with back pain have pelvic floor muscle tenderness or weakness that must be addressed to resolve their pain.

Very often, you might suffer from discomfort that seems unrelated to your pelvic floor when in fact it's a direct result of pelvic floor dysfunction. Consider the case of my patient Catherine, who came for help because she felt burning when she peed. Every time she sat down to pee, she felt a sharp pain at the opening of her urethra. She found herself putting off peeing because she dreaded the sensation. When she finally went, she had to grip the wall and hold her breath because of the extraordinary pain she felt when her stream started. Her physician ran a urine culture, which was negative for a urinary tract infection, but still he gave her antibiotics (just in case). She took the medication, unsure if it was helpful but willing to try anything. The antibiotics then led to a yeast infection, which then led to taking an antifungal medication to treat that.

After a month, her pain wasn't better, and she went back to her doctor. He again ran a culture, which was negative, and prescribed her antibiotics, which again led to a yeast infection. She cycled on and off medication for eleven months until finding her way to pelvic floor therapy, which she only discovered from an online deep dive into her symptoms. As it turns out, Catherine had *pelvic floor muscle spasm*, which can mimic a urinary tract infection and cause this exact issue of burning with urination. After just a handful of sessions teaching Catherine stretches to relax her pelvic floor muscles, breathing techniques to help start her urine stream without tensing, and instructions to use a vaginal massage wand to release tight muscles, she had almost full relief of her symptoms—after nearly a year of suffering.

This is just one example of how women can struggle with a pelvic floor issue, and the road to improvement is actually quite simple. The sad fact is that many medical providers are not aware that our pelvic muscles are a piece of the puzzle. There are many more symptoms and complaints we'll dive into throughout this book, but the point is that the pelvic floor plays a critical role in the healthy functioning of our bodies. If your pelvic floor is a problem for you, then it's a problem. Don't let anyone (even yourself) try to convince you that you don't deserve to get care.

Your Pelvic Floor Is Connected to . . . Your Whole Body

While this book is dedicated to these small but mighty muscles, the pelvic floor does not work in isolation, nor can it be treated in isolation. Yes, medications, procedures, and surgeries, along with exercise and lifestyle changes, can be pieces of the puzzle to address common pelvic floor disorders, but sometimes we have to go beyond the pelvic floor muscles if there's a pelvic floor problem. Why?

Thirty-six muscles attach to your pelvic bones, many of which work together with other parts of your body. These muscles are responsible for everything from going to the bathroom to running a race to birthing a baby to twerking on the dance floor.

Remember when we talked about layers of the onion? When we experience pain or limitations, we have to also consider those outer layers of the onion, muscles like your abdominals, glutes, thighs, and hip muscles, as contributors. If they are tight or unbalanced, they are likely creating tightness or dysfunction in our pelvic floor too.

Pelvic floor dysfunction is related to back pain, breathing challenges, jaw clenching, foot pain, hip pain, and so much more. Fifty percent of women with pelvic organ prolapse experience low back pain. Hip pain can contribute to constipation. Abdominal muscle tension can lead to incomplete bladder emptying. Our pelvic floor muscles are connected to other parts of our anatomy.

But remember that night when you couldn't sleep because you were ruminating about that issue at work that's been haunting you for weeks? And then you woke up the next morning and couldn't start your urine stream or strained to poop? Our physical well-being is also only part of the puzzle.

Your Pelvic Floor Is Connected to . . . Your Mind

When I was pregnant with my son, my husband asked whom I wanted to call when I went into labor. The list was short. There was no one. I was living in Dallas at the time close to my in-laws, while my parents and siblings were in the neighboring state. Planning for an unmedicated birth, I hoped to go into labor without being induced, labor at home as long as possible, then drive to the hospital and safely have our baby.

My husband and I are both people pleasers. We want everyone in our presence to feel comfortable, have what they need, not be upset, and feel included. But I also knew that to have any chance at an unmedicated birth, I needed to stay as relaxed as possible. Birth was not the time to try to please others. If my family was at the hospital waiting for me to give birth, some part of me would have felt like I or my husband had to check on them. While I knew our family would respect our wishes to not come to the hospital, I didn't even want to have to send text updates or messages about what centimeter dilated I was. So my husband and I informed no one while I was in labor and made phone calls only *after* my son was born. These measures gave me the space I needed to birth our son without interruption. I know what stress does to my body. It causes me to tense up. And I also know what stress does to the pelvic floor. It causes the entire region to tense up.

Have you ever been in a super stressful meeting and checked your jaw? *Is it clenched?*
Have you ever been sitting in traffic and checked your butt? *Is it tightened up?*
Ever watched a scary movie and checked your thighs? *Are you squeezing them together?*

Whether you are aware of it or not, your body holds on to tension, and this tension can settle in your . . . you guessed it . . . pelvic floor. Tension can even become habitual. There have been studies showing that watching a violent movie—not sexually violent, just violent—actually causes tension in the pelvic floor muscles. Considering current-day stressors, like parenting, working, healthcare, politics, and the environment, it's no wonder that our bodies and pelvic floors can easily settle into a chronic state of tension. So have compassion for your body—and also, trust it. Your symptoms are not ever "all in your head," as so many patients say they have been told by others. Our mental, emotional, and psychological states influence our body and pelvic floor.

A patient named Elizabeth was never able to have an orgasm with her partner due to her pelvic floor tension. After a course of therapy and experiencing her first orgasm, she sent me flowers. "I've never felt more like a woman than I did at that moment," her card read. Another patient named Ester came to see me for abdominal pain on her C-section scar. As I performed a gentle massage to release the restriction surrounding her scar, tears streamed down her face as her emotions rose to the surface from my touch. Our pelvic area holds enormous emotional intensity. Many people carry a sense of shame in the area, while some find it to be a source of tremendous power and strength. Therefore, when addressing pelvic floor health, we have to consider our body *and* our mind.

Our pelvic floor health is helped by consistent and reliable support from a pelvic floor therapist, regular exercise and adequate sleep, and yoga, meditation, or breathing exercises in our daily practices, all of which also promote mind–body well-being. And the well-being of our pelvic floor—from the muscles to the tissues—is central to our overall health. One of the best, easiest, and cheapest ways to regulate your nervous system, release muscle tension, and care for your pelvic floor is to breathe.

You'll find throughout this book that I remind you to breathe for two reasons. Your diaphragm muscle, which controls your breathing, and your pelvic floor muscles work together. If you are holding your breath, your pelvic floor muscles will be limited in their ability to relax and contract. Deep breathing has been shown to slow your heart rate and reduce your body temperature, but it also assists in pelvic floor relaxation and pain management. Additionally, connecting your breath to your pelvic floor exercises can support better and stronger contractions. So, just like I tell my son when he is nervous going up to bat during a baseball game: use your superpower, buddy. Just breathe.

You Want Me to Put My Finger Where?

Throughout this book, I am going to encourage you to get comfortable with your nether regions—your vagina, your anus, your perineum, and every part of your pelvic floor. It might be helpful for me to explain what a pelvic floor therapist does and how they do it. As a pelvic floor physical therapist, I am trained to work on the muscles, tissues, and nerves in the pelvic region of the body. Your muscles contract and relax or maintain tension to create movement. Your nerves are the messengers from your brain to your muscles to communicate exactly what action you need to perform. Your tissues sort of bind your muscles and nerves together, like Saran Wrap around a sandwich. When I meet with patients, my first step is to get a sense of their needs and any problems they are having, but the next first step is to examine all three of these components (muscles, nerves, and tissues).

Your pelvic floor muscles are *internal* structures in your body, which we can't see to assess. This is likely why pelvic floor problems are also easy to ignore or dismiss. But in order to properly assess and treat these structures, we have to examine them, just as we would a biceps or hamstring muscle. And the way we do so is by performing an internal pelvic floor muscle examination through your vagina or anus. A typical pelvic floor muscle assessment performed by a pelvic health therapist (who should have short fingernails) entails something similar to a pelvic examination at a gynecologist, but with fewer clunky metal objects, zero stirrups, and your butt won't be falling off the table.

First, we assess how your hips and pelvis move and test the strength of your abdominal and hip muscles (clothes on for that part). Then we perform an internal pelvic floor muscle examination with your consent to determine if your pelvic floor muscles are weak, tense, uncoordinated, or already doing a darn good job (bottoms off for that part). Then we go to the next step—where I educate you on this part of your body. To be the expert of your body, you need to know the anatomy of what's right and the anatomy of what is wrong. How can we care for a part of ourselves if we don't even know what exactly it is, what it does, or how it works? And finally, I coach you with the best exercises and lifestyle tips to help manage your problems or prevent them in the future.

You may be thinking, "Okay, Sara, I don't have a pelvic floor therapist handy at the moment, but I want to know what's going on down there." It is your body, and I encourage you to get familiar with it. There is absolutely no reason why you shouldn't and can't get a better sense of these muscles yourself.

EXPLORE YOUR FLOOR

Your pelvic floor does so much for you. There's a lot to love. Here are three ways you can self-examine your pelvic floor. You'll need a mirror, your finger, and an attitude of appreciation and acceptance toward your amazing body. Take some notes as you follow the guide below, which will give you information about your pelvic floor muscle performance and which treatment pathway to follow in this book. In Chapter 2, we will look at general pathways for care—and in the subsequent chapters, we will look at more specific protocols for problems that can arise.

IDENTIFY YOUR EXTERNAL VULVA

Lie down on your bed, undressed from the waist down, with your legs relaxed open. Use a pillow to support your head and one underneath each knee to help your hips relax. With a mirror between your legs, start by spreading your labia and just look.

1. Can you identify your labia minora (hairless) inside the labia majora (with hair)?
2. Can you identify your clitoris?
3. Can you identify the vaginal opening?

OBSERVE YOUR EXTERNAL PELVIC FLOOR MOVEMENTS

Watch your contraction using the mirror between your legs. Perform what you would consider a pelvic floor contraction, or a Kegel.

1. Do your vaginal opening, anal opening, and perineum (between your vagina and anus) lift up toward your head? *That is a proper Kegel of the superficial pelvic floor muscles.*
2. Can you hold the contractions for five seconds, or does it let go right away? *Holding for five seconds is a sign of endurance of the deeper pelvic floor muscle layer.*
3. Do you feel your muscles fully relax afterwards, or does it feel like they are stuck once you tighten and contract? *Your muscles should naturally relax back to resting after a contraction.*
4. Are your butt muscles tightening and lifting you off the bed? *For a Kegel, your butt should stay relaxed.*

Next, watch your relaxation using the mirror between your legs. Push out like you are trying to poop, birth a baby, or lay an egg.

1. Does your perineum lift up again or not move—or does it push down toward your feet? *Moving toward your feet is the proper direction for bulging and relaxation.*
2. Are you holding your breath to push or exhaling out? *Ideally you should be breathing instead of holding your breath.*
3. Are you seeing any movement at all or contracting and tightening again? *You should see movement down while pushing out your pelvic floor.*

EXAMINE YOUR INTERNAL PELVIC FLOOR MUSCLES

Now check your pelvic floor muscles internally. No mirror is needed here, just your finger with a trimmed fingernail and a medical glove if you would like. You can stay in the same position as above or lie on your side with a pillow placed between your knees. First, place your index finger (or your index and middle fingers together) at the opening to the vagina, which you ideally identified above with a mirror. Slowly and gently insert your finger into the vaginal opening up to your first knuckle. Here you are at the layer of your superficial muscles.

1. Perform a Kegel contraction. Can you feel these muscles tighten? *Tightening is a contraction of the pelvic floor muscles.*
2. Apply gentle pressure to the bottom or either side. Do you feel burning or tenderness? *Burning or tenderness can be a sign of muscle tension.*

Second, slide your finger in up to your second knuckle and rest the pad of your finger on the side wall of the vagina. The tip of your finger is at the level of your deeper pelvic floor muscles.

1. Contract or Kegel. Can you feel your muscles tighten around your finger? *Tightening is a Kegel.*
2. Can you contract and hold for five seconds, and then your muscles completely relax? *Again, holding for five seconds is a sign of endurance.*
3. Apply gentle pressure with your fingertip to the left and right side walls of your vagina. Do you notice any tenderness, or does one side feel more tender than the other? *Tenderness can be a sign of muscle tension.* (Also, if this pressure makes you feel like you need to poop, well, you probably need to poop.)

Third, slide your finger in until your third knuckle, and your finger is completely inserted up to the pelvic bowl of muscles.

1. Bend your fingertips. Do you feel a cliff that your finger goes over? *If you find this, you are in the bowl of your pelvic floor, the deeper muscles called the levator ani.*
2. Repeat the above steps to contract, relax. Can you contract and hold for five seconds, and then your muscles completely relax? *This is a Kegel contraction, testing the endurance of the muscles and then relaxation of the muscles.*
3. Then press on the side walls. Does it feel tight like a trampoline, soft and mushy and your finger sinks in, or tender like you are pressing on a bruise? *If you have tenderness, it can be a sign of pelvic floor muscle tension.*

4. Last, remove your finger, wash your hands, and then give yourself a pat on the back for performing your first pelvic floor muscle self-exam!

PUT IT ALL TOGETHER

I remember the first time I explored my own pelvic floor. I was on my way to my pelvic floor therapy continuing education class and knew that internal pelvic floor examinations would be performed *by me* and *on me* by another therapist. Before I went, I thought, "Well, I want to see what mine feels like before I test it on another person." And as expected, it was no big deal. As a physical therapist, it is just examining a body part like I would a foot or an ankle, except I really don't like feet, so it was actually better than a foot exam.

And I encourage you to get to know this part of your body as well. See it. Explore it. Assess it. This is the first step. From this self-exploration and examination, my hope is that you not only connect with a part of your body often deemed mystical, foreign, or off-limits but also determine the condition of your pelvic floor to follow the tips and perform the exercises shared in this book.

For example, if you have difficulty relaxing your pelvic floor or you experience tenderness with pressure at the opening or deeper layers, you likely have pelvic floor muscle tension or overactivity. If you have difficulty contracting your pelvic floor muscles or are unable to hold a Kegel contraction for five seconds, you likely have pelvic floor muscle weakness or underactivity. In the chapter that follows, I cover what you need to do with the pelvic floor discoveries you just made along with the general guidelines all people should know for pelvic floor care. If I could put these tips on the inside of every bathroom stall door, I would. But for now, the next chapter will suffice. Let's turn to the ins and outs of care for your floor.

CHAPTER 2

Pelvic Floor Health 101

As a pelvic floor therapist, I get *a lot* of vagina questions from patients, friends, family members, and even people I randomly meet at my kids' baseball park.

"Lately I've been peeing four or five times a night. I might as well sleep on the bathroom floor. Is this normal?"

"I knew hot flashes were part of menopause, but didn't know painful sex was too. Am I the only middle-aged woman who hates sex now because it hurts?"

"Why does my vagina smell different after having a baby?"

People want to know what's normal and what's not—from how their vagina feels to how it looks and smells. There are no questions that are off-limits for me, and I love when people feel comfortable asking questions and having these conversations. Do many women experience peeing throughout the night? A hundred percent. Is it normal? Sadly, many medical professionals will say yes, leaving women feeling hopeless and demoralized. But in truth, it's not normal to go more than twice, and you can improve symptoms like these.

In my many years as a PT, I've realized that vulvar and vaginal care are often talked about as part of the wellness industry, in the same bucket as beauty. And because physical therapy is associated with fitness, pelvic floor care is not taken as seriously as it ought to be. But true pelvic floor care goes beyond fitness and beauty—it is *healthcare*.

Healthcare is essential to one's overall function and well-being, whereas wellness is like what we call here in New Orleans *lagniappe*, meaning "a little something extra." It might help you look better or feel better, but it doesn't necessarily help you function better. Seeing a pelvic floor therapist is the equivalent of seeing your primary care doctor, gynecologist, or dentist. It should be part of your standard health maintenance.

This book is focused on healthcare—and on giving you exercises, new habits, and tools to care for your pelvic floor and to advocate for your pelvic floor needs. While at times it is best to see a pelvic floor professional, there are a ton of things you can do to set your pelvic floor up to be healthy all the way through your elder years. Think of it this way: if you brush your teeth, you are far less likely to have cavities and rotting teeth down the road. If you do some basic pelvic floor care, you are far less likely to have pelvic floor problems down the road. So let's start with some guidelines to set yourself up for optimal pelvic floor health. Throughout the book, I refer to many of these guidelines, exercises, and practices. These are pages you will want to bookmark or dog-ear.

The Fundamentals for Your Floor

If I don't have my perfect pillow to sleep on at night, I wake up with a cramp in my neck and can only turn a few degrees to the right before I start to wince. My neck muscles easily get out of whack with something as simple as a pillow change. Then I need a good thirty minutes of yoga, massage to my shoulders, and a round of acupuncture before I am pain-free and back to sleeping well. Similar to other muscles in our bodies, our pelvic floor muscles are affected by something as simple as a long plane ride or a bout of constipation, or as serious as a traumatic event or a childbirth (the list goes on). Our pelvic floor health can change in small ways over time until a larger problem presents, or it can go through a dramatic shift quickly, setting off sirens. Our pelvic floors need maintenance for optimal day-to-day function, and when a season of life arrives like puberty, pregnancy, or meno-pause, our care routine needs to shift to support our bodies.

It's important to know the basics: the brushing and flossing equivalent for our pelvic floors. Here are my basic guidelines for better pelvic floor health. I go into much greater detail in the following chapters, but by incorporating some of these funda-mental guidelines, you set yourself up for optimal pelvic floor health. You can weave these basics into your daily life at any age—the younger, the better.

CHECK YOUR POSTURE

The positions in which you sit, sleep, and stand affect the position of your pelvis and therefore influence your pelvic floor. Good posture places your muscles and joints in optimal alignment and will help you avoid overtensing or overstretching your muscles, ligaments, and joints. Just like when you develop a tech neck looking down at your phone for too long, you can develop problems in your pelvic floor assuming a position for too long. Posture is something we have so much control over—and some simple habits can be hugely helpful in terms of preventing pelvic floor issues (and these habits can improve issues that we might already have).

SLEEPING POSTURE

While sleeping, keep your posture in a neutral alignment as much as possible. I prefer sleeping on a firm mattress as that feels best for my back, but whichever mattress you get the best sleep on is the best mattress for you. Here are tips for getting into the optimal alignment in whichever position is most similar to your natural sleeping position.

Lying on your side, stack your hips so they are in alignment with one another. Placing a body-length (emotional support) pillow that runs from your thighs to your ankles between your knees will help. The alignment of your hips supports a more relaxed position for your pelvic floor. Avoid bringing one knee up to your chest as that can tug on your pelvic joints and over time can lead to pain.

Lying on your back, place a pillow under your knees to take pressure off your low back. Pressure on your low back can lead to tight hip muscles and pelvic floor muscle tension.

Lying on your stomach, aim to keep your body straight instead of hiking one knee up toward your chest. Again, hiking your knee up places undue strain on your pelvic joints and leads to asymmetry of your pelvic floor muscles, both of which can lead to problems over time.

STANDING POSTURE

When you stand, you likely shift your weight quite a bit, which in fact is an excellent way to prevent muscles from getting overly tight or tense versus being in a static position. Allow yourself to shift. When standing, we also want to be in a neutral alignment. Balance your weight evenly between both legs instead of popping one hip out to the side. Keep your head over your shoulders and your hips, with your knees and ankles falling into straight lines.

Very often when someone has pelvic floor muscle tension, I see butt clenching, which tightens your pelvic floor and anal sphincter. Over time this can lead to tailbone pain or impede the outflow of poop. I also see people stick their butt out, which causes the bowl of your floor to tilt forward, also increasing tension to hip muscles. Tune in to your standing posture. To see if you are standing in a neutral position, try this posture assessment.

Stand with your back, shoulders, and heels against the wall. Tuck your chin so your ears are over your shoulders. Check that your hips, knees, and ankles are in alignment. Assess the space between your low back and the wall. If your back is completely flat and there is no space, tilt your pelvis slightly forward. If your back has a wide gap, tilt your pelvis slightly back. Ideally, and depending on the size of your bum, we want a small gap between the wall and your back, not an exaggerated curve but not completely flat against the wall either. This positions your ribs over your pelvis in a neutral alignment to untuck your butt and let that booty tension go.

Look at yourself from the side in a mirror to confirm that you are standing in an optimal posture. Observe to see if you are hanging your head forward or sticking your butt out. Notice what it feels like to make minor corrections.

SITTING POSTURE

Most of us sit way too long and way too often. I am in awe when I see babies and toddlers leaning forward to touch their toes or bringing their feet to their mouths with ease. Once kids become school-aged and sit in desks for six to seven hours a day, we see their shoulders start to round and their hamstrings become tight, and the flexibility and freedom of movement they had diminishes. And it usually gets worse from there. After years of school, commuting, and then possibly working at a desk for hours a day, our pelvic floor muscles get tight and tense from lack of movement and blood flow.

Learn how to "sit better." Many of us twist our legs like a pretzel, turn our knees and thighs inward, or tilt our pelvis back, called sacral sitting, all of which can create tension in your pelvic floor muscles. When sitting, your back should reach the back of the chair (use a pillow behind you if needed for low back support), and your feet should be placed flat on the floor (use a stool if your feet do not touch the ground). Crossing your ankles is a better option than crossing your knees, because it does not shorten and tighten your pelvic floor muscles, leading to over-activity over time. If you are sitting on the floor, a cross-legged position is also fine. Aim to take a break from sitting every thirty minutes to an hour.

Can wearing high heels negatively affect my pelvic floor?

Absolutely. Wearing high heels places your ankles in a plantarflexed position (pointing your toes), which can alter the position of your pelvis, increase the activation of your abdominal and gluteal muscles, and contribute to pelvic floor muscle tension. Increased force from walking in high heels can also further activate the pelvic floor. Additionally, heels that are too high or too narrow can cause us to feel unsteady, which has a negative effect on balance, stability, and pelvic floor function. In an ideal world, wear flats that are comfortable or shoes with a three- to five-centimeter heel height (about 1.5 to two inches) to protect your pelvic floor.

EXERCISE

Motion is lotion, and movement is essential for the health of our pelvic floor. When patients ask me what is the best exercise they can do, I tell them to walk. It's free. It's low-strain on your joints. It has a low impact on your pelvic floor. It's weight-bearing and excellent for bone density. And it promotes circulation through-out your pelvic floor (and the rest of your body). Generally, all exercise is good for a healthy pelvic floor, but some guidelines exist in the case of pelvic floor function.

If you experience pelvic floor pain or tension, exercises that tighten or place prolonged pressure on your pelvic floor can exacerbate those tension symptoms. For example, cycling can increase pelvic floor tension due to prolonged pressure from the saddle on the pelvic floor muscles and nerves. Weightlifting can bring on pelvic floor tension due to chronic shortening of your pelvic floor muscles during lifting. And it might sound counter-intuitive, but Pilates and barre classes tighten your pelvic floor for prolonged periods—which can lead to long-term tension if not followed with relaxation. These are not "bad" per se, but they need to be balanced with exercises that promote pelvic floor relaxation. I walk you through relaxation stretches in the pelvic floor relaxation protocol in the coming pages. If you are a cyclist, weightlifter, or Pilates practitioner, take note to add these to your post-workout cooldown.

Additionally, if your pelvic floor muscles are weak, high-impact exercises like running, jumping, and heavy weightlifting may further compromise your pelvic floor function—and so exercises that strengthen your pelvic floor will be useful (and it might be wise to go slowly with the high-impact movement until things improve). Swimming or seated rowing might be a good option if you are dealing with leakage or pressure during high-impact exercise. But again, exercise is generally a win for your pelvic floor and should be part of your pelvic floor maintenance.

EXHALE

As a general rule of thumb, holding your breath isn't great for your pelvic floor. Breathing is good for you. But this is especially important for your pelvic floor when you are exerting yourself. As you breathe, your diaphragm moves up and down and creates a piston effect with your pelvic floor, giving it space to contract and relax. When you hold your breath, it locks pressure in your abdominal cavity. When you carry a heavy piece of luggage, lift weights at the gym, or even strain to poop while holding your breath, the pressure created in your pelvis doesn't have a place to go, so it will find the path of least resistance. For people with vaginas, that often means that pressure goes down toward your pelvic floor, contributing to pelvic floor weakness, pelvic organ prolapse, hemorrhoids, and urinary leakage.

Every time I lift my son into the car, I make a habit of saying, "Okay, buddy, one, two, three, breathe." I exhale as I lift him into the car. I repeat this same process when I lift him out of the bathtub, when I lift a heavy box of groceries out of my trunk, and even when I push furniture around my living room to rearrange it for the eighth time. Make a habit of exhaling when you exert yourself. It is hugely protective for your pelvic floor.

NUTRITION AND DIET

I don't need to give a huge ten-page paper on how to eat well. But it wouldn't be right to skip over it entirely. What you eat and drink affects the health of your pelvic floor. So I will sum it up in three points.

EASY ON THE PROCESSED FOODS

Processed foods (pretty much anything in a wrapper or box) are convenient, but they also limit the amount of natural fiber from fruits, vegetables, and whole grains we get in our diets. Not only do these dense, starchy, and difficult-to-digest processed foods contribute to constipation, but they also lack vitamins and minerals that help keep our immune systems healthy and blood sugar balanced. A diet lower in fats and processed foods and higher in fruit and fiber is way friendlier to our pelvic floor functioning and is associated with less constipation and abdominal discomfort.

LIMIT BLADDER IRRITANTS

Bladder irritants are pretty much everything I consider fabulous, such as coffee, carbonated drinks (including sparkling water), caffeinated drinks, and alcohol. Foods include spicy foods and citrus or acidic foods and juices. These can either irritate the bladder, making it want to empty its contents more quickly, or rush to your bladder, giving you a strong, sudden urge to pee. You don't *have* to avoid these, but if you find yourself struggling with frequent bathroom trips or occasional leakage, you may want to go easy on them.

CUT BACK ON THE SWEETS

I would skip dinner for dessert any day. But sugar, and even artificial sugars and sweeteners, can contribute to bladder irritation, urinary tract infections, and even weight gain, which is linked to increased risk of urinary incontinence. Absolutely do not feel like you have to cut all sugar and sweeteners out completely, but for your pelvic health (and health in general), cutting back on sugar is never a bad thing.

TAKE A BREAK

Stress wreaks havoc on our bodies and nervous systems and doesn't spare our pelvic floors. We all need to make de-stressing part of our routine. Whether it's taking a walk, getting outside in nature, pausing for a few minutes of deep breathing, or sliding into a warm bath with a cup of tea at the end of a long day, taking a beat to de-stress on a daily basis benefits your pelvic floor in the long run.

NOW THAT YOU KNOW WHAT YOUR PELVIC FLOOR IS, HOW YOUR PELVIC floor functions, and some basics on how to care for it, you're set, right? Unfortunately, no. Many of us aren't taught the core exercises for pelvic floor maintenance. And when we have issues, we aren't given the tools to improve those conditions. Let's begin with the pelvic floor exercise many women are told is the holy grail of pelvic floor care (it is not) . . . a Kegel. Kegels are useful and even important—but they are not everything for pelvic floor care.

Kegel Was Just One Man

Whether you grew up in the eighties and nineties like I did or found yourself reading women's health and fitness magazines over the past four decades, all you may have read or heard regarding the care of your pelvic floor goes something like this:

Want better sex? *Do Kegels!*
Looking for stronger orgasms? *Try Kegels!*
Trying to get your body back after having a baby? *Put Kegels on the list!*
Leak when you laugh? *You guessed it . . . Kegels!*

A Kegel is simply a pelvic floor muscle contraction. The name derives from Arnold Kegel, an American gynecologist who in the 1940s developed a machine to measure pelvic floor muscle strength and labeled the contraction of the muscles a Kegel. It is hard to believe that decades later, the name of a vaginal or pelvic floor contraction is still named after a male doctor from the mid-1900s, but I digress. I'll use the term now, as so many are familiar with it, but I hope this eventually changes. (A friend recommended we start calling them puss-ups.)

STOP YOUR URINE STREAM

While a Kegel has been widely used to describe a pelvic floor contraction recommended to strengthen the pelvic floor muscles, it falls short. Telling women to do Kegels for pelvic floor weakness is like telling someone with back pain to just do a bunch of crunches. Treatment for pelvic floor issues is not a one-size-fits-all approach. I've heard outrageous recommendations like doing 2,000 Kegels a day or employing a routine called the Cup Method where you walk around naked, tighten your pelvic floor muscles in a constant Kegel, and hold a cup between your legs to catch any urine leaks. While heroic levels of Kegels might offer relief to one individual, a much different protocol might be needed for another.

Practicing Kegels isn't just a matter of knowing when to do them—it is also a matter of knowing *how*. If you have pelvic floor *weakness*, Kegels can be a great starting point. But many people don't know how to do them correctly. They don't know how to use them progressively to actually strengthen the pelvic floor and vaginal walls. And doing Kegels can actually make some problems worse. Throughout the following chapters, I offer guidance on when to use Kegels—and when to lay off them. But because we will be visiting them frequently in the book, let's go over the basics now.

A Kegel is a small, subtle contraction that can be held for different lengths of time (one-second holds up to ten- or twenty-second holds). We can do them sitting and standing, and we can employ them when doing a range of day-to-day functions like before picking up a heavy box or baby, before lifting weights at the gym, or even before coughing or sneezing.

A Kegel activates the front and back parts of your pelvic floor muscles together. Imagine you are stopping your urine stream, holding in a fart in an elevator, picking up a blueberry with your vagina, or sucking up a thick smoothie with your vagina (my personal fave). Wherever you are reading or listening to this now, take a moment to practice a Kegel.

Sit up tall with your feet supported on the ground. Inhale and exhale to help all of your muscles let go and your nervous system quiet down.

1. Squeeze the front of your pelvic floor muscles at your urinary sphincter like you are trying to stop your urine stream. Relax.
2. Squeeze the back of your pelvic floor muscles at your anal sphincter (aka butthole) like you are trying to not pass gas. Relax.
3. Squeeze the front and back together simultaneously and think of squeezing and lifting those muscles up toward your pubic bone. Relax. (Avoid tightening your butt muscles as this is not the same as contracting your pelvic floor. If this occurs because you find yourself lifting off your seat, relax and try again without squeezing your butt.)

If you feel like you are squeezing the same way for all of the above, that's actually a good thing and totally fine. A Kegel engages both the front and back parts of the pelvic floor, and the options above just give you different ways to connect with the muscle and perform the contraction. Even after all this, how do you know if you are doing them correctly and not just squeezing your butt? First I'm going a bit into how to relax your pelvic floor and then walking you step-by-step through how to assess your Kegel. Get excited. It's going to be fun!

LAY AN EGG

For years I had the tendency of leaning over my phone and my computer, sometimes for hours throughout the day. Imagine rounded shoulders, forward head, tight neck muscles . . . terrible posture. I started getting headaches and worked with an acupuncturist and did yoga to help release a lot of the tension in this area, which helped. I bring this up because the pelvic floor muscles are similar to the muscles in our neck, and to all of the other muscles throughout our body. Tense muscles don't need more tightening; that only makes the problem worse. Focus needs to be more on relaxation of the muscles versus tightening and contracting.

Just as important as a pelvic floor contraction or Kegel for strengthening our pelvic floors is the idea of relaxing the pelvic floor. We touched on the full range of motion of your pelvic floor muscles earlier, and how fully relaxing these muscles is necessary contracting. This is why Kegels cannot *and should not* be the blanket exercise for any pelvic floor issue, which they have been for so long.

Since your pelvic floor is working all throughout the day, ideally to hold in pee and poop and support your organs, to fully lengthen and relax your muscles takes a bit of connection. For this, imagine yourself *laying an egg.* Try this to see if you can feel your pelvic floor muscles lengthen or bulge.

1. Sit up tall with your feet supported on the ground. Inhale and exhale to help all of your muscles let go and your nervous system quiet down. On the next exhale, imagine you are laying an egg and bulge your perineum down toward the seat underneath you. Release. Your pelvic floor should lengthen and open up as you do this, versus tighten and squeeze.

2. Try this again, imagining you are pushing out poop on the toilet or birthing a baby through your vagina. This should feel the same as the above and is just another way to imagine the same movement.

3. You can also try sitting on a toilet or lying on your side and place your hand over your perineum and anal opening. This may give you the sensation of something to push against.

STRENGTHEN OR LENGTHEN

In future chapters, I offer my expertise on whether you likely need to strengthen or lengthen your pelvic floor based on issues you are experiencing. I go through symptoms and conditions that *most* often align with pelvic floor muscles that need strengthening and *most* often need relaxation. That said, I also encourage you to take matters into your own hands and try to determine this for yourself. If you can sense when you contract and when you relax, this is a great first step to connecting with your pelvic floor—and to knowing what to do when issues arise. Furthermore, Kegels and laying an egg alone aren't the only ways to strengthen or lengthen. Along with basic tips and habits we've already been through (think posture, breath, movement, diet, and de-stressing), incorporating the lengthening and/or strengthening pathways below can help you prevent or overcome pelvic floor problems.

Find Your Pelvic Floor Pathway

Before you put together a plan to address a pelvic floor problem, identify whether it is more a result of pelvic floor weakness or tension. If your pelvic floor is weak, focus more on the strengthening suggestions throughout the book. And if it is tense, the relaxation protocols are for you. See the two lists below that describe the most common symptoms of pelvic floor weakness and tension. Take note of the symptoms that apply to you.

Common symptoms if you have pelvic floor weakness/underactivity:

- Leaking urine (any amount)
- Leaking urine with a cough/sneeze/jump/exercise
- Leaking urine with a strong urge to pee
- Heaviness in your vagina that is worse at the end of the day
- Smearing of poop in underwear
- Feeling like something is falling out of your vagina
- Feeling like something is falling out of your anal opening
- Decreased sensation with sex
- Weak orgasms

Common symptoms if you have pelvic floor tension/overactivity:

- Difficulty starting your urine stream
- Feeling like you do not empty your bladder completely
- Pain or burning with urination
- Frequent urinary tract infections
- Urine stream sprays in different directions or starts and stops
- Strain during bowel movements
- Not feeling completely empty after bowel movements
- Hemorrhoids or anal fissures
- Painful sex
- Difficulty achieving orgasms
- Painful orgasms
- Vaginal pain, rectal pain, abdominal pain, or tailbone pain

These lists are not exhaustive, but they contain clusters of symptoms to help you pick your starting point to address your pelvic floor problem. If your issues align with the pelvic floor weakness category, start the strengthening protocol. If your issues fall into the pelvic floor tension category, follow the relaxation protocol. If you are not experiencing any of the above and are here for prevention, proactively work through the strengthening protocol. As you work your way through this book, you will see that I offer guidance for how to use these protocols for every condition or symptom.

THE PELVIC FLOOR STRENGTHENING PROTOCOL

Increased pressure on the pelvic floor (from a baby or heavy lifting or excess weight), weak muscles and ligaments, and hormonal changes with aging and pregnancy can all contribute to pelvic floor weakness. Throughout the book, I go into issues that stem from weakness, and in many of those cases, I recommend this strengthening protocol. (In some cases, I will suggest amendments to this basic protocol.)

KEGEL ME THIS

Overall, strengthening your pelvic floor involves more than performing Kegels while you sit at a stoplight or in a Zoom meeting. You must perform them in a variety of positions for different lengths of time and incorporate them into activities. Although Kegels are not the only exercise that will strengthen your pelvic floor, they are a fundamental exercise and an excellent place to start.

Long Holds and Quick Flicks. Your pelvic floor muscles have two separate types of muscle fibers: marathon muscle fibers and sprint muscle fibers. Marathon or slow-twitch muscle fibers make up 70% of your pelvic floor and are primarily responsible for endurance (like holding the urge to poop as you are walking from the back of Target to the restroom in the front of the store) or maintaining muscle tone throughout the day (as when standing in line and supporting your bladder to prevent the constant drip of urine). Your sprint or fast-twitch muscle fibers make up 30% of your pelvic floor musculature and turn on strongly and quickly to prevent urinary leakage during a cough or quick sidestep. In order to work both types of muscle fibers to strengthen the entirety of your pelvic floor, perform both quick contractions (also called quick-flick Kegels) holding for just one second and longer-hold contractions (also called endurance Kegels) holding for five to ten seconds.

Change Positions. Perform Kegels in all of the positions you need the muscle to work, like when lying down, kneeling, standing, upside down on a roller coaster, or on hands and knees. Also, try to integrate them into all your normal activities, like during exercise, when standing up from a chair, while walking to the bathroom to pee, or before a cough or sneeze.

Relax Between Contractions. Just like with a biceps curl, you don't want to go halfway down and then curl up again. Following a pelvic floor contraction, fully relax your pelvic floor. If you can't tell when you are fully relaxing, take a deep breath in and out between contractions, and your muscles will naturally let go.

Gradually Build Up the Intensity. If you are looking to prevent leakage with a cough or sneeze, a simple strengthening regimen followed by daily maintenance exercises may suffice. But if you are looking to run five miles without leaking, your program needs to look different. Train your muscles for what you are asking them to do.

Once you get the basics of performing pelvic floor contractions, increase your hold time of Kegel contractions or gradually add weights or resistance bands to your workouts.

KEGEL BEFORE YOU COUGH

This is one that you must remember, and it's called "The Knack." The term first used by researcher James Ashton-Miller, because the English word "knack" implies the use of a trick or skill. In the case of urinary incontinence, "The Knack" is a pre-contraction of your pelvic floor (doing a Kegel) before a cough or sneeze to help prevent anticipated leakage. This teaches your pelvic floor muscles to turn on when you need them, and as your muscles get stronger and more effective at closing your urethra, you can actually prevent leaks. Now, this may not work right away, but train yourself and your pelvic floor to pre-contract so it becomes almost automatic with a cough or sneeze. And eventually you will find this can help prevent leaks.

STAY UNDER YOUR TISSUE THRESHOLD

Even if you are a straight-A student doing the strengthening protocol every day, sometimes you will be in the middle of your exercise routine (say, running) and all of a sudden—yikes!—you leak. If this happens, you've hit your tissue threshold, which means you've pushed yourself beyond what your muscles and tissues can take. Perhaps you've run a bit too far or you've lifted too much weight or done one too many reps.

If you ever hit a point where you start leaking, stop, modify your workout, or scale back. Pushing into leakage isn't going to help all your hard strengthening work. It's going to potentially make matters worse. Stay under the threshold of what your pelvic floor can handle. This may fluctuate depending on how full your bladder is, the time of day you are working out, or even the day of the month in your menstrual cycle. But listen to what your pelvic floor is reporting. It might be telling you it isn't quite strong enough for those thirty pounds added to your squats. Take a pause.

AVOID STRAINING

Straining does not equal strengthening. Period. Straining during pooping can weaken your pelvic floor muscles over time—and that can lead to all sorts of problems. As part of your protocol, don't strain. Ever. (Later in the book, we will get to techniques that will help you if you've been relying on straining when you go to the bathroom.)

CONSIDER PELVIC FLOOR WEIGHTS

Ben Wa balls, yoni eggs, and Kegel weights promise everything from more intense orgasms to fewer symptoms of incontinence, increased sexual satisfaction, and even balanced hormones. These devices all differ but suggest that inserting the ball/egg/weight into your vagina for a period of time will lead to stronger pelvic floor muscles. But if you use them as often instructed by popular wellness sites (just pop into your vag and hold tight for a while), your pelvic floor muscles can end up in a chronic state of tension, which is why instruction on how to properly and effectively use them is key. The general guidelines I suggest are as follows:

1. Wash the devices with mild soap and water before and after use.
2. Lubricant is not typically necessary for insertion.
3. Insert lying down on your back and practice a pelvic floor contraction followed by full relaxation afterwards. Perform three sets of ten quick contractions and three sets of longer five- to ten-second hold contractions, relaxing between each contraction.
4. Once performing the exercises lying down feels relatively easy, at a future session, progress to performing in different positions (standing, kneeling, sitting) and with varying activities (think mini squat, taking a step forward or to the side).
5. Gradually increase the amount of weight inserted as your muscles become stronger.
6. Go slowly. No need to exhaust your muscles like they tell you in weightlifting class. A session can be as short as five to ten minutes performed two or three times a week.
7. If you experience pain or an increase in symptoms, stop and check in with a pelvic therapist.

Your pelvic floor can get stronger by lifting weights, but using these devices won't give you more energy, calmness, or vagina superpowers as many claim. So this activity can be help-ful for some but are not a must for all.

MAINTAIN A MAINTENANCE PROGRAM

You don't have to do a rigorous Kegel program for the rest of your life, but you also can't do nothing and expect your incontinence or prolapse to be cured forever. I've compared strengthening your pelvic floor to flossing and brushing your teeth. You don't have to do it, but if you don't, it usually leads to a return of some of the issues you just worked so hard to improve. Studies show performing thirty Kegels per day five times a week can help maintain muscle strength. So, if you don't want a cavity in your pelvic floor, stick with the program. Below are basic exercises in addition to pelvic floor contractions you can do to strengthen your pelvic floor. *For instructional videos of the exercises below, please check my YouTube channel: https://www.youtube.com/ @thevaginawhisperer*

Bridges. Lie on your back with your knees bent and feet flat on the floor. Contract your pelvic floor with a Kegel, then engage your core by drawing your belly button in toward your spine. Squeeze your buttocks and lift your hips off the floor until they are in alignment with your knees and shoulders. Hold for five seconds, maintaining a pelvic floor and core contraction while tightening the buttocks. Slowly lower back to starting position and release pelvic floor and core contraction.

Ball Squeezes. Lie on your back with your knees bent and feet flat on the floor with a soft ball (about the size of a soccer ball) between your knees. Contract your pelvic floor with a Kegel, then engage your core and pull your belly button in toward your spine. Squeeze the ball with your inner thighs, maintaining a pelvic floor and core contraction, and hold for five seconds, then release.

Modified Bird Dogs. Get into a hands-and-knees position. Contract your core and pelvic floor muscles, and slide the tips of your left toes back until your leg is straight as you lift the opposite arm to shoulder height. Keep your back flat and core engaged. Lift your toes six to twelve inches off the floor and lower back down. Slowly return back to the starting position, release pelvic floor and core contraction, and repeat on the opposite side. If you are experiencing wrist pain or carpal tunnel syndrome, use a closed fist instead of a flat hand. If your back is arching or you have difficulty maintaining balance, stretch your leg back without lifting until balance improves.

Squats. Get into a standing position with your feet slightly wider than hip-distance apart. Contract your pelvic floor and exhale as you squat down and stick your buttocks back and keep your chest upright. Keep your pelvic floor contracted through the entire squat up and down. Slowly return back to starting position and release pelvic floor and core contraction.

Lunges. Get into a standing position with feet shoulder-width apart, toes pointing forward. Contract your pelvic floor and deep core muscles and take a long step forward with your right leg, lowering your left knee toward the ground until your right front knee is bent at 90 degrees and your right thigh is parallel with the ground. Step backward with your right leg, returning back to starting position, and release pelvic floor and core contraction.

THE PELVIC FLOOR RELAXATION PROTOCOL

As I mentioned, relaxation of your pelvic floor is just as important as strengthening your pelvic floor, if not more. And laying an egg isn't the only way to relax your pelvic floor muscles. In the chapters to come, I often recommend you incorporate the following relaxation protocol into your days. A number of the problems women face down there—from painful sex to tailbone pain—require that we simply *let go*.

BREATHE

Your diaphragm, the breathing muscle under your ribs, and your pelvic floor work in harmony. You may find yourself holding your breath throughout the day unknowingly, which in turn keeps your diaphragm in a stuck position, leading your pelvic floor to get stuck too. Deep diaphragmatic breaths can help return mobility and relaxation to your pelvic floor.

Place your hands on the sides of your rib cage. As you inhale, imagine the air expanding your ribs, opening them up like an umbrella. Your hands can give you a place to focus your breath as you breathe into your ribs. This will naturally help your pelvic floor become less tense and let go. Schedule these breaths throughout the day: in the shower, when you are stressed after a meeting, while waiting in line, or before bedtime. Deep breaths help your muscles get used to being in a more relaxed position instead of a chronically tight tense position.

RELEASE YOUR EXTERNAL MUSCLES

Working externally on your abdominal wall, buttock muscles, hips, and thighs can promote relaxation of external pelvic muscles, which in turn promotes relaxation of internal muscles. Ball massage or foam rolling can provide a way for you to self-massage and release tight muscles at home. Place a tennis, lacrosse, or firm yoga ball against the wall and gently press your outer buttock muscles into it, holding for four or five breaths as any tenderness slowly decreases. Move around to another tender area and hold. Using a foam roller, you can do the same lying on the ground.

Cupping is also a relatively easy technique that can be performed at home. Using silicone cups and a small amount of lotion or oil, a gentle amount of suction can be used as you glide these cups over an area of restricted or tight tissues like your abdominal wall, inner thighs, or outer buttocks.

MASSAGE THE PERINEUM

Perineal massage is most often used during pregnancy to prepare the perineum for vaginal birth in an effort to minimize the risk of severe tearing and postpartum pain. This technique can also be used postpartum after your perineal scar has completely healed, as early as six to eight weeks following birth, but it can be performed even months or years later if painful sex or scar restriction persists. Perform this massage three times a week for five to ten minutes each session. Prior to starting perineal massage, perform gentle diaphragmatic breaths and pelvic floor relaxation stretches. After perineal massage, you use vaginal dilators if those are in your pelvic floor toolkit.

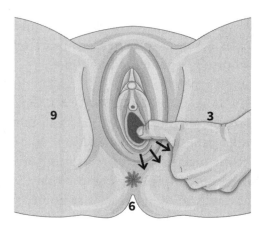

Perineal massage: thumb inserted into vaginal opening, applying pressure toward three o'clock

INSERT VAGINAL OR RECTAL DILATORS

Just like you get a massage to decrease shoulder and neck tension, you can do the same to release pelvic floor muscles. Vaginal dilators are plastic or silicone medical devices that look like tampons of different sizes. Anal dilators are similar to vaginal dilators but are inserted into the anus to release muscle tension toward your backside, which can be helpful for those with tailbone pain, rectal pain, or pooping challenges.

Typically dilators come in a set of four to eight and progressively increase in size by length and diameter. These should be inserted into the vaginal or anal opening in a manner that does not produce pain but rather helps you maintain relaxation of the pelvic floor. These can help release muscle tension upon insertion, with gentle stretching at the opening and with movement. Once one size feels comfortable and pain-free, you can progress to the next largest size. Details on how to use vaginal dilators are included in Chapter 6 on sex, and anal dilators are discussed in Chapter 4 on pooping.

USE A TRIGGER POINT WAND

Trigger point wands are curved devices that help target a particular tender spot in the pelvic floor that needs to relax. These are typically the diameter of the index finger and help women locate nodules of discomfort or tension in the pelvic

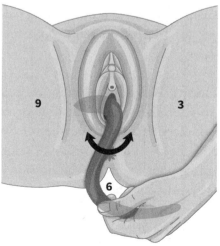

Trigger point wand inserted into vaginal opening
with pressure applied at nine o'clock

floor musculature. They are used internally to sustain gentle pressure in order to promote relaxation of that muscle. These can be used in the vagina or anus, but once you pick a hole to use with the device, stick with that hole. Putting something into your anus and then into your vagina can transfer bacteria.

Once inserted, press the tip of the wand toward your pelvic floor muscles, searching for a sensitive spot. Hold the pressure as you breathe and the tenderness decreases. Typically, a five- to ten-minute session two or three times a week is plenty for trigger point release.

STRETCH IT OUT

Stretches can help lengthen and relax the pelvic floor muscles. Set a time for stretch breaks or find a way to work them into your day, like doing a deep squat while brushing your teeth or a modified downward-facing dog at your desk. Performing stretches for pelvic floor relaxation will help reset your muscles to a more relaxed state. I've found in my practice that the following stretches are the very best for relaxing the pelvic floor muscles. Perform each of the following once a day, holding the stretch for five deep breaths. *For instructional videos of the stretches below, please check my YouTube channel: https://www.youtube.com/ @thevaginawhisperer*

Modified Happy Baby Pose. Lying on your back, bring both knees to your chest and separate your knees wider than your shoulders. Hold and breathe for five breaths. To increase stretch, hold on to the inside of your ankles instead of knees or place your hands on the outside of your feet and bring them toward your chest.

Child's Pose. In hands-and-knees position, touch your toes together and separate your knees wide. Rock back onto your heels, resting your butt on your heels, and stretch your arms forward. Hold for five breaths.

Figure 4 Stretch Lying Down. Lie down on your back with knees bent and feet hips-width apart. Cross your right ankle over your left knee and pull the left leg toward your chest, holding on to the back of the left thigh with both hands. Hold for five breaths, then repeat on the left side.

Figure 4 Stretch Sitting. Sitting in a chair, cross your right ankle over your left knee. Press your right knee down and lean forward with a flat back. Take five deep breaths and switch sides.

Hip Flexor Stretch Sitting. Sitting in a chair without arm rests, turn so you are sitting sideways. Let one leg stretch toward the back and keep the front leg bent with your foot on the ground so you are in a seated lunge position. Take five deep breaths. Switch sides.

Cat–Cow Pose. In hands-and-knees position, place your hands shoulder-width apart and your knees directly below your hips. Inhale deeply and arch your lower back, bringing your head up and tilting your pelvis forward. Exhale deeply and round your back, bringing your head and pelvis down. Take five deep breaths.

Shin-Box Stretch. Seated on the floor with one leg in front of you with your shin at a 90-degree angle, the other leg behind you also bent at 90 degrees. Lean over the front knee with your back straight to feel the stretch in your hip. Take five deep breaths and switch sides.

Thread the Needle. Begin in hands-and-knees position with your wrists directly under your shoulders and your knees directly under your hips. On your exhale, slide your right arm, palm up, underneath your left arm. Let your shoulder rest on the mat if possible. Soften and relax your lower back and feel a stretch around your right shoulder, ribs, and waist. Hold for five deep breaths. Press your left hand into the floor and slide your right arm out, and return to starting position. Repeat on the other side.

Modified Downward-Facing Dog. Stand behind a chair or elevated surface. Place hands on the back of the chair and push hips back until your upper and lower body make an L shape. Your back is flat and parallel to the ground as you feel the stretch on the backs of your thighs. To increase the stretch, walk feet slightly forward and press chest to the floor. Take five deep breaths.

Deep Squat Stretch. Begin by standing with feet slightly wider than shoulder-width apart and toes pointed slightly out. Slowly bend your knees and push your bottom back, as if you're about to sit down. Keep your chest lifted and your back straight. Your heels can be flat on the floor, or you can place a rolled towel or yoga mat under your heels for more support. Hold the pose for five slow breaths, then slowly rise. I encourage people to work this into their day, like when brushing your teeth in the morning and evening or when reheating your coffee for the second or fifth time in a day.

The protocols above are guidelines that will help you relieve pelvic floor tension or weakness (or both) if you are experiencing pelvic floor issues or hoping to prevent them. But as with all things in healthcare, every individual is different, and there is no one-size-fits-all approach. If you follow the guidelines above, and your symptoms worsen or do not improve, check with an in-person pelvic health therapist to determine the appropriate pathway for you and return to these protocols when you have additional information specific to your needs.

When to Consider Other Options

Sometimes it just takes more than exercise, proper posture, and muscle training to improve or resolve a pelvic floor issue. Solving these common and complex problems is more like putting together a puzzle, and sometimes therapy is not enough. Physicians who specialize in pelvic health conditions include the following:

- Urologist (bladder and sexual healthcare)
- Urogynecologist (bladder doctor specializing in female anatomy)
- Gastroenterologist (stomach, liver, and digestive issues)
- Colorectal surgeon (advanced butt stuff including colon, rectum, and anus issues)
- Obstetrician (delivers babies and provides reproductive healthcare)
- Gynecologist (reproductive and sexual healthcare)
- Physical medicine and rehabilitation physician (muscles and nerves)
- Neurologist (brain and nerve issues)
- Pain management physician (chronic pain)

More comprehensive tests can be performed, medications and procedures can help manage or improve symptoms, and in many cases, surgery can offer women the relief they have been seeking. Therapy is performed alongside these additional treatment options to address the symptoms *but also the root cause* of a pelvic floor problem. You are empowered with tools and techniques to manage your symptoms and also knowledge of where to go if additional support is needed. A team approach is the best approach, and if your symptoms do not improve with the guidance provided in this book, see a provider for additional support.

The Dentist for Your Pelvic Floor

Many women who visit my office believe that when it comes to their pelvic health, they are coming too late. First things first: it's *never* too late. *Never.* Learning about your body, implementing healthy lifestyle changes, and working to overcome or prevent pelvic floor issues does not have an expiration date. You can weave the basic practices from this chapter into your life at any age or life stage, and I guarantee you it will make a difference.

While I wish we all learned pelvic floor care sooner, there is so much we can do now to make up for lost time. As we launch into the chapters where I address specific problems, I encourage you to not be hard on yourself or place blame on yourself. This education needs to be integrated into our healthcare system so women get it when they're young and then continuously across their lifespans. We don't know what we don't know. You are here to change that. Changing your habits takes discipline, but it can be done over time with commitment and practice. This information can change your future and, when shared with others, can change theirs.

Let me end Part 1 with a story. After practicing for almost ten years, I started seeing a lot of women who previously had mesh surgically implanted into their vaginas to treat urinary leakage or pelvic organ prolapse. Mesh surgery was and still is a common procedure for fixing prolapse issues. One day, when I examined one of these women, it was clear that the surgically implanted mesh to support her vaginal walls was eroding in her vagina. This was the source of her pelvic pain, which led to an infection and repeated surgeries to remove disintegrating tiny mesh threads throughout her pelvic floor.

While I was grateful to be a trusted resource and help her manage her pain with exercises and massage, I was also disheartened by the pain that she and so many other women with mesh complications experienced. After she finally had the mesh pieces removed and completed pelvic floor therapy, she was 80% pain-free. But I wish her experience had never even occurred.

So many pelvic health issues are treatable, and the right

education and training can prevent them from ever occurring. For example, better labor and childbirth practices can minimize the risk of postpartum challenges, including unnecessary cesarean section surgeries and common pelvic floor problems like leakage, pain, and prolapse. What if these women who had that mesh surgery were coached on optimal birthing practices or given postpartum exercises and training or received therapy heading into menopause to strengthen their pelvic floors? Perhaps they wouldn't have needed that surgery in the first place, and their incredibly painful experience could have been avoided.

I believe this preventative pelvic healthcare system can exist, because it already exists in other disciplines in our healthcare system, like going to the dentist. Around toddler age, you start seeing a dentist regularly every six months to learn how to properly clean your teeth with regular flossing and brushing. You also receive a checkup from the dentist to make sure there are no cavities, decay, gum recession, or teething issues warranting monitoring or addressing. We receive this ongoing care for our teeth and gums for the rest of our lives, and treatment occurs as needed to address any problems that arise. To top it off, *it's covered by insurance.* Dental care is woven into our lives seamlessly and routinely as a normal part of healthcare.

Imagine if pelvic healthcare was woven seamlessly into your life, like dental care. When toddlers are learning to pee and poop, parents would be educated on optimal toileting habits. They could consult with a pediatric pelvic floor therapist if their kids experienced bedwetting, incontinence, or constipation, all common pediatric pelvic floor concerns. At puberty, what if young women had routine checkups with a pelvic floor therapist to explain things as simple as instructions for tampon or menstrual disc insertion, abnormal symptoms of painful menstruation (which can be an early indicator of endometriosis), or urinary leakage with exercise (which 45% of female high school athletes experience)?

During annual primary care or gynecologist visits, questions could be asked about peeing and pooping habits, vaginal pain or burning, pain with sex, premenstrual symptoms or period pain, bladder symptoms during sports, and knowledge of family history of pelvic health issues. Appropriate referrals to a pelvic health therapist could be made to address bladder or bowel symptoms, pelvic pain, or painful intercourse.

Pregnant women should be automatically referred to pelvic floor therapy for exercise training and to address aches and pains, which are common but also totally treatable. A postpartum visit to the doctor or midwife after six weeks isn't enough; there should also be a visit to a pelvic health PT and ongoing care until Mom has returned to work, exercise, sex, and life without pain, peeing, or pooping problems. During perimenopause and menopause, women should be seeing a pelvic health therapist to learn exercises to strengthen their pelvic floors, which weaken over time with age and decreased estrogen and testosterone levels.

Pelvic health conversations from medical providers should be incorporated early and consistently as a standard part of women's healthcare during every season of life. This comprehensive approach addresses not just the symptoms someone experiences (for example, peeing her pants when laughing) but also the contributing factors to the issue (pelvic floor weakness after childbirth) and how to improve them (strengthening or relaxing the pelvic floor). This is not an outlandish healthcare model, because it already exists . . . for our teeth. Vaginas everywhere would benefit from a similar model.

In the next two sections of the book, we will explore each of the individual systems related to your pelvic floor—and we will look at the different seasons of life when pelvic floor changes commonly occur. Again, you may be here for a specific issue or just general learning about your body, but I encourage you to read through *all* of the chapters of this book. You will truly understand how your body works, get insight and guidance to address any pelvic floor issues, and learn to prevent problems down the line. Let's get down to the real business by tackling my two favorite topics first: peeing and pooping.

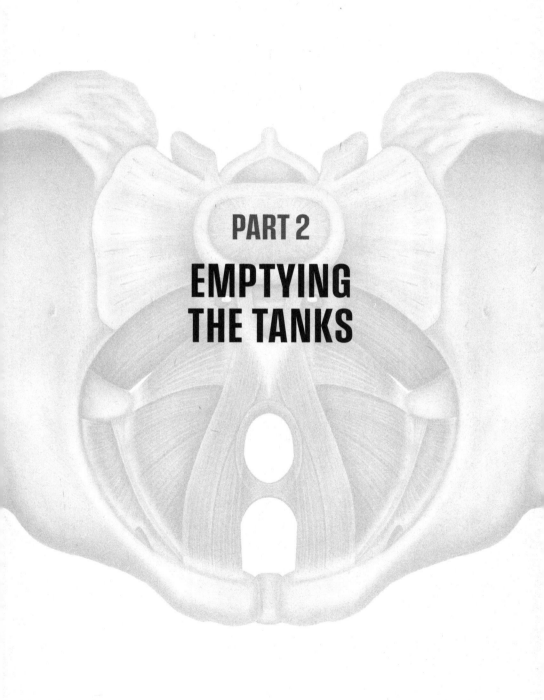

PART 2

EMPTYING THE TANKS

CHAPTER 3

Taming the Tinkler

Sandra, excited about her upcoming retirement as a teacher, always looked forward to her Saturday morning walks with her best friend. She had been doing her two laps around City Park in New Orleans rain or shine for over twenty years. But as her retirement day approached, her frequent urges to pee started affecting her routine. "I reluctantly cut out my morning coffee on Saturdays, I avoided drinking water before heading out, and I peed right before I left and when I passed the bathroom after each lap. Then I'd be good . . . for a while."

Sandra's strategies helped her maintain her Saturday morning walking routine, but the problem grew worse. Soon she couldn't complete even one lap without fighting the urge to pee. With only one bathroom available at the start of her walk, she wore a pad "just in case," and on several occasions that pad came in handy. And then the day came when she couldn't hold it. By the time she made it to the bathroom, not only was her pad completely saturated with urine, but pee dripped down her leg. Mortified and discouraged, Sandra pondered giving up her walks altogether. She could handle giving up her morning coffee, but the idea of missing her Saturday exercise routine with her friend for fear of wetting her pants was devastating.

Peeing seems like such a basic human function, so we expect it to be straightforward. From our diaper days as newborn babies through early childhood and into adulthood, we don't really think about how we pee. We have the urge, we hold it until we get to the bathroom, we sit on the toilet (or hover if it's gross), and then the pee comes out. Easy pee-sy, right? However, during certain seasons of our lives, these basic functions can start to change. Peeing problems can happen at any age—but as the years pass, problems with the plumbing are more likely. The truth is, many women suffer from peeing issues at some point during their lifetimes. But almost always, it is not *just* a peeing issue but *also* a pelvic floor issue.

The relationship between peeing and our pelvic floors is complicated—but preventing peeing problems, and knowing how to heal them, is achievable for all of us, once we have an understanding of how our pelvic floor and bladder work together. Before we discuss what to do when your bladder and pelvic floor are not working together optimally, let's look at how your bladder works and the important role your pelvic floor plays in the peeing process (*hint*: it helps keep pee in and let pee out).

How the Pelvic Floor and Peeing Work Together

When my boys were little, they played with train tracks. They would set up mini stations along the track that circled our living room floor where their train would stop before it reached its final destination under the couch. Similar to these train tracks, your urine has a few stops between where it's made and its final destination . . . the toilet.

First stop: your kidneys. We all know what kidney beans look like (in New Orleans we call them red beans and traditionally cook and eat them on Mondays with rice); kidney beans mirror the shape of your kidneys, which are positioned between your mid- and low-back region and measure a bit larger than the palm of your hand. You have two of them, and they filter your blood, remove waste products, and produce urine.

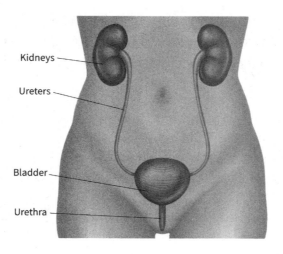

Female urinary system: front view of the kidneys,
ureters, bladder, and urethra

Second stop: your bladder. Urine flows continuously from each kidney, via a tube called your ureter, to your bladder in your lower pelvic area, where it is stored until it leaves your body. As your bladder fills with urine, its muscular walls stretch and send a signal to the brain saying, "Whoa, I'm getting *really* full." To keep pee in, your pelvic floor muscles (remember that urinary sphincter we talked about in Chapter 1) tighten up until you are ready to empty your bladder.

Third (and final) stop: your toilet. Your urine travels from your bladder out of your body through a five-centimeter-long tube called the urethra, originating at the base of your bladder and carrying urine through the pelvic floor and urinary sphincter to exit out to your urethral opening.

Finally, the route is complete. Pee is in the toilet or wherever its final destination may be. During this process, your pelvic floor muscles play two roles: to compress and close your urinary sphincter to keep pee inside your bladder as it fills, and to relax your urinary sphincter to let pee out. This is the way it's *supposed* to work. But unfortunately, things don't always go as planned. Here are just a handful of the complaints and confessions women have presented to me over the years.

> "Every time I laugh, I leak."
> "I have to push to get my stream started."
> "I pee five times a night, and I am losing sleep."
> "My stream splashes my thighs when I pee ever since I had kids."
> "Every time I do jumping jacks, I feel like I'm going to pee my pants."

Our pelvic floors and bladders are interconnected. Just like when a member of my home isn't happy (usually it's me), everyone in the household suffers (my husband and kids). When you have a pelvic floor muscle issue (weakness, tension, or incoordination), your bladder function is affected too (leakage, pain, straining, incomplete emptying, etc.).

My patient Karissa was a university student and cheerleader when she came to see me for help with urinary leakage. Karissa had never been pregnant or given birth. In fact, she had just a handful of sexual experiences since starting college. She shared that she noticed occasional leaks of urine in high school when she did jumps and flips. Not thinking much of it, she wore black tights during practice and a panty liner when she performed at games so she wouldn't be embarrassed if it happened. In college, her leaks became more frequent and her uniforms were green, so dark-colored clothing was no longer an option to mask any moisture. She didn't want to quit cheerleading— but she also didn't want to deal with possibly leaking and having everyone see.

Many female athletes and young women who have never been pregnant leak urine, because pelvic floor–related peeing issues can be due to any number of reasons, and often ones we don't even think of, such as:

- High-intensity exercise that increases pressure on your bladder over time
- Prolonged pushing during childbirth, which stretches your pelvic floor muscles and ligaments and can cause nerve damage
- Decreased estrogen levels, which thin the vaginal walls that support the urethra and bladder
- Frequently delaying the urge to pee, causing pelvic floor muscle tension and difficulty emptying your bladder
- Chronic straining when pooping that weakens your pelvic floor muscles and affects bladder support

In the grocery store or pharmacy, there is an entire section devoted to incontinence products. If you've been in the position of having to purchase these items, did you place them at the top of your cart for all to see, or did you hope to hide them under a head of lettuce and a cereal box? If the former, congratulations! I love your confidence. But for most people, it's the latter. I love that these products are so accessible, but the social stigma around them is unfortunate given how commonly they're used. Does this mean that all women are doomed to pee their pants or pee too often at some point in their lives? And do we just deal with it and hide it? Are adult diapers the destiny for all vagina owners? The answer: *no*.

Karissa and Sandra both needed some vagina whispering, as do many of us at some point in our lifetimes. Even if right now you pee just fine and nothing seems to be amiss, if you have a pelvic floor (that's everyone), then peeing issues can occur when you least expect them. This is why knowing the proper way to pee, tips for prevention, and understanding how to incorporate pelvic floor therapy into your life can do you (and your pelvic floor) a world of good.

The Proper Way to Pee

Believe it or not, there is a right way to pee. I wish I could pass along this info to every little girl at the moment she uses the big-girl potty, and she could carry it with her into adult life. The guidelines below walk you through the best practices for peeing to optimize your pelvic floor health *right now*. After you put these into practice, teach your kids, parents, friends, partners, and patients these six tips, as this simple education will save a lot of pelvic floors.

SIT AND DON'T SQUAT

I like to sit . . . a lot. Ask my husband or my kids. If we head to a park, I will be the first to find a bench to sit on. Maybe because I am often on my feet when working with patients or my tired mom bones will take any break they can, I like to sit. And fortunately for me and my pelvic floor, another great time to sit is when I pee.

Sitting down on a toilet seat to pee helps your pelvic floor and urinary sphincters relax so your bladder can fully empty. Place your feet flat on the floor, lean forward, and rest your forearms on

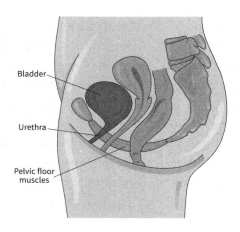

Bladder

Urethra

Pelvic floor muscles

Female bladder: a view from the side

your knees. You might even feel your pelvic floor muscles relax in this position. This is the optimal position to pee.

Some of you may be thinking, "Oh no, Sara! I will *not* sit on a public toilet seat!" But hear me out. When you hover over the toilet seat to pee, your pelvic floor muscles don't fully relax, and your bladder may not empty, leading you to strain or to need to pee again minutes later, neither of which is ideal. If you can find it in your soul to wipe the toilet seat, clean it with a cleansing wipe, or line the seat with toilet paper, please do so and sit down.

But what should you do if you *have* to stand up to pee? In New Orleans, where I live, we have Mardi Gras, which is not actually a single day, but rather a *season* stretching two weeks long and filled with block parties, parades, music, drinking, and very few clean bathrooms. If you attend a parade, you will undoubtedly find yourself with a full bladder, and the only restroom available is a smelly porta potty on a street corner. In this situation, sitting down to pee is just not an option.

If a similar circumstance arises, you can hover your butt over the toilet, lean forward, and rest some of your body weight onto your elbows (I call this the forward squat). This position is your plan B if a toilet is unsuitable for sitting. And what about when you are camping, at an outdoor concert, or wading into the ocean water and need to pee? If a toilet is *not* available, assume the same squat position and place one hand on a wall or tree behind you to rest your body weight and lean back (I call this the lean-back), use one hand in front to hold on to a tree branch or post (the one-hander), or if in the water, squat down and rest your weight on your forearms. In all of these situations, take some deep breaths, relax your pelvic floor muscles, and let your stream flow. If there is no toilet paper (or none suitable for using), a little booty shake at the end gets out those last few sprinkles.

JUST SAY NO TO POWER-PEEING

If you push when you pee (aka power-pee), you're not alone, but there is a better way. The bladder wall is a muscle that pushes your pee out for you. There is *no need* for you to push to empty your bladder. The additional pressure from pushing can stretch your pelvic floor muscles and ligaments over time and lead to pelvic floor weakness, urinary leakage, and even pelvic organ prolapse.

Is it okay if I just push out those last few drops? I don't feel empty unless I do that.

Your kidneys are constantly filtering blood, which constantly creates urine. Your bladder is *always* collecting urine. Hypothetically you could push drops of pee out all day as there will always be more urine trickling into your bladder. A normal amount of urine that remains in the bladder after you pee (called residual volume) is around fifty milliliters of pee, about one fourth of a cup. If you feel like you have to push out those last few drops, try shaking your hips side to side and rocking forward and backward a few times. Or try double-voiding, which entails peeing, wiping, standing up, and then sitting back down again to release any remaining drops. If nothing comes out, get up and walk away knowing you did all you could to empty your bladder without pushing.

DON'T DO KEGELS WHEN YOU PEE

Kegels, as we know, strengthen your pelvic floor muscles. By performing Kegels when you pee, you are tightening and contracting your pelvic floor muscles instead of relaxing them to empty your bladder. Contracting your pelvic floor muscles while peeing sends a mixed message to your brain and prevents your bladder from completely emptying. Peeing is the time for relaxing your pelvic floor muscles, not tightening by doing Kegels.

There is one exception *and only one exception* to this rule. Many therapists, myself included, instruct patients to try to do a Kegel contraction *one time* while peeing to see if they can stop their urine stream. This can be an effective way to test if you are doing a Kegel properly and if you have adequate pelvic floor muscle contraction to hold in your urine. So you can try this once as a test. Then don't do Kegels when you pee ever again.

PEE WHEN YOU HAVE THE URGE

You don't want to miss any of the movie, you don't want to stop at the gas station, you don't want to lose your place in line, so you hold it in. But holding in your pee when you have the strong urge to go causes stress and tension in your pelvic floor. Normal frequency to pee is every two to four hours during the daytime and zero to two times during sleeping hours at night. If you delay the urge to pee, extending past four hours, or frequently throughout the day, your pelvic floor muscles can go into a state of chronic tension, and you may have difficulty relaxing when you eventually go. Also, your bladder becomes overfilled to accommodate a large volume of urine and is less efficient in emptying, which leads to incomplete bladder emptying and possibly even urinary tract infections.

AVOID PEEING JUST IN CASE

"I should probably pee before we go." These words have likely crossed your lips at some point in time when you won't be near a toilet. While this may seem like a good decision, it actually isn't good for your pelvic floor. Typically your bladder stretches as it fills with urine, and nerves in your bladder wall communicate with your brain that it's getting full and you will have to empty it soon. If you regularly pee just in case and empty your bladder before that stretch signal occurs, your bladder can become more sensitive and signal the urge to pee more frequently. Before you know it, you find yourself having the urge to pee all of the time. This is common and totally reversible. Later in this chapter, I share techniques on urge suppression to help you delay the urge to pee to get your bladder back to normal.

Is it okay to pee standing in the shower? Is this bad for my pelvic floor?

Peeing in the shower can be convenient, and great for the environment, but there has been some controversy over whether it would actually damage your pelvic floor or cause a pelvic floor problem. As a seasoned shower pee-er and board-certified pelvic floor therapist, I can assure you it will not cause harm *as long as* you avoid pushing your pee out. Sometimes peeing in the shower can even be helpful; when women have a hard time peeing or if they experience pelvic floor muscle tension after surgery or childbirth, getting in a warm shower and taking some deep breaths can help them pee. One caveat: if you have a bladder urgency issue and running water makes you feel an uncontrollable urge to pee, the running shower may trigger and exacerbate the problem, even causing leakage. Otherwise, feel free to shower-pee away.

HYDRATE BUT DON'T OVERHYDRATE

Many of us will avoid drinking fluids in the hopes it decreases the likelihood of peeing or leaking during an important day or event. But without adequate hydration, your urine becomes *too* concentrated (like that dark yellow urine in your first morning pee), you have to pee more frequently, and you have an increased risk of a urinary tract infection. Dehydration can also cause constipation. Hard poops hanging out in your pelvis can put pressure on your bladder and also lead to more urgency or leakage of pee. So the instruction is simple: stay hydrated. Proper hydration has huge implications for your pelvic floor. Sip water throughout the day instead of chugging a full glass all at once, and avoid drinking beverages that may cause more urgency to pee (all the good stuff: coffee, alcohol, sparkling water, and carbonated drinks). Also, avoid overhydration. Filling your bladder *too much* can cause you to pee too often. If your urine is crystal clear and you are going über-frequently, it's okay to decrease your water intake.

WE MIGHT THINK THAT THESE LITTLE DETAILS—DRINKING LESS WATER, peeing just because we are near a toilet, waiting until the next stop to go if we have the urge—are no biggie. But over time, these small decisions can become a very big deal for your pelvic floor. I recall my twenty-five-year-old patient Maya, a teacher, who often delayed the urge to pee because she couldn't leave her kids in the classroom unattended. As a result, when Maya finally had the opportunity to go to the bathroom, she had a hard time starting her urine stream. Her pelvic floor muscles were so tense from holding back the urge to pee that she needed to push to start her stream until her bladder felt completely empty.

Because she chronically delayed bathroom trips, she developed pelvic floor muscle tension and had to strain to pee, which then led to stretching of her pelvic floor muscles, which ultimately led to bladder prolapse. Essentially, the front part of Maya's vaginal wall, which supports her bladder, became so weak from straining when she peed that her bladder pushed into that wall and out of her vaginal opening. As devastating as this can be for a woman of any age, this was especially challenging for a woman Maya's age.

After I worked with Maya in therapy for three months, she learned the root cause of her problem—how delaying the urge to pee led to her bladder prolapse. This understanding allowed Maya to recognize the importance of going when she needed to go, so she scheduled an assistant to come mid-morning to give her a bathroom break. Without holding in and developing more tension in her pelvic floor muscles, she was able to relax to start her urine stream. She no longer strained. With exercise and some lifestyle changes, Maya's prolapse improved. Maya's story is an example of why these six peeing habits above are foundational for preventing pelvic floor issues and for overcoming them. (It is also proof that teachers need more bathroom breaks.)

When Tinkle Troubles Arise

Now that you know how the bladder and pelvic floor work together, and how to pee, hopefully you have a better understanding of how problems can arise. For some women, issues can come on quite suddenly, and for others, symptoms gradually progress from an occasional sneeze-pee to requiring incontinence pads and liners on a regular basis.

If you are experiencing an issue, one of your first steps is to determine whether your pelvic floor is too tight or too relaxed. Return to Chapter 2 to help determine if your pelvic floor leans toward too tense or too weak. That information will help guide you a bit as you read through any of the problems you might be experiencing in the next pages.

URINARY LEAKAGE

Urinary leakage, also called urinary incontinence, is the loss of urine at an inconvenient or inappropriate time. Leakage can be as mild as losing a few drops of pee when you cough or laugh and as severe as complete loss of your bladder contents when making your way to the bathroom. But no matter how mild or severe your symptoms, peeing your pants just plain sucks. One out of two of us will experience incontinence in our lifetime, and it can limit our ability to socialize, exercise, have sex, and even travel. It affects our mental and emotional health, consuming our brain space with thoughts of "Do I smell?" or "Can you see it through my pants?" or "Where is the closest bathroom already?"

Recently I took up tennis as a reason to get together weekly with a dear group of friends and go outside for exercise. One evening during a match, I jumped up and to the side to return a ball, and I felt a little squirt from my bladder. "Oh, shit," I thought. Not only was I swirling with concerns about a visible wet spot on the crotch of my pink leggings, but for the remainder of my game, I was reluctant to make quick moves or jumps because I didn't want it to happen again. And I lost. Even worse, I am the self-proclaimed Vagina Whisperer. If I am leaking while exercising, what does that say about me? Well, my friends, it says that pelvic floor dysfunction and urinary leakage can happen to anyone, including me, and I educate about peeing, pooping, and pelvic floors all day. My body is changing. I am trying new sports and asking different things of my body. And just like so many of you and the women I work with, my pelvic floor also needs TLC. Let's break down incontinence into three categories:

SNEEZE-PEES: STRESS INCONTINENCE

Leakage that occurs when you cough, sneeze, laugh, jump, run, or throw up is called stress incontinence. Ultimately the pressure on your bladder is greater than the ability of your urinary sphincters and pelvic floor to hold in your pee. So you leak. Karissa, the college cheerleader who came to see me because she leaked, experienced stress incontinence. This is hands-down the most common type of incontinence women experience and the one most often brushed off as normal. But no amount of urine leakage—even from a sneeze—is something to brush off.

Stress incontinence is often due to pelvic floor muscle weakness or *underactivity*, and pelvic floor strengthening exercises like Kegels are the solution. However, leakage also occurs with pelvic floor muscle *overactivity*, when pelvic floor muscles are too tense and Kegels can make leakage worse. So again, before you start squeezing away to improve your pee problems, determining whether you have pelvic floor muscle weakness (underactivity) or tension (overactivity) is essential for you to know which pelvic floor pathway is right for you.

If you have stress incontinence and have pelvic floor muscle weakness, this is a pretty straightforward protocol to increase the strength and support of your vaginal walls and pelvic floor.

Perform Pelvic Floor Strengthening Exercises.
Depending on whether you are trying to stop a leak when you sneeze or stay dry during a five-mile run, you want to train your pelvic floor muscles for what you need them to do. Follow the basic strengthening protocol by starting with quick pelvic floor contractions (three sets of ten repetitions) and longer five- to ten-second holds (three sets of ten repetitions) but pausing if you lose your form or can't hold the contraction without holding your breath, squeezing your butt and thighs, or even curling your toes (toe strength will not help you prevent leaks). If you are working to improve leakage with high-intensity exercises, you can perform these pelvic floor contractions with more dynamic movements like small hops, squats, and lunges and ultimately incorporate that pelvic floor/Kegel contraction and relaxation into every strengthening repetition.

Squeeze Before You Sneeze. Every time I feel a sneeze come on, I cross my legs and perform "The Knack" (discussed on page 62) to prevent a leak. This pre-contraction of your pelvic floor teaches your pelvic floor to turn on when you need to prevent leaks. Now, this may not work right away or every time, but by training yourself to "squeeze before you sneeze" or "Kegel before you cough," you can eventually prevent those little leaks . . . whether you cross your legs or not.

Stay Under Your Tissue Threshold. Once you return to working out, running, or jumping, you may do your first ten jumping jacks and think, "Yay, no leakage. It's working!" But then, on your eleventh jumping jack, you pee your pants. This means your pelvic floor is showing up, but after so long, it's getting fatigued and working past the threshold of what it can handle at that time. The same goes for running or lifting weights if you start leaking when you hit a distance or a weight threshold. Stay under the threshold of what your pelvic floor can handle. This may fluctuate depending on how full your bladder is, the time of day you are working out, or even the day of the month in your menstrual cycle. But listen to what your pelvic floor is reporting and take a pause.

Use a Bladder Support if Needed. Stress incontinence occurs when pressure from above, say with a cough or sneeze, is more than your pelvic floor muscles can support from below and leakage occurs. Placing an internal bladder support into your vagina can take the pressure off the urethra and vagina to minimize leaks. Internal supports can be as DIY as inserting a tampon into the vagina or more advanced like using an over-the-counter or a prescription bladder support like a pessary. These supports can be temporary to help minimize leakage and prolapse while you are working to regain your muscle strength, or permanent solutions to delay surgery and prevent leakage or prolapse from worsening. They can be used only during an activity that may cause you to leak or for all-day support. Be sure to follow removal instructions depending on which support you decide to use. For example, a tampon has to be changed every eight hours, while some pessaries can be worn for several days straight.

I GOTTA GO, I GOTTA GO: URGE INCONTINENCE

Urge incontinence is leakage that occurs with the urge to pee. Sandra, who leaked when she walked with her friend in the park, had urge incontinence. If you experience a strong urge to pee when you wash your hands or hear running water, and before you know it, pee is running down your leg, you have urge incontinence. As mentioned above, peeing in the shower will not cause a pelvic floor problem, but getting a strong urge to pee when you turn the shower on can be an indicator of urinary urgency and a pelvic floor issue.

Treatment for urge incontinence focuses on developing relaxed yet strong and coordinated pelvic floor muscles to help you delay the urge to pee, communicate with your bladder to chill out, and hold in urine to get to the restroom. Women and even men who have urge incontinence often pee just in case to avoid getting an urge to go as they fear they can't make it to a restroom in time.

Suppress the Urge with Breathing. Your diaphragm, the breathing muscle under your ribs, and your pelvic floor work in harmony. Taking deep diaphragmatic breaths can help relax your pelvic floor. Place your hands on the sides of your rib cage. As you inhale, imagine the air expanding your ribs, opening them up like an umbrella. Your hands can give you a place to focus your breath to naturally help your pelvic floor let go. Schedule these breaths throughout the day: in the shower, when you are stressed after a meeting or waiting in line, or before bedtime.

Suppress the Urge with Kegels. When urgency occurs, stop moving, sit down (if possible), and squeeze your pelvic floor muscles (Kegel) quickly and tightly about ten times. This communicates with your bladder to stop sending the urgency signal. Once urgency disappears, continue what you are doing or calmly make your way to the toilet. If urgency reappears, repeat this process again. If the urge comes right as you are pulling your undies down, pause and squeeze your pelvic floor tightly as you sit down to pee. Once seated, take deep breaths to help your pelvic floor relax to start your stream.

Suppress the Urge with Distraction. Distraction helps us take our minds off something, and although often inconvenient, in the case of forgetting about the urge to pee, it can be quite helpful. Earlier I advised you to pee only when you need to pee, and distracting yourself and delaying the urge here contradicts that. But because urge incontinence often causes you to pee too frequently when you don't really need to go, distract yourself by checking your email, making a phone call, going for a walk, or simply focusing on your breathing to take your mind off of the "I gotta go, I gotta go" that's on repeat in your mind.

Avoid Foods and Drinks that Bring on Urgency. If you experience the frequent urge to pee, limiting the foods and drinks that can cause urgency may help. These are pretty much everything we consider fabulous, such as coffee, carbonated drinks such as sparkling water, caffeinated drinks, and alcohol. Foods include spicy foods and citrus or acidic foods and juices. These can irritate the bladder, making it want to empty its contents more quickly, or they might rush to your bladder, giving you a strong, sudden urge.

Manage Your Constipation. I know this part of the book is about peeing, but we can't talk about peeing without talking about pooping. Here's why: these organs are neighbors in your pelvis and affect one another. If your rectum is full of poop because you are constipated, it takes up more space in your pelvic cavity and puts pressure on your bladder, making you have to pee more often or leading to urinary leakage. Additionally, straining during bowel movements weakens your pelvic floor muscles over time. So a top tip to help your bladder is to take care of your bowels. More on this in the next chapter.

MIXING IT UP: MIXED INCONTINENCE

Finally, there is mixed incontinence. If you experience *both* stress incontinence and urge incontinence, you fall into the mixed incontinence category. This pretty much means you leak with a cough or sneeze *and* if you have a strong urge to go . . . not-so-lucky you. Treatment for mixed incontinence entails using both of the recommendations above for stress and urge incontinence, but I suggest that you start by addressing the one that is most troublesome for you. If you find yourself having urgency and leaking more often than a sneeze-pee, you may consider medication for urgency while you work on strengthening your pelvic floor. If leakage occasionally happens with running water but always happens when you run, focus more on the strengthening protocol and strategies for stress incontinence.

FREQUENT PEEING DURING THE DAYTIME

As mentioned earlier, the normal frequency to pee is every two to four hours during the daytime. Frequent urination is often due to a condition called overactive bladder syndrome (OAB), which causes a frequent and sudden urge to pee that's hard to control. Frequent urination can also result in leakage if you can't make it to the restroom in time. Frequent pee-ers, try not to stress; here are a number of things you can do to alleviate the issue.

USE URGE SUPPRESSION TECHNIQUES

If you find yourself going frequently because you have a constant urge to pee, utilize the urge suppression techniques outlined in this chapter.

TIME YOUR PEE BREAKS DURING THE DAY

Try incorporating "timed voids"—a strategy to help you gradually increase time between your pee breaks. Set a timer and go pee whenever that timer goes off. If you get the urge to go before the timer goes off use the urge suppression techniques to delay the urge to go. If the timer goes off and you don't really have the urge to go, go anyway. Then reset the timer and wait until the next time it goes off to pee. The goal of this is to train your bladder to have a consistent filling and emptying schedule.

Say you start this timer going off every thirty minutes. Once you're able to consistently go every thirty minutes, increase the

TAMING THE TINKLER   *99*

voiding interval by fifteen minutes to go off every forty-five minutes. Continue this pattern until you can bump it up to every sixty minutes. Increase the intervals gradually to train your bladder to hold more capacity. However, if fifteen minutes feels impossible, you can just do five-minute increases. Your goal is to get between the two-hour and four-hour marks of peeing breaks. Once you can confidently hold it for two-plus hours during the daytime, you can stop the timed void and start going when you have the urge to go.

FREQUENT PEEING WHILE SLEEPING

Many of us wake at night to pee, and if it's once or twice, that's normal. But with pregnancy, aging, hormonal changes, side effects of medication, overhydrating at night, or just suboptimal bladder habits, some women are losing sleep because they're up several times a night. You shouldn't be getting up more than twice a night to pee; it's not good for your overall health. Try these tips to decrease your nighttime peeing and help you get that much-needed rest.

MANAGE THE BEFORE-BED PEES

If you lie down to go to sleep and have to pee even though you just peed, do Kegels several times in an attempt to suppress the urge. Then take a few deep breaths to help relax your nervous system and your bladder urgency. If the urge persists, distract yourself, read a book, scroll on your phone, listen to a meditation—anything that takes your mind off the urge to pee.

SET AN ALARM

If you are waking multiple times during the night, use an alarm strategy to allow your bladder to gradually learn to stretch. Start by setting a timer to wake every two hours, then stretch it to three hours until you are only waking once at night.

FRONT-LOAD YOUR FLUIDS

If you find yourself peeing multiple times before bed, or if you are waking multiple times at night, plan to drink 50 to 70% of your fluids before noon and stop your fluid intake two hours before bedtime. This gives your bladder time to fill and empty a few times before going to sleep.

DIFFICULTY STARTING YOUR URINE STREAM

Challenges starting your stream are often caused by pelvic floor muscle tension. Also referred to as urinary hesitancy or bladder retention, difficulty starting your stream can be due to aging-related causes, pelvic floor muscle tension, diseases such as diabetes, side effects of medication or surgery, outlet obstruction, impaired nerve function, and more. In the case of pelvic floor tension, focus on relaxation for improvement.

USE THE PELVIC FLOOR MUSCLE RELAXATION PROTOCOL

Using the protocol outlined in Chapter 2 will help relax your pelvic floor muscles. Focus on the stretches that aid in releasing hip and pelvic floor tension, such as the figure 4 stretch, child's pose, and modified happy baby pose.

AVOID HOLDING YOUR PEE FOR TOO LONG

Chronically holding your pee for an extended period (more than four hours during the day) can lead to pelvic floor tension and overstretching your bladder. That tension will result in difficulty relaxing your pelvic floor when it's time to pee. Aim to pee within the normal time frames of every two to four hours during the day and zero to two times at night, for six to eight total pees during the day.

SIT TO PEE

Sitting, as I mentioned earlier, is the optimal posture for peeing. It helps your pelvic floor muscles relax to start your stream.

SPRITZ AWAY

Spritz warm water at the opening of your urethral opening with a peri bottle (a plastic bottle designed to help you cleanse your perineal area) as you breathe and wait for your stream to start. If you still need more help, run the faucet or shower water. This is not a climate-friendly option, but hearing running water can trigger urgency to help your pelvic floor relax.

BREATHE

As you sit, take those big, deep diaphragmatic breaths to help your pelvic floor muscles let go.

What if I feel like my bladder is frozen? No matter what I do, I cannot pee in a public place or outside of my home.

Shy Bladder Syndrome is a more severe experience of difficulty starting your urine stream because the bladder "freezes up." The medical term is *paruresis*, the inability to urinate in the presence of others or the fear of being able to initiate or sustain urination when other people are nearby. This is more likely to occur in public places or if people are around, but it can even occur when someone is in their own home and fears someone hearing their urine stream. Pelvic floor therapy alone typically isn't adequate to effectively resolve it; sometimes a catheter is required to help empty your bladder. If you think you are suffering from this condition, make an appointment with a physician and work with a mental health therapist to address the anxiety surrounding urination, as talk therapy, medication, and meditation have been proven to help.

SPLAYED OR STACCATO STREAM

After giving birth to her daughter, a friend confided in me that the angle of her urine changed, and every time she peed, urine sprayed forward and to the side. Never having struggled with this before, she found if she leaned forward and to the side while peeing, her urine would hit the toilet water instead of spray all over her thighs. "A splayed stream" or "staccato stream" can occur if your urinary sphincter is tense or tight as your bladder is eliminating your urine. Think of when you turn on a hose and place your thumb over the opening, and water either trickles out or sprays in a bunch of directions. Similarly, if your bladder is contracting to eliminate urine but meets resistance of a tight urinary sphincter or tense pelvic floor muscles, your urinary stream may splay in a bunch of different directions or start and stop. Check with a medical provider, typically a urologist or urogynecologist, to rule out a more serious condition, but pelvic floor muscle tension is likely to blame.

ASSUME THE PROPER PEEING POSITION

As mentioned earlier in the proper peeing tips section, remember to always sit down to pee to help your pelvic floor and urinary sphincter relax.

DON'T DELAY THE URGE TO PEE

The longer you hold in your pee, the more tense your pelvic floor muscles get. When you have the urge to pee, pause what you are doing and go.

PRACTICE PELVIC FLOOR MUSCLE RELAXATION

Use the pelvic floor muscle relaxation protocol in Chapter 2 to help relax your pelvic floor muscles on a more consistent basis. Focus on the stretches that aid in relaxing the pelvic floor muscles, like cat–cow pose, child's pose, and modified happy baby pose.

My pee comes out powerfully when I pee. Sometimes I have to tighten my muscles to slow it down. Is this similar to splayed peeing, and should I be relaxing or strengthening my pelvic floor?

What's likely happening is your bladder is really full, and once you relax your pelvic floor muscles, your bladder wall (which is a muscle) is squeezing your urine out so quickly and forcefully it feels like a firehose between your legs. If it's been longer than two hours, empty your bladder when you first have the urge to go and avoid delaying or holding your pee for a prolonged period of time. If you are going frequently (less than every two hours) and this is still happening, your bladder needs to be "stretched" using the tips in the "Frequent Peeing during the Daytime" section above.

BURNING DURING PEEING

Burning when you pee can be a sign of a number of things. First and foremost, it can be a sign of a bacterial infection, yeast infection, urinary tract infection, or sexually transmitted infection. In the case of burning, check in with a medical provider first to make sure you don't have an infection. If you do, treat the infection first. If burning persists, your pelvic floor muscles are likely involved.

Have you ever banged your elbow and felt a sharp shooting pain down your forearm into your pinky and fourth finger? We often say, "I hit my funny bone," but in actuality it's not funny at all, and you've just compressed your ulnar nerve, which resulted in a strange burning or tingling sensation down into your hand where the nerve ends. Similarly, you can compress or irritate a nerve in any part of your body, including your pelvic floor. Tense muscles and tissues along the pathway of your pelvic nerves can result in burning or pain at your urethral opening where your pee exits. To relieve burning, we want to release tension along the entire length of the nerve in addition to focusing on pelvic floor muscle relaxation.

SIT, CHILL, AND BREATHE WHEN YOU PEE

When we anticipate pain, we often tense our bodies to guard or protect against an unwanted sensation. If we have experienced burning with urination in the past, we may anticipate that pain and tense up while we are simultaneously trying to relax our muscles to pee. When you are attempting to start your stream, sit down and take deep breaths to relax your nervous system and your pelvic floor. As your stream starts, even if it burns, continue to take deep breaths to help your pelvic floor and sphincter stay relaxed.

MASSAGE YOUR BOOTY MUSCLES

It's all connected. Tension in your glutes and other muscles attaching to your pelvis can also increase tension in your pelvic floor. Place a firm ball like a tennis ball, lacrosse ball, or yoga ball against the wall and press your butt into the ball. Roll your hips side to side and up and down until you feel a tender spot and hold the ball in that spot for several breaths. Repeat on both sides of your glutes for three to five minutes on each side once a day.

STRETCH IT OUT

Stretching can soften and lengthen the muscles in the pelvic floor, which will help alleviate burning. In the pelvic floor relaxation protocol, focus on child's pose, modified happy baby, and figure 4 stretch lying down to release tense hip muscles. These can be found in more detail in Chapter 2.

BLADDER PAIN/PAINFUL BLADDER SYNDROME

From the time I started practicing as a pelvic health PT through today, I have seen a lot of women (and men) who have bladder pain that is only relieved when they empty their bladder of urine. But when the bladder gradually fills again, their pain returns. So these people pee ten to fifteen times an hour in an effort to get any relief. This condition, after urinary tract infections or more severe bladder disease is ruled out, is known as interstitial cystitis (IC) or painful bladder syndrome (PBS). It is similar to irritable bowel syndrome (IBS) but for your bladder. A urologist typically makes this diagnosis in their office, and treatment includes medication, electrical stimulation to your muscles or nerves, or even surgery. But there's a very clear connection between bladder pain and your pelvic floor muscles.

Overactive or hypertonic pelvic floor muscles are present in almost all patients with painful bladder syndrome/interstitial cystitis, and treating the pelvic floor is an absolute necessity for relieving these debilitating symptoms. Since the pelvic floor is typically tense or overactive with pain conditions, you want to follow the pelvic floor muscle relaxation protocol in Chapter 2, but you may also want to try some of the following.

CHECK IN WITH YOUR BODY AND BOOTY

People with painful bladder syndrome often tense their butt and pelvic floor muscles unknowingly. Because this chronic tension leads to pain, check in to see if you are butt-clenching throughout the day. Set a timer on your phone or place a little red dot sticker on your computer monitor, and every time that timer goes off or you notice the red dot, notice if you are clenching. Take a deep breath, wiggle your hips, and change positions to help those muscles let go.

USE A TRIGGER POINT WAND

In Chapter 2, I covered how to use a trigger point wand to release pelvic floor trigger points or taut bands in your muscles. For the case of painful bladder syndrome, address the side muscles of your pelvic floor but also the tissues internally surrounding your urethra. These spots will be located when the wand is hooked

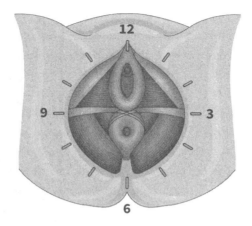

Diagram of pelvic clock over pelvic floor muscles

past your pubic bone and at one and eleven o'clock if you envision twelve o'clock is the position of your urethra.

STRETCH YOUR ABDOMINALS

Tension in your lower abdomen can also contribute to bladder pain. Stretches like thread the needle and modified downward-facing dog and cat–cow (see Chapter 2) are important parts of a daily stretch routine for bladder pain.

HEAT UP

Use heating pads or patches over the abdominal wall can soothe discomfort. A heating pad should not be left on the skin for longer than thirty minutes at a time and should not be overly hot as it can burn your skin.

INCOMPLETE BLADDER EMPTYING

Your bladder sits like a deflated balloon on top of your pelvic floor. If you fill a balloon with air until it's about to pop, you create a lot of pressure inside of that balloon. Similarly, as your bladder fills with urine, it stretches as it fills, and pressure is created inside. This is called bladder pressure. To prevent urine from leaking out, your urinary sphincter tightens at the base of your bladder to meet the pressure inside the bladder. When you pee, your urinary sphincter relaxes, and your bladder walls, which are muscular, squeeze to create pressure to empty the urine.

Similar to an orchestra, if one instrument is out of tune, the music won't sound right. In the case of peeing, if you have too much pelvic floor tension and your sphincter is not relaxing sufficiently or your bladder walls are weak and you don't create adequate squeeze pressure, your urine may not empty well. All of the pieces have to work together properly for things to flow.

LET IT FLOW

If you feel like you are not emptying your bladder, your instinct will be to push while you pee or to get out those last few drops at the end. Even if your stream is weak, pushing will weaken your pelvic floor over time. Instead, sit and take some deep breaths and let your stream flow.

DOUBLE-VOID

Once you have finished urinating but before you stand from the toilet, rock your hips forward and backward and then side to side a few times. Then wipe, stand up, and sit down again, and relax your pelvic floor muscles to see if additional drops come out. This technique is called double-voiding. If a few more drops come out, great. If not, stand up and walk away feeling confident your bladder is empty.

FOCUS ON PELVIC FLOOR MUSCLE RELAXATION

Use the pelvic floor muscle relaxation protocol listed in Chapter 2. Focus on the stretches aimed at releasing pelvic floor muscle tension, like child's pose and modified happy baby pose.

Sometimes if I squeeze and release my vaginal muscles a few times, a few additional drops will come out. Is that a good thing to do or a bad thing?

This is a totally fine maneuver as long as you are not pushing out those last few drops. Squeezing your vaginal muscles is essentially a Kegel contraction, and doing three or four Kegels after you are completely finished urinating can release additional drops of urine still hanging out in your urethra. This is useful if you tend to dribble a little urine on the toilet seat or into your undies after trips to the bathroom. Just make sure you are doing a Kegel instead of pushing out.

Pee Like a Pro

As I mentioned earlier in this chapter, peeing issues typically start small. Maybe it's a little leak here or there and an occasional change of underwear. Perhaps you pee just in case before leaving to drop your kids at school and then again when you return home. Sometimes you feel the urge when you water your garden. Then it becomes every time you wash your hands. But over time, these small inconveniences become bigger problems and more to manage.

When you next head to the bathroom, observe how you are peeing. Are you relaxing or power-peeing? Do you truly have an urge, or are you going just in case? Now that you are armed with tips to tackle these common issues, you have what it takes to pee like a pro so you can absolutely live your best life.

CHAPTER 4

The Scoop on Poop

After struggling with constipation on and off for years, Lashona, a hospital administrator and mother to a seven-year-old son, came to me for therapy because she was experiencing pain with bowel movements (BM). In the course of a few years, she had a harder time emptying, and she endured a sharp, shooting pain with every attempt to poop: "It feels like an ice pick is stabbing me in my butthole," she told me. She started working from home so she could have easy access to her bathtub and heating pad to soothe her aching bottom after her daily business. "At first it was just happening every once in a while, and I thought it would eventually go away, but it's been months now. I wake up every day dreading going to the bathroom."

Whether you strain to empty, leak stool, have persistent hemorrhoids, or experience pain with bowel movements, your pelvic floor is involved. Recall your pelvic floor anatomy from Chapter 1. The female pelvic floor has three openings: the vaginal opening, the urethral opening where urine empties, and the anal opening where stool and gas exit your body. Your anal sphincter (aka your butthole) and your urethral opening (your pee hole) are neighbors. Just as peeing problems often have a pelvic floor component, so do pooping problems.

Number two has been a big part of my life. Not just by taking poops, cleaning up my kids' poops, and talking about poops at my dinner table, but also by educating people about how pooping problems are often a sign that there are issues with one's pelvic floor muscles. I aim to empower people to poop better—because how you empty is a huge factor in protecting your pelvic floor. From hemorrhoids and fissures to farting and constipation, many of these gastrointestinal challenges can be treated through pelvic floor therapy that we can do in our own homes. But before we dig into how to properly poop and improve these conditions, I have one PSA: if you are experiencing weight loss, decreased appetite, abdominal pain, bleeding with bowel movements, or a sudden change in your bowel movements, I encourage you to first check in with your general doc. You want to rule out conditions or diseases that could be more systemic and severe.

How the Pelvic Floor and Pooping Work Together

Do you ever feel bloated after a big meal or a vacation? If you're lucky, the next morning you will wake up, drink a cup of coffee, do a little online shopping, and then BAM—the urge will hit, and you will have a huge bowel movement. Then you will feel like a million bucks for the rest of the day. Having a solid and complete number two, such that we feel empty and relaxed afterwards, can make our day. But constipation, pain with bowel movements, or incomplete elimination can leave us feeling grumpy, tired, and uncomfortable, and wreak havoc on our pelvic floors.

Poop is waste, and its path begins after food enters your mouth. Your food travels through your esophagus and empties into your stomach. In your stomach, acids break down the food, and then it empties into your small intestine, which is actually not small considering it measures twenty-two feet in length on average. In the small intestine, nutrients are absorbed from your churned-up food particles, and all the rest empties into

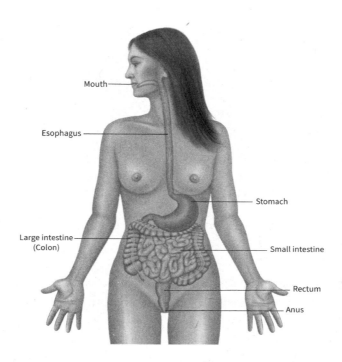

Female digestive system: front view of the intestines, colon, rectum, and anus

your large intestine, also known as your colon. The large intestine is shorter than the small intestine, measuring just five feet in comparison, but it's about five centimeters wide, a smidge smaller than the top of a soda can. Your colon is where all the magic happens. It receives the digested food from your small intestine, dehydrates it, and forms poo. Muscular contractions of your colon move the waste down until it eventually reaches your rectum.

The rectum serves as a passageway between the colon and your anal sphincter, where poo exits the body. Once a small amount of waste or gas hits the rectum, your brain determines whether it's air and you just need to squeak out a fart, or it's poo and you need to make your way to the toilet. Your pelvic floor responds by contracting to support what's in your rectum and tightens up to help prevent your poo from coming out. The

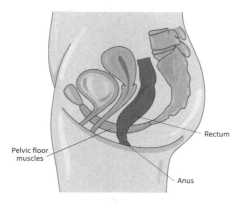

Pelvic floor
muscles

Rectum

Anus

Female rectum: a view from the side

specific muscles in your pelvic floor responsible for maintaining bowel control are your puborectalis muscle and your anal sphincter.

The puborectalis muscle slings around the bottom of your rectum and kinks it like a hose as it fills. The very bottom portion of your digestive tract is your anus, a short canal after the rectum that serves as the final passage of poo from your body. The anus has two sphincters, the internal anal sphincter and the external sphincter, which work as additional mechanisms to hold in poo and relax to let it out. They are like the backup dancers in the pooping show.

In order for stool to exit your body, your puborectalis muscle relaxes, and a gentle bearing down creates pressure to relax your anal sphincters and release poop to its final destination. *Note this difference from peeing.* With pooping, you *should* push to empty, but you want to be sure to exhale and breathe as you do so. With peeing, you should not push to empty as the bladder with its muscular walls pushes pee out as you relax.

The entire digestive process from mouth to butthole takes anywhere from one to three days. What you eat (meats and cheese are harder to break down than fruits and veggies), your hydration (not getting enough water slows this process), how

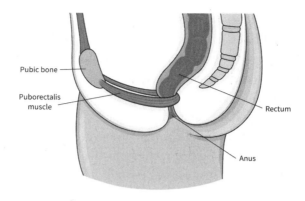

Pubic bone

Puborectalis
muscle

Rectum

Anus

Side view of puborectalis muscle sling, which tightens rectum to hold in stool

quickly or slowly your colon contracts to propel your food (certain medications or conditions can slow this down), and the ability of your pelvic floor muscles relax to empty (pelvic floor muscle tension or incoordination can prevent emptying) all play a role. One way to test your digestion is with corn, which does not break down well and will end up in the toilet. Eat a bowl of corn or corn on the cob and watch for when the corn kernels appear in your poop. The amount of time between eating the corn and the arrival of your corn-poop can give you a decent sense of how long it takes you to digest food.

Your entire gastrointestinal system is related to your pelvic floor health, from the types of foods you eat to when you eat them and how your stomach and colon are processing them. That's also not the only system that affects your bowel health, as is the case with many pelvic health matters.

One of my very first patients, a young college-aged woman named Shannon, complained of difficulty emptying her bladder. (This is a chapter about pooping, not peeing, but stay with me.) When she came in, I inquired about her general pelvic health, as I do with all my patients. How were her bladder habits, menstrual cycle, pooping schedule, and sexual health? She shared she had struggled with constipation since she was a kid. She remembered not wanting to poop at school, so she would hold it all day until she got home. Then it would hurt to empty her bowels, so she avoided it, often going several days without bowel movements. This led her to strain when she tried to poop, which over time led to a weakening in her pelvic floor muscles, which then caused a mild bladder prolapse. All this prevented her from completely emptying her bladder. So although she presented with a bladder issue, it was a pooping problem that was the culprit.

Shannon's issue is just one of many I often hear about in my office. And while there are entire books written about elimination and gut health, they often don't focus on the role of our pelvic floor in the issues that arise. Many of the common gastrointestinal complaints can be related to pelvic floor issues:

> "I feel poop is stuck in a pocket right at the opening, and I can't get it out."
>
> "My poops are really skinny and I feel like I don't empty all the way."
>
> "My poops are like hard rocks, and I only go once or twice a week if I'm lucky."
>
> "I have to sit for thirty to forty-five minutes to get things going."
>
> "I have stains in my underwear no matter how well I clean."
>
> "I feel like I'm not going to make it to the bathroom in time when I get the urge to go."

Why does something so natural go awry? Our modern world goes fast; we move through the day not paying attention to what we eat and drink (and *how* we eat and drink). We don't always carve out enough time for exercise. We rush our bathroom breaks, sometimes forcing ourselves to go (or putting off when we need to go). And we don't practice good elimination habits. All of these behaviors cause stress to the pelvic floor and interfere with our ability to take nice, soft, consistent poops.

When you can't or don't poop, you pretty much feel like . . . poop. So let's do something about it.

The Proper Way to Poop

A really long time ago, folks squatted over a hole in the ground to empty their bowels. Over time, outhouses were created for people to pee and poop in one location *and* to move smelly poop away from homes. Eventually, these outhouses evolved to include a chair with a "toilet seat" that allowed people to sit instead of squat. And as running water became available, toilets moved from outside to inside homes so folks no longer had to walk in the cold or dark to use the restroom. This is how we came to our modern toileting situation, which is cozier and more comfortable, but not necessarily the optimal position for pooping. In short, as the world has evolved, we've actually moved further away from the best way to poop. Turns out we had it right from the very beginning.

ASSUME THE OPTIMAL POOPING POSITION

In terms of pelvic floor health, you need to squat. Remember that puborectalis muscle we mentioned a few pages back? The squatting position relaxes and lengthens that muscle, essentially straightening your rectum and anus so your poop has a straight shot out instead of having to make a tricky and often challenging turn. The squat position is the first rule of the proper way to poop.

Since most of us don't have a hole in the ground for elimination, nor do we want one, there are still ways to mimic the squatting position when pooping. Sit down on the toilet seat and place your feet on a step stool or pooping stool so your knees are positioned above your hip level. Getting your knees higher than your hips will improve emptying, decrease straining, and increase efficiency.

Thanks to some proponents of this proper poop form, a

Sitting   Squatting

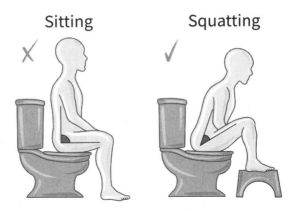

Sitting upright on toilet compared to sitting with feet elevated and leaning forward to relax pelvic floor

number of footstools you can buy have revolutionized better poops using modern-day toilets. These poop stools are available online and in stores, but you can also do it yourself by placing yoga blocks or any other prop of similar height under your feet. Just make sure your feet are elevated at least seven inches.

AVOID STRAINING

When we have the urge to poop and just can't get it out, we feel the desire to strain and push super hard to get those pesky poops out. Breathe out with a forceful exhale to aid emptying without overtightening your pelvic floor. These breaths should be long and slow, not overly aggressive. Some ways to do this as you bear down are to exhale as if you are blowing out fifty candles, blow through a straw (a great one for kids), puff your cheeks and pretend you are blowing bubbles, or grunt and make a *grr, moo,* or *hmm* sound. You may have to perform them several times as you bear down while pooping, and that's okay. Holding your breath or straining to empty actually makes pooping harder and less efficient, and causes *more* pelvic floor tension, obstructing your ability to empty. I mentioned earlier that some pushing and bearing down is recommended to eliminate, but the key here is to *not* hold your breath and cause more pressure on your pelvic floor.

Are bidets okay to use after bowel movements? I heard they can cause infections.

Bidets can be an excellent butt and vulva washer, and I particularly like them for use after bowel movements, during menstruation, and immediately postpartum. Several bidet units are available that are easily installed onto your home toilet, offering different angles of spray, intensity of spray, and even options for warm or cold water. Bidets have not been found to increase the likelihood of getting vaginal or urinary infections, hemorrhoids, or fissures and can actually help minimize aggressive wiping if you experience discomfort. They have been found to increase anal itching if overused, and bacteria do hang out on the actual sprayer, so it needs to be disinfected and cleaned along with your toilet bowl. Otherwise, I'm a fan.

CREATE A ROUTINE AS MUCH AS POSSIBLE

Have you noticed that sometimes the urge to poop comes maybe thirty minutes after a meal? Your digestive system likes a routine, and eating meals at similar times of day and around the same size allows your digestive system and organs to get into a rhythm that can facilitate an optimal pooping process.

Many people eat, then have to go. I am envious of these people as their systems are pretty regular and predictable. When something goes in, something comes out. Eating triggers the gastrocolic reflex, which causes muscular contractions of your colon to push poop toward your rectum, then signal the urge to poop. Often if we are constipated, we avoid eating because we feel so full, but having a little something to eat can actually help get things moving. If your schedule allows, get into a rhythm of eating meals around the same time every day, and you can anticipate this reflex to trigger thirty to forty-five minutes after eating to help you poop. You may have to wake earlier if the reflex happens in the morning so you have adequate time to handle your business before you head to your place of business.

DON'T DELAY THE URGE

The ideal frequency to have a bowel movement is a range between three times a day and three times a week. Despite the conventional norm of a regular once-daily bowel habit, very few people actually have that practice, and pooping every other day still keeps you in a normal range of motility.

Some folks avoid pooping in public places or when away from home. And many folks, myself included, simply can't stop when the urge presents because we are busy, preoccupied in a meeting, or teaching a classroom of students. Whenever I can't stop my appointment, I hold, and the urge eventually goes away. It comes back later, but by that time, my poops are hard, requiring more force and straining, which can weaken my pelvic floor over time. Additionally, when poop stays in the rectum for a prolonged period over and over again, the rectum stretches, becomes floppy, and is less effective in expelling poop.

Chronically delaying the urge can lead to bigger challenges, like complete impaction of stool, which requires more aggressive treatments to empty. The take-home message? Don't delay the urge if you can help it. And plan your schedule so if you typically have the urge in the morning or after a meal, you have adequate time to empty the tank.

KEEP YOUR POOP SOFT-SERVE SOFT

Your poop should be soft like soft-serve when it comes out. Poop that is too soft can be problematic as it is more difficult to hold in, leading to more urgency and even leakage getting to the bathroom. To firm up your stools if they are too soft, add bulking foods to your diet like potatoes, white rice and white bread, apples, and bananas.

If it's too hard, it is likely to cause damage to your pelvic floor, and you may never feel empty. To soften your stools, boost your fresh fruits and veggies, decrease your processed foods and dairy, stay hydrated, and start "prune-chasers," as one of my patients who struggled with constipation during her pregnancy called them. After every meal, she ate one or two prunes to give her body a little fiber boost throughout the day and help her poop.

Amazingly, there is a chart you can use, called the Bristol Stool Form Scale, to compare your poops and see what you may need. When you next go to the bathroom, bring in this book and check your poops with the photo below.

If your stools are type 1 or 2 and harder lumps, you need to soften your stool. If they fall between type 3 and 4 and come out smooth like soft-serve ice cream, keep up the great work. If they are type 5, these are a little on the soft side, and you may need to add a bit of fiber. Types 6 and 7 are diarrhea and indicate your bowels are irritable, inflamed bowels, and your stool needs bulking.

UNTUCK YOUR BUTT

Remember the rules of posture in Chapter 2? The way you sit and stand affects your pelvic floor and how you poop. Standing with your butt sticking out (tilting your pelvis forward) or tucking your butt under (tilting your pelvis backward) influences

Bristol Stool Chart

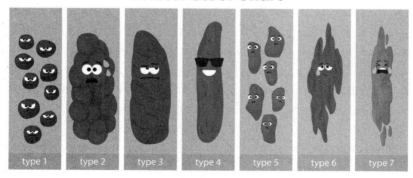

Bristol Stool Form Scale

the tension and function of your pelvic floor muscles needed for elimination. Again, neutral alignment is best. I find a lot of folks with pooping problems are butt-clenchers, so check in with your tush while sitting and standing and assume the best postures to avoid overtightening your backside.

MANAGE YOUR STRESS

Just about every morning, I wake up, get my kids' school lunches packed, hustle my groggy kiddos out the door, chow a granola bar, and chug a cup of coffee on my drive to school drop-off. My nervous system is far from rested, and my butthole is far from relaxed. These are not ideal conditions for when the urge to poop strikes.

The pooping process is stimulated by a "rest and digest" state in our nervous systems. In a highly anxious world, our "fight or flight" sense may often be on guard—and being on guard prevents us from getting into the relaxed state required for a good, healthy poop. You've likely heard the term "tight-ass" for an anxious or tightly wound person. A tense person can quite literally have a tight butthole, which inhibits the ability to poop. "Tight-ass" is in fact a pretty accurate term to describe these folks. On the flip side, when our nervous systems are calm, our colons can work their magic to relax the pelvic floor muscles and anal sphincters to empty.

To get in a rhythm of regular emptying, you must also manage your stress levels. Exercise, adequate sleep, healthy meals, screen-free downtime, close connections with family or friends, acupuncture, therapy, and a whole list of other self-care routines can help. But whatever works to help you manage your stress, do it. Not just for your poops, but also for your entire pelvic floor, your overall health, and your quality of life.

IF YOU FOLLOW THE SEVEN TIPS ABOVE, YOU ARE WELL ON YOUR WAY to pooping properly and minimizing your risk of pelvic floor problems. And even then—given that there is a world of things

THE SCOOP ON POOP   *121*

that can impact our pelvic floors—problems still can arise. And there's a lot we can do for that, too.

I've struggled with constipation since I was a kid. Is that causing my pelvic floor problems now?

Many, many kiddos struggle with bowel disorders as kids. Kids often delay going because they are too busy playing. They feel embarrassed or too shy to poop at school or in public places. They sit on high toilets, which prevents their ability to get into a squatting position. All of these habits likely play a role in childhood constipation. Eventually poops left for a prolonged period in the rectum become hard and painful to empty, leading kids to not want to poop at all. These kids often turn into my adult patients who come in reporting they have suffered from constipation most of their lives and are now struggling with pelvic floor problems. A full rectum can also lead to chronic bedwetting and incontinence in kids and weakening pelvic floor muscles due to chronic straining.

When Poop Problems Arise

Margaret first came to see me for abdominal pain and bloating. The pain had begun years earlier when she started traveling more consistently for work. As a business consultant, she boarded a flight every Monday morning, then had a jam-packed week of meetings, happy hours, and work dinners. She returned home late on Thursday evenings. Rarely did she have a week at home, unless she took vacation.

She did not know if pelvic therapy was what she needed, but after years of seeing gastroenterologists, making dietary changes, and taking medications, her discomfort was next-level unbearable. When she came to see me, we talked about her routine—and quickly took note of the fact that she had fallen out of sync with exercise, consistently ate meals out, and raced to early-morning meetings, leaving little time upon waking to tend to the urge to poop if it arose. She wasn't able to leave her meetings, and by the time she got back to her hotel room at the end of the day, her pants were tight, her abdomen was bloated, and her abdominal pain was borderline unbearable. This cycle continued for months.

I asked her what had happened in her care before she came to me. She said she had sought help from a physician who prescribed fiber supplements and recommended drinking more water. After a few days of fiber, she was gassy and even more bloated and stopped taking the supplements. She'd then tried over-the-counter medications to help with bloating and gas, which were minimally effective. So she took another medication to get some pain relief, but that caused even more constipation. After several months of no relief, she noticed blood in the toilet after bowel movements and had sharp pain in her rectum when having a bowel movement. Her third gastroenterologist took an X-ray of her abdomen and found she was completely backed up with stool. That's when her physician suggested pelvic floor therapy, as it was a treatment she had not yet tried.

As you can imagine, Margaret was no longer just desperate. She was intensely concerned. I told her that if she could commit to doing regular pelvic floor therapy care, she would be able to turn around many of her symptoms. And with that, she made a promise to herself to do just that: for the next four months, she made her therapy appointment work with her busy travel schedule. She integrated massage techniques for her abdomen, stretches to help relieve abdominal discomfort and pelvic floor tension, and better eating and exercise routines when away from home into her daily lifestyle. Sure enough, her symptoms improved. Her pain was less, she was having two or three bowel movements a week (an improvement from once a week), and she knew how to get things back on track if she started feeling pain or discomfort again.

Margaret is not alone. Many of us struggle with pooping problems and don't have the awareness, tools, or tips to improve them. Let's address the most common challenges with tips to help.

CONSTIPATION

Constipation is the number one gastrointestinal complaint in our country, and it can manifest in a number of ways. Constipation is the chronic condition of having hard bowel movements that require straining to empty, of incomplete emptying, of pooping less than three times a week, and straining every time you need to go. To make this pooping dilemma even more interesting, there are three main types of constipation.

SOOOOO SLEEPY: SLOW TRANSIT CONSTIPATION

Slow transit constipation occurs when the involuntary contractions of your colon are not effective or efficient in moving your stool down to your rectum to empty. This slower transit time causes your stool to harden, making it more difficult to pass. Most people experience slow transit constipation at some point. Whether it's when you vacation and you suddenly don't have a bowel movement for a week, you ate too many cheddar cheese cubes at a birthday party, you are ovulating and your progesterone is surging, or you are dehydrated from the summer spikes in temperature, slow movement through your gut is common.

I'M STUCK AND I CAN'T GET OUT: OUTLET OBSTRUCTION CONSTIPATION

Does your poop feel stuck at the opening, like it gets through your colon but no matter how hard you strain or struggle to empty, it just doesn't want to come out? Outlet obstruction constipation is a situation in which your stool moves through your colon just fine and reaches your rectum, but once in the rectum, it can't "get out" due to the impaired ability to relax your pelvic floor muscles or incoordination of your pelvic floor muscles. While it might not feel like it, your pelvic floor muscles are not relaxing or coordinating properly to get it all out.

Is it safe for me to manually remove a hard stool in my rectum?

In the case of severe constipation when poop is so packed in that you can't empty it, some folks have the urge to insert their finger into their anus to remove it. This technique, called manual evacuation or disimpaction, requires inserting an index finger (ideally lubricated and gloved) into the rectum, gently breaking up the stool using a scissoring motion, then removing it in a circular manner. This maneuver is repeated until the rectum is cleared of hardened stool. This manual evacuation can be appropriate as an emergency technique (I had to perform it on my kiddo once during a severe bout of constipation on a family vacation) but should not be relied upon as a regular method to remove stool as it can damage your tissue and sphincter with constant finger poking in the area. Ideally, your system can regulate to promote emptying without a manual assist. Instead, check in with a gastroenterologist or pelvic floor therapist.

MIXING IT UP: SLOW TRANSIT AND OUTLET OBSTRUCTION CONSTIPATION

There are a lucky few who have both types of constipation: slow transit and outlet obstruction. These two forms can easily over-lap. If this is you, your belly likely feels bloated and full, *and* you feel like poop is stuck in your rectum and just won't come out.

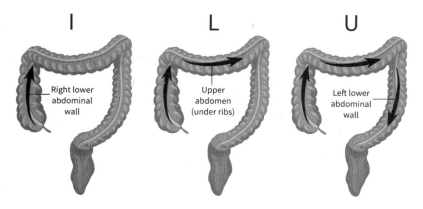

Abdominal massage along course of colon from right to left

FOR ALL THREE FORMS OF CONSTIPATION, I RECOMMEND THE FOLLOW-ing pelvic floor therapy strategies:

Utilize Abdominal Massage. The colon is positioned like an upside-down U in the abdominal cavity. Performed daily for fifteen minutes with moderate pressure (one to two centimeters deep) for four to eight weeks, abdominal massage reduces bloating, shortens transit time, decreases fecal incontinence, and decreases constipation. It can also stimulate your parasympathetic nervous system, which is responsible for helping you empty your bowels. Abdominal massage is free and can be performed on yourself, and there are no negative side effects.

To perform, lie flat on your back with your abdomen exposed. Place one hand on the lower right side of your abdomen. With moderate firm pressure, move your finger in a circular motion, performing a deep massage. Perform five to ten circles and work your way higher up the right side toward your ribs, like in the shape of an I, and repeat. When you reach the upper right side of your abdomen, but below your ribs, move toward your left side, creating the shape of an L, massaging the upper abdomen underneath the rib cage. When you reach the upper left side of your abdomen, work your way down toward the left lower abdomen, creating a U shape. You are massaging with firm pressure in the I–L–U course along your abdominal wall. Once at the left lower abdominal wall, you can repeat this process for a total of ten minutes of massage.

Perform Daily Stretches. If your pelvic floor muscles are part of your pooping problem, follow the relaxation protocol in Chapter 2. Just make sure you clear the room of loved ones, because you will likely release some gas during these stretches. The best position to relax the pelvic floor and puborectalis is the squatting position, or getting your knees elevated above hip level. Perform these stretches daily in the morning or evening and after any exercise or workouts:

- Child's pose
- Happy baby pose
- Deep squat stretch

Breathe. I can't tell you how many times I've instructed my boys to "take a deep breath, buddy," knowing fairly well this should be something I say to myself throughout the day. There is no question about it—taking slow, deep breaths helps quiet your nervous system, decrease pain, and improve stool consistency and frequency of bowel movements. Perform thirty minutes of slow, deep breathing, five days a week, inhaling for four seconds and exhaling for six seconds.

Use Proper Pooping Mechanics. Proper pooping posture is essential for folks who struggle to empty. Go grab your footstool (or poop stool) and follow my instructions above on how to assume the optimal position for pooping to help you empty more completely when you go.

Support Your Perineum. Sitting on the toilet, wrap toilet paper around your fingers and place your finger on your perineum, facing upward. With firm pressure up from your fingers onto your perineum, perform a bearing-down maneuver to have a bowel movement. Bearing down is the "laying an egg" exercise from Chapter 2. Try this maneuver while sitting on the toilet with feet flat on the floor, and then try with feet elevated on a toilet stool. Feel your perineum press down into your fingertips and work on that slowly and gently, performing five to ten times until you feel confident you can recreate this maneuver while bearing down to have a bowel movement.

Try an Anal Dilator. When you have outlet obstruction, you likely have tension or tightness in the puborectalis muscle, which leads to poor or uncoordinated relaxation when attempting to empty. This can be treated with yoga poses and stretching as mentioned above, but manual release of these muscles, by stretching and performing deep pressure point massage inside your butthole, can also help. An effective way to do this on your own is with an anal dilator. Dilators look like tampons and come in progressively larger sizes. Often used vaginally for pelvic floor muscle relaxation and desensitization, they can also be used rectally.

Two things to note for correct use: First, once you use them rectally, don't put them back in the vagina, and vice versa. Pick a hole and stick with it. There are dilators specifically for anorectal use that have a longer handle and more comfortable design for insertion into your bum. Second, use a lot of lubricant. If you are using a latex condom, do not use an oil-based lubricant. If you are using a silicone lubricant, do not use a silicone dilator. Water-based lubricant is typically safe for use with anal dilators. Details on dilator use are in Chapter 2's relaxation protocol.

Every time I travel, my bowel movements slow down. Is vacation constipation a real thing?

Nothing beats returning home to your toilet after not having a bowel movement for four days during a trip. Vacation constipation is actually super common for a lot of people due to dietary changes, sitting for prolonged periods of time, and decreased water intake. Even changing time zones can have an impact (literally). To help maintain good poops while traveling, stay hydrated and bring along probiotics, prunes, or magnesium citrate supplements, which can help keep your stool soft and easier to pass. Consider bringing a step stool with you or place your suitcase or a trash can under your feet while pooping to get into that optimal squatting position. Also, get up every hour on long plane rides and stop every two on long car rides.

FECAL INCONTINENCE

On three occasions, I almost pooped my pants. In 2007, I was headed into my first day of work in Austin, Texas. To say I was nervous would be an understatement. The entire twenty-minute drive, I could feel my stomach churning. I looked at my MapQuest printout (in the days before iPhones and map apps), and sweat started to bead on my forehead as I got closer. I had to go . . . badly. Fortunately, as I turned onto the access road just a half mile to my new workplace, a bright light and haven appeared: Starbucks. I swerved into the parking lot, parked, and waddled inside as I cautiously tried to clench my butthole to prevent an accident. I finally reached the toilet and swiftly pulled down my pants, sat down, and proceeded to take a massive poop. And after a few minutes and sweet relief, I cleaned up and headed the remaining half mile to my new clinic to start my career as a pelvic PT. Most of us, at some point in our lives, will experience something like this, or worse.

Fecal incontinence is defined as the urgent, accidental, and involuntary loss of stool or gas. Although less than 10% of women report this, it's more likely upwards of 20%, and many of us might have an incident at some point in our lives, as I did in Austin that day. Those who experience fecal incontinence often feel embarrassed, which leads to social isolation, poor self-image, and inability to work, and it is one of the leading reasons for admission to a nursing home. If you have ever experienced this, you know the frustration and humiliation one feels.

Urgency, loose stools, and limited access to a toilet can all be contributing factors that lead to fecal incontinence. Our muscle mass decreases with aging, and just as with urinary leakage, having difficulty holding in gas or stool can occur. Women who have recently given birth, have experienced a third- or fourth-degree perineal tear during birth, have had pelvic organ prolapse, have undergone a colon resection or pelvic radiation, or have nerve injury are all at a higher risk.

The ability to hold in a bowel movement and make it to the bathroom in time is aided by three mechanisms: the internal anal sphincter, external sphincter, and pelvic floor muscles (including the puborectalis). Typically with fecal incontinence, there is a deficit or weakness in one or several of these areas. We talked a lot about the importance of the puborectalis muscle with regards to constipation, but if this muscle is weak and not kinking the hose (rectum) effectively, stool slides on through to the anus without much of a barrier. And if the anal sphincter is also weak, then it's really challenging to hold it in. Looser stools make it even harder. To address fecal incontinence, start here:

PLAN FOR EASY ACCESS TO A BATHROOM

Make sure you have easy access to a bathroom if you suffer from incontinence. It is a key lifestyle modification while you begin to implement some of the strategies below. At home, make sure there is a clear pathway to the bathroom should urgency or leakage occur. Choose a side of the bed that's closest to the restroom. Have a nightlight or well-lit path to walk there. And even have a towel on your nightstand or side table should you need it. Consider a bedside commode if the walk to the bathroom is farther than what's manageable. Addressing incontinence is not always about making it go away. It's also about implementing strategies to make life easier and more manageable. When traveling on an airplane or train, use the restroom before boarding and choose an aisle seat should you need to use the restroom in flight.

STRENGTHEN YOUR PELVIC FLOOR

Start with the pelvic floor strengthening protocol in Chapter 2. As your muscles get stronger and you can hold a Kegel contraction in the lying down or sitting position for a longer period of time, about ten seconds, progress to performing Kegel contractions in a standing position. Working up to ten seconds while standing and slowly increasing the time to twenty seconds will improve your pelvic floor muscle endurance to help you walk to the bathroom.

When the urge to have a bowel movement arises, contract your pelvic floor for ten to twenty seconds while you are standing next to the toilet before sitting down to have a bowel movement. The next time, hold it for ten to twenty seconds at the door to the bathroom. Then practice holding it for ten to twenty seconds down the hallway from the restroom. Holding the urge successfully without leakage will help you feel more confident in your ability to prevent leakage with fecal urgency when away from home.

BULK UP YOUR BOWEL MOVEMENTS

Holding a bunch of rocks in your hands, the equivalent of holding harder pieces of poop in your rectum, is pretty easy to manage. Then imagine holding applesauce in your hands. The applesauce will likely seep out through your fingers and is more challenging to contain. The difficulty when you combine soft stools and weak pelvic floor muscles is it's hard to hold them in. This can result in a strong urgency to poop, difficulty making it to the bathroom in time, or staining and seepage in your underwear. Firming up your stools can help.

Get the consistency right. Closer to firm without being overly hard will help, as if it's too soft it may not come out at once. Between types 3 and 4 on the stool chart is ideal. If you are taking a stool softener or magnesium, you may want to decrease intake. Additionally, tracking what you eat and drink can help identify any triggers that can lead to looser stools. These often include greasy foods, fatty foods, dairy, gluten, spicy foods, and caffeine. Limiting the intake of these can help. If that's not sufficient, eating foods that bulk up your stools, including rice, breads, white potatoes, and oatmeal, can help. You can also try an over-the-counter fiber supplement like Metamucil. These can sometimes cause gassiness, so they might not be optimal for some.

EMPTY COMPLETELY

If you are pooping multiple times a day (more than three), you may not be emptying at your first attempt, and this can lead to more urgency or frequent bathroom trips later, which is more likely to cause incontinence. To empty, sit down, elevate your feet on a stool or squatty potty, lean forward, and blow out slowly as you bear down.

CHECK YOUR DIET

Certain foods are more likely to contribute to loose stools. When I lived in Texas, cheese was abundant, and queso was as common as ketchup on a table. It also did a number on my digestive tract. The following morning, after I delighted in chips and queso the night before, I would have loose stools. And it did not get better until I moved out of Texas, because avoiding chips and queso there is near impossible. Other dietary items known to contribute to loose stools and gastrointestinal upset are coffee, spicy foods, and greasy foods. Some are also sensitive to gluten or dairy. To figure out what foods might be causing your loose stools, try implementing an elimination diet. Start by cutting out the most potentially irritating foods and then add them back in one at a time to see how your body reacts. This can help you determine the culprit for irritable or loose bowel movements.

MAINTAIN GOOD HYGIENE

This tip won't necessarily fix your pooping problem, but it is essential for those experiencing fecal incontinence, smearing, and staining. Having moisture on our skin for a prolonged period of time can cause skin irritation and breakdown. Use incontinence pads for any type of leakage versus a maxi pad or period liner. Incontinence pads are superior in wicking moisture away from your skin. Change your pads frequently. If any amount of leakage occurs, change the pad. A pro tip: if you wear incontinence underwear, place an incontinence pad inside the incontinence underwear. So if leakage occurs and is contained to the pad, just take out the pad and replace with a fresh one instead of having to take off your bottoms and put on a whole new pair of incontinence underwear. You'll thank me for this tip if you ever use it in the middle of the night.

Using a bidet or spritzing water on your bottom to cleanse will spare you from frequent wiping, and you can even get a travel bidet that can fit in your bag or purse. If skin irritation does occur, try to go without wearing incontinence underwear or a pad for a part of the day to let the skin breathe and use an over-the-counter barrier cream to protect tissues. Bring a change of underwear and clothes along with a plastic bag for any dirties should an accident occur.

Although incontinence can be inconvenient and affect your daily life, I hope that implementing some of these methods will help you mitigate it so that you can continue to enjoy your life and do the things you enjoy.

I have streaks or skid marks in my underwear. Does this mean I have fecal incontinence and pelvic floor weakness?

Also known as fecal staining, skid marks in your undies often occur with incontinence. But it can also happen when you're constipated. When you see skid marks, it is often because liquid seeps around the hard pieces of poop and comes out on your underwear, or you are not emptying well and need to clean your bottom better. In this situation, if you clear up the constipation, the staining should be improved.

Follow the tips for constipation including using the proper position to have a bowel movement with your feet elevated and make sure your stool is soft but also not overly mushy. After a bowel movement, contract your pelvic floor by contracting your anal sphincter to maneuver any additional stool toward the anal opening. Clean the anal area with water afterwards using a bidet or peri bottle or pat dry with a moist wipe or toilet paper.

HEMORRHOIDS AND ANAL FISSURES

Hemorrhoids exist in everyone's butthole and are only problematic when they become enlarged or uncomfortable. Commonly called piles from the Latin word *pila*, which literally means "balls," hemorrhoids can feel like little balls popping out of your booty hole. Depending on the type of hemorrhoid you have, internal or external, you may feel anal itching, swelling, pain while sitting, or pain during and after bowel movements, or notice blood when wiping or in the toilet water. If you have any bleeding with your bowel movements, please consult with a gastrointestinal or colorectal surgeon to make sure it's not something more serious.

Hemorrhoids are prolapsed veins in your anus and rectum that are a result of chronic straining, constipation, lots of heavy lifting, or increased pelvic pressure like during pregnancy or childbirth. They are usually treated with medication and pain relief (and in more severe cases, surgery), but pelvic floor exercises and education on proper pooping mechanics are necessary to decrease your discomfort and prevent your hemorrhoids from chronically occurring. Hemorrhoids frequently reoccur because of straining. For long-term hemorrhoid relief, you need to minimize straining, make sure you are emptying your bowels completely, and implement tactics to soothe sensitive tissues for pain relief.

Anal fissures are different from hemorrhoids and more like paper cuts near the external sphincter that cause pain and bleeding with bowel movements. Think of when you are putting on a shirt with a tight neck hole that you can't fit your head through. You tug at it, and a seam ends up ripping to accommodate your noggin. Same thing happens with the skin around your anal opening. Small tears in the anal tissues occur, commonly from activities like pushing out hard stools or from anal insertion during intercourse. Women who have increased pelvic floor tension (read: tighter buttholes) are more at risk because their anal sphincter muscles can't relax well, and therefore these tiny tears occur when something is trying to enter or exit their butthole. Treatment for fissures is similar to that of hemorrhoids as the focus is on pelvic floor muscle (especially on the backside) relaxation.

COOL IT OFF

To get some relief from hemorrhoids or fissures, ice can be your friend. If you've ever given birth vaginally and placed an ice pack in your undies, then this is no different but will be placed closer to your bottom. Gently wedge a covered ice pack (avoid putting cold packs directly on skin) between your butt cheeks for twenty minutes several times a day. The general rule of thumb for icing is twenty minutes on and twenty minutes off to give your tissues some time to get blood flow back.

SOOTHE YOUR BOTTOM

A sitz bath, which is essentially sitting your bum in a tub or seat of water, can provide comfort. Although cold water can help shrink swollen hemorrhoids, you may find a warm sitz bath with Epsom salts can be helpful for managing pain. Try both to see what works better for you. Also try using witch hazel wipes (name-brand Tucks pads) to wipe, or you can even use a cold one from the fridge to wedge between your butt cheeks. Last, an over-the-counter (or prescription) medication will help soothe symptoms. Think Preparation H. A favorite of mine is a Chinese medicine called Mayinglong Musk ointment.

USE A CUSHION TO SIT

Sitting can become a real pain when your hemorrhoids are flared. Using a donut cushion to sit can help, but instead of an inflatable one, opt for a dense foam one with a center cutout. It's a little more supportive and comfortable to sit on. Pro tip: if you want to keep your hemorrhoid issue a bit more clandestine, get a cushion that fits inside a canvas shoulder bag, and you don't even need to take it out of the bag. Just place the bag on the seat and sit.

BE GENTLE

Avoid sitting on the toilet longer than five minutes, as prolonged pressure on your anal sphincter can aggravate your symptoms. You may find that *not* using a squatty potty or pooping stool is preferred when hemorrhoids are inflamed. Exhale when you are bearing down to avoid excess pressure on hemorrhoids, and clean afterwards with a spritz from a bidet or peri bottle. Dabbing wet toilet paper on the area instead of abrasive wiping can also help.

KEEP YOUR POOP SOFT

Often it's a hard stool that causes a tear, so make sure to hydrate, eat fiber-rich and unprocessed foods, and use a stool softener or an all-natural supplement to get your stool soft.

RELAX YOUR BOOTY

Typically hemorrhoids and fissures occur with a tight anal sphincter, tight glutes, or both. Of the relaxation stretches in Chapter 2, you can perform cat–cow stretch or figure 4 stretch, or massage a ball on your hip and glute muscles to release external tension. Don't forget to check for butt clenching throughout the day.

PENCIL-THIN POOPS

Poops that look stringy and pencil-thin are often a sign of pelvic floor muscle tension. Like squeezing toothpaste from a tube, if the opening (your anal sphincter) is too small, your bowel movement comes out very thin and long. You are getting some good stuff out, but the challenge is you often do not empty completely in this situation. The solution is to open your door.

RELAX YOUR PELVIC FLOOR

Utilizing the pelvic floor relaxation protocol will help you release tension in your anal sphincter and pelvic floor.

RELEASE YOUR GLUTES

Tension in your glutes can also increase tension in your pelvic floor. Place a firm ball like a tennis ball, lacrosse ball, or yoga ball against the wall and press the side of your buttock muscles, either left or right, into the ball. Roll your hips side to side and up and down until you feel a tender spot and hold the ball in that spot for several breaths. Repeat on both sides of your glutes for three to five minutes on each side once a day.

SQUAT

The more you squat, the more relaxation you will have to your pelvic floor and anal sphincter specifically. Hold a deep squat or child's pose for a solid sixty seconds, taking big, deep, relaxing breaths as you hold your pelvic floor in a relaxed position.

FIND YOUR BEST POOP POSTURE

Squatting is hands-down the best plan if you have pencil-thin poops. Again, posture can make a big difference in how we empty. If you are struggling with pencil-thin poops, there are toilet seats that have foot platforms you can stand on and squat so your bum is over the toilet bowl. It might feel weird at first, but no one is watching. I say go for it!

FOR MANY, PELVIC FLOOR EDUCATION, SOME NEW HABITS, AND EXERCISE are sufficient to turn a pooping problem around, but pelvic floor therapy is often one piece of the puzzle. Other treatments for bowel issues may include electrical stimulation, biofeedback, surgery, Botox, or implantation of a stimulation device. Continuing to work on your pelvic floor along with these other treatment options is essential, but other measures are available if therapy is not enough. If you utilize these techniques and your symptoms do not improve or worsen, if pain wakes you at night when sleeping, if you have weight loss or weight gain, or your symptoms are impacting you emotionally and psychologically, check in with a gastroenterologist and colorectal surgeon.

Poop Like a Pro

Sometimes children carry inherent wisdom—and it is helpful to be reminded of this basic truth. When my son was two, he started crawling out of his crib every morning. My youngest was just six months old, I was incredibly exhausted, and I was not ready to sacrifice another minute of rest for my agile toddler. After looking online for solutions (placing a net over the top of the crib or switching him to a "big boy bed," neither of which I was prepared to do), I decided to turn the doorknob around in his room so it locked from the outside instead of the inside. I figured if he crawled out and the doorknob was locked, he couldn't open the door and would at least stay in his room, but I would be able to hear him on the monitor if there was an emergency. Perhaps not the best parenting hack, but sleep deprivation makes parents make drastic choices.

It seemed to be a beautiful solution. Many nights, immediately after leaving his room, I would hear the thud of his feet hitting the ground, followed by him wiggling the doorknob, attempting to open it. Minutes later I could hear him retreat back to his crib, defeated. "Sweet victory," I would think as I happily walked to my room to get much-needed rest. This plan worked for weeks, until one morning.

It was a Saturday, and I'd enjoyed seven straight hours of luxurious sleep. But when I woke, I noticed he was unusually quiet in his room (always a suspicious situation for a toddler). I rushed down the hallway, unlocked his bedroom door, swung it open, and saw *and smelled* poop *everywhere*. My son had reached into his diaper, taken his poop, and smeared it on his walls, floors, dresser drawers, door, and toys. The entire room reeked. As one does when defeated by a toddler, I sighed (maybe wept a tiny bit), put on rubber gloves, and got to work. I dunked him into a tub and washed him thoroughly, then scrubbed, wiped, and bleached every inch of his bedroom floor and walls. And can you guess what he was doing as I was on my hands and knees, scrubbing every inch of his room? He was smiling.

And then I remembered—*oh yeah, it isn't healthy for us to hold it in.* He went because he had to go. Pooping is natural, but it's not always easy, convenient, or straightforward. No matter the situation, it will always eventually find its way out, but hopefully in a manner that is comfortable and a little less messy.

My parting words of wisdom from this story: commit to healthy pooping habits, as they will all support your floor for years to come. Observe yourself while emptying your bowels. Are you exhaling when you have a bowel movement? Do you empty better with your feet on a stool or on the ground? Look at your stool. Is it soft like soft-serve or hard balls floating in the water? Pelvic floor–related pooping problems can start small, but they can become chronic issues over time. To maintain optimal health, use the tips and exercises in this chapter. Stay committed, and get your bowels into a routine. And if nothing else, get yourself a pooping stool. I promise, it will change your life for the better.

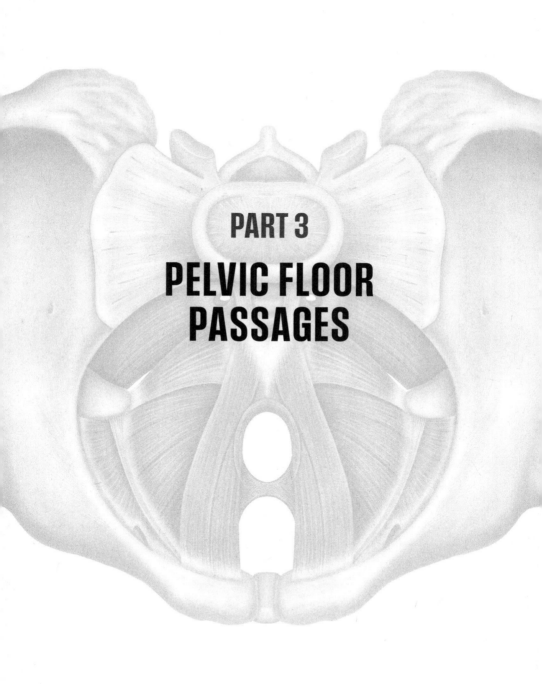

PART 3

PELVIC FLOOR PASSAGES

CHAPTER 5

The Power of Your Period

We pee and poop throughout our entire lives—but between the ages of ten and sixteen, a natural change comes along that has titanic-sized implications for our pelvic floors: our periods. The day a young woman gets her first period is a day she will likely remember. I was ten years old and about to get braces at the orthodontist's office. Just before the procedure started, I made a quick dash to the bathroom where I peed, wiped, and saw blood on the toilet paper.

"Moooooom!" I yelped, hoping she was still just outside my bathroom stall. I was panicking, as any ten-year-old would.

"Yes, Sara?" she responded, cool and collected.

Phew, I thought. Help is here!

"I think I just started my period!" I said, staring at the pink smear on the toilet paper.

"Shoot. Well, honey, I don't have anything with me. You're just going to have to wait until we get home," she said.

It was not the response I had hoped for . . . or needed. There really aren't words to capture the surprise, awe, and freak-out that a girl feels when she first meets Aunt Flo. Nervous and confused about what to do, I wadded up toilet paper, stuck it in the crotch of my underwear, and hoped for the best. Already nervous about getting braces, I spent the next three hours in the orthodontist's chair, staring at the ceiling tiles and praying that I wasn't bleeding through my favorite Esprit shorts. Later that afternoon, my mom came into my bedroom, gave me a book on periods and a box of maxi pads, and said, "Let me know if you have questions." Then she walked out the door. That was my education on reproductive health. My schooling on menstruation. My entry into womanhood.

In the years that followed, one week out of every month I used a large maxi pad (always with wings) and worried someone would hear the crinkle when I sat down in a chair. When I was on my period, I brought a sweater to school just in case I needed to tie it around my waist to cover bloodstains. My experience was pretty standard for a young woman growing up in the nineties, left to fend for herself at one of life's most significant developmental transitions. You would think, and hope, that as decades passed, this coming-of-age experience would be more instructional, supportive, and ceremonious. Unfortunately, this is not the case. The same women who were sitting on toilets reading the sides of a tampon box are the ones raising children now—and based on my discussions with friends and clients, the trend of being tight-lipped about discussing menstrual health continues. And there is virtually zero education about how our periods impact our pelvic floor.

Adolescent and teen girls look to their mothers, aunts, doctors, and other trusted adult women for guidance on the ins and outs of their periods and how to care for their bodies and pelvic floors. When these topics are discussed in hushed tones, or never discussed at all, women are clouded in feelings of bodily shame and embarrassment from the start. They may experience pain, discomfort, or pelvic floor symptoms without knowing where to go for help or that help is even available.

On average young women start menstruating at twelve years old, meaning we can have about four hundred fifty menstrual cycles in our lifetime. Half of the world's population menstruates, yet discussion of this topic in virtually all cultures is uncomfortable and often avoided. Education should really start when we are young girls, so we understand what is coming.

Discussions on puberty need to be more in-depth than scanning a brochure at the pediatrician's office. Tampons and pads need to be available like toilet paper in public bathrooms. Women need accurate information about their own menstrual and pelvic health—and then they can pass it on to the next generation of women at a time in their lives when their attitudes about menstrual health are still being formed. In order for young women to develop positive feelings about their bodies, this mindset needs to be modeled.

The first menstrual cycle, known as menarche, occurs during puberty, which is a transitional time of physical, hormonal, and emotional changes for adolescent girls. Puberty typically occurs between the ages of eight and thirteen, and menarche is the central event of that life transition. *Menarche*, Greek for "moon" and "beginning," signifies a young girl's transition into becoming a young woman. Some cultures and countries celebrate menarche as a significant milestone. In parts of India, for example, a girl's parents invite close friends and relatives for a party to celebrate or host a ceremony to mark her passage into womanhood. In some cultures, menstruation is considered sacred, and menstrual blood is considered a source of feminine strength and power. Young women in these cultures feel more empowered in their bodies, and their culture's view of the transition supports their growing confidence. But these viewpoints are, for the most part, outliers.

In many countries, including the United States, menstruation can be regarded as something unclean, dirty, and inappropriate for public discussion. Some young women miss school during their periods due to pelvic pain or lack of menstrual hygiene products. In some cultures, women are not allowed to visit religious temples and must sleep separately from their husbands during menstruation. There are many who believe women should be banned from having sex with their husbands during their periods because it is viewed as repulsive or unclean. In some traditions, women aren't allowed to worship, cook, socialize, or undertake certain household chores when they are bleeding. While the original intention may have been an effort to allow rest, it promotes feelings of shame, fear, and anxiety.

Navigating our periods is hard—even *with* resources, education, and access to period products. But the silence around our periods is uniquely damaging, because it creates a culture of silence around our own bodies. It shuts us down from listening to our bodies, trusting our bodies, and seeking answers when we experience pain or discomfort in our pelvic floors. Feelings of secrecy and shame hover over menstrual cycles, which can lead to missed days of school or work and widen the gender and education gap even further. In short, *how* we talk about our periods when we are young will shape how we approach our bodies and our pelvic floors when we are older. We need to bring our periods out of the dark to discern what's normal, what's not, and how to get help when period problems arise.

Period problems are inextricably linked to pelvic floor problems. Hormonal fluctuations during our cycle influence vaginal lubrication, the consistency and frequency of bowel movements, and pelvic floor strength. And the state of our pelvic floor muscles can limit which menstrual health products we use. In this chapter, I aim to educate you about your cycle during your menstruating years as it impacts your pelvic floor—but I also hope to help you embrace and take proud ownership over your cycle. This natural process of your body is nothing to be ashamed of. When we are empowered to understand and care for our bodies during our cycle, we can even begin to appreciate and celebrate it for its magic.

How the Pelvic Floor and Periods Work Together

Have you ever been asked by your doctor, "What was the first day of your last menstrual cycle?" Many of us may scratch our heads in response. Not only does it seem like a big ask to recall that day of the month, but we may not even recall what week it was. And what is the true start day anyway? Is it the cramping day before you see blood? Or is it the day you spot before the blood really begins flowing?

Your menstrual cycle officially starts on the day that bleeding begins. This is considered day one, and your menstrual cycle ends the day before your next period begins. An entire menstrual cycle typically lasts twenty-four to thirty-eight days. This range can vary throughout your life. For instance, it may be shorter when you are younger and longer when you are nearing menopause. Further, the number of days varies from person to person as it's influenced by genetics, geography, disease, lifestyle, medications, and even race. Your cycle is the result of a symphony of communication between your brain, your hormones, and your reproductive organs. This symphony differs for every individual, and if one member of that orchestra is off-key, it influences the entire experience.

The primary organs in this symphony are the ovaries, where your hormones are produced and eggs are released, and your uterus, where the lining builds up and then sheds if no egg is

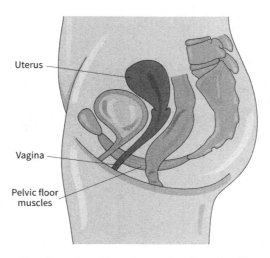

Female uterus and vagina: a view from the side

implanted. The hormones that are produced affect the strength, relaxation, and tone of your pelvic floor along with vaginal lubrication. The uterus and ovaries have separate yet intertwined roles in this monthly cycle. Let's start with the uterus.

WHAT'S HAPPENING IN THE UTERUS

A hollow, pear-shaped organ, the uterus sits in the female pelvis and is responsible for pregnancy, menstruation, labor, and birth. The word *uterus* originates from the Latin word for "womb." It's worth noting that the Greek word *hysteria* also means "uterus" and is the same word used to describe a female suffering from psychological distress (historically thought to be caused by dysfunction of the uterus). In other words, in ancient times, being a woman with pain or anguish was often equated with having a psychological condition. *Read: we are not suffering from a condition or disorder; the natural state of our bodies is to have hormonal fluctuations that affect our mood.*

The uterine cycle has three phases: menstruation (when you bleed), the proliferative phase (after you bleed until you ovulate), and the secretory phase (after you ovulate until you bleed again). During each phase, changes in your uterus, pelvic floor, and body occur, and your hormones are a bit of a roller coaster.

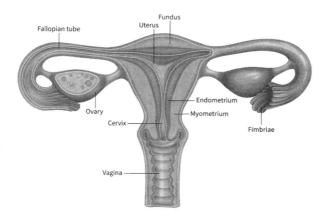

Female reproductive system: uterus, vagina, ovaries, and fallopian tubes

MENSTRUATION: I'M BLOATED AND BLEEDING PHASE

Menstruation, also known as menses or a period, is the time from the start of menstrual bleeding to when it ends. This lasts an average of four to six days but can range anywhere between three and eight days. Prior to menstruation, the lining inside the uterus thickens in preparation for implantation of a fertilized egg. If a fertilized egg doesn't implant into the uterine lining, no pregnancy occurs—and at that time, menstruation occurs, and the lining sloughs off and out as blood.

Menstrual blood is a combination of blood and this uterine lining, also called the endometrium, which sheds from the uterus through the cervix and out of the body through the vagina. A normal amount of menstrual blood for an entire menstrual cycle is between thirty and eighty milliliters per period, which is the equivalent of a stick of butter. Your pelvic floor muscle tone, the ability to contract your pelvic floor to prevent leakage or support your pelvic organs, is at its lowest during menstruation due to lower estrogen levels. So this amount of blood combined with low pelvic floor tone can cause increased pressure and heaviness in your pelvis and vagina during this time. And if you've ever felt like a bowling ball was coming out of your vagina on day one of bleeding, you know exactly what I'm talking about.

During menstruation, the hormone levels of estrogen and progesterone are at their lowest. Low levels of estrogen during menstruation not only reduce pelvic floor tone but also lead to symptoms of fatigue, headaches, irregular sleep, irritability, and a decreased sex drive. (This explains why on the first day of my period, I find myself exhausted with a headache and want to crawl into bed by 8:00 p.m.) And low progesterone levels are often the culprit for loose poops during your period.

Many women report experiencing increased pelvic floor symptoms leading up to and during menstruation. These include heaviness or pressure in the vagina, pelvic pain, and pain with urination and with bowel movements. Some research suggests decreased pelvic floor muscle performance and endurance during your period. So, while you are bleeding, you may want to rest, chill, hydrate, and put your pelvic floor exercises on hold until after your period passes.

When a woman has lower estrogen levels early postpartum, lactating, heading into menopause, and even during certain times in her monthly menstrual cycle, there is a less-than-optimal influence on the pelvic floor: we have less strength and support. We will address the effect of hormones and your pelvic floor in the menopause chapter also, but know this: hormones are key players in pelvic floor health.

PROLIFERATIVE PHASE: LET'S GET IT ON PHASE

After menstruation, we enter the proliferative phase, which occurs from the last day of bleeding until ovulation, when a mature egg is released from one of the ovaries. This mature egg travels from the ovary down into the fallopian tube, where it hangs out for about twelve to twenty-four hours, waiting for fertilization by a sperm. During this phase, estrogen levels steadily increase, triggering the uterine lining to proliferate by building up a thick inner lining in preparation for implantation of a fertilized egg. If a fertilized egg *does* implant in the uterine lining, pregnancy occurs. If a fertilized egg *does not* implant, the lining sheds, menstruation occurs, and you bleed, and the process repeats in the next cycle.

When estrogen peaks just before ovulation, your cervical mucus becomes thinner and more slippery. This would have been a helpful fact to know when I was a confused teenager and saw what I thought were egg whites in my underwear once a month. So, to my young self, and all other young selves out there: it is normal. And it is healthy. Increased estrogen also contributes to pelvic floor muscle tone and strength and increases your vaginal wall thickness during this pre-ovulation spike. You may also have increased sexual desire and libido. So this phase is not only a great time to get your pelvic floor strengthening exercises in, it's also a great time to get busy (with protection, if you don't want to get pregnant). The rise in estrogen also triggers spikes in two more additional hormones, luteinizing hormone (LH) and follicle-stimulating hormone (FSH), which ultimately stimulate ovulation to occur. Progesterone stays low throughout the entire proliferative phase until after ovulation. The total time of menstruation and proliferation is about fourteen days based on the average of a twenty-eight-day cycle.

SECRETORY PHASE: LEAVE ME ALONE, DON'T TOUCH ME, I'M TIRED PHASE

The last phase in the uterine cycle is the secretory phase. It begins when an egg is released from your ovaries (ovulation) and ends when menstruation begins again. This phase lasts about fourteen days and completes your full menstrual cycle. During this phase, the uterine lining is waiting for implantation of a fertilized egg into the uterine wall. If that occurs, you're pregnant; if not, the uterine lining starts to break down and gets ready to shed during your next period.

The biggest hormonal player during the secretory phase is progesterone. Progesterone rises during the secretory phase to prepare for implantation of a fertilized egg into the uterine lining. This rise also leads to those unenjoyable premenstrual symptoms of feeling bloated, sluggish, sad, and constipated. So if you are wondering why your jeans are super tight and your poop is as hard as rocks before your period, it's due to progesterone. During the secretory phase, estrogen levels are generally low, causing cervical mucus to decrease, leading to less discharge and vaginal dryness. Estrogen has one more spike in the middle of this fourteen-day phase, leading to another point in your menstrual cycle when pelvic floor strength and tone are greatest.

I ran a marathon, my only one ever, when I was twenty-six years old living in Austin, Texas. I trained for six months, waking early on Saturdays for morning runs with my training group followed by cold plunges into Barton Springs and then a plate full of pancakes at Kirbey Lane. The training and the race were some of the hardest physical and mental feats I've accomplished (pregnancy and childbirth being the hardest). And while training, I discovered that right before and during my period, I had my worst workout days, when I felt like my feet were bricks and I could not find my groove during the run.

The days after my period, I often felt like I was flying and had a burst of energy giving me my best run in weeks. I had been told that sleep and nutrition played a role in my workouts and recovery, but discovered on my own that my menstrual cycle also had an influence. Knowing this now, I choose gentler and more restorative workouts like yoga, walking, or easy cycling during my period. The days following my period when I am most energetic, I love a higher-intensity workout or longer ride on my spin bike. The takeaway is, our body is in a constant cycle during our menstruating years. And understanding this cycle and the hormones at play can help us work with the rhythms of our body instead of against it.

I have a young daughter. How early should I start teaching her about the menstrual cycle?

It is never too early to talk about it. It is the act of *not* talking about it that sends the message to girls that it is shameful or taboo. For example, if your daughter is five and asks about pads, tampons, or even birth control pills that they see in your bathroom, explain what they are. If they inquire about why you are wiping blood, tell them that when Mom isn't pregnant with a baby, her uterus sheds its lining. Answer their questions as they come to you, letting them know they can talk to you about it openly. And you can trickle in additional information along the way, perhaps as you notice changes in their body odor, body hair, breasts, or genitals. Use resources like books, videos, and even social media.

We need to normalize these conversations not just for young girls, but for boys as well. My sons are familiar with my pelvic floor and vulva models casually lying around my home, and when questions pop up around their bodies or mine, they are answered instead of shut down with a "we don't talk about that." There is no "perfect" age or time to have a conversation about menstruation. Crack the door open bit by bit and make sure your children know they have the freedom, safety, and comfort to come knock when they need to.

WHAT IS HAPPENING WITH YOUR OVARIES

Your ovaries are a pair of small, oval-shaped glands located on both the left and right side of your uterus, attached via ligaments. The word *ovary* comes from the Latin word *ovum*, meaning "egg." The ovaries produce, store, and finally release your eggs during the midpoint of your menstrual cycle at ovulation. These glands can range from the size of a grape to the size of a kiwi during your fertile years and shrink after menopause to the size of a kidney bean.

Think of the female ovaries as the equivalent of male testicles when it comes to hormone production. Besides storing and releasing eggs, ovaries also bear the super important role of producing the hormones estrogen, progesterone, and androgens, which include testosterone. When ovulation becomes less frequent and eventually stops during menopause, these hormones are no longer produced by the ovaries, and you pretty much become a hormonal desert, which wreaks havoc on your pelvic floor. The ovarian cycle has two phases. The first phase is the follicular phase, which occurs before ovulation. This phase overlaps with menstruation and the proliferative phases of the uterus. The second phase is the luteal phase, which occurs after ovulation and overlaps with the secretory phase of the uterus.

FOLLICULAR PHASE: I'M BLEEDING, THEN FEELING PRETTY GOOD PHASE

The follicular phase occurs from day one of your period until ovulation. Every woman is born with a set number of eggs that are housed inside of follicles in the ovaries. Follicles are fluid-filled sacs about the size of a grain of sand, and at birth, a female can have between one and two million follicles in her ovaries. By the time of her first menstruation, she will have around 200,000 to 300,000 follicles. Each year, follicles slowly die off and are reabsorbed into the body. The follicles and eggs you are born with are the only ones you will have. It's pretty wild to think that at the time you are born, your body holds the cells that could become your future potential children.

During the follicular phase, one follicle grows faster and reaches the size of an average grape, then releases a mature egg around day fourteen of the menstrual cycle at ovulation. Some women don't feel ovulation occur at all, while others may feel a sharp or dull cramp, lower abdominal pain, or a twinge on one side of the abdomen. One egg is released every menstrual cycle from your first period to your last period. (In rare cases, two eggs can be released, leading to fraternal twins if both are fertilized.) When ovulation eventually stops (from certain forms of birth control, after surgical removal of the ovaries, or when menopause occurs), you stop releasing eggs, and pregnancy can no longer occur. By the time of menopause, a woman may have fewer than 1,000 eggs, and any remaining eggs die off.

Progesterone stays low, and estrogen is really the star in the follicular phase. Estrogen, which is made within the ovaries, stays at a low level until the very end when a rapid spike prompts a surge in LH, signaling the end of the follicular phase and beginning of ovulation. That rapid surge in estrogen increases your sex drive, makes your vagina sperm-friendly, and increases your cervical fluid (aka discharge). You have thirty times more cervical fluid during the late follicular phase, when estrogen levels rise, compared to the early follicular phase, when estrogen levels are lower. This rise in estrogen around day seven of your cycle correlates with stronger pelvic floor muscle contractions and increased pelvic floor muscle tone. Again, we see the power of estrogen and its influence on our pelvic floor.

LUTEAL PHASE: GIVE ME STRETCHY PANTS AND A BAR OF CHOCOLATE PHASE

The luteal phase follows the follicular phase and lasts from the time of ovulation until the start of your next period. This phase overlaps with the secretory phase of the uterine cycle and lasts on average fourteen days but can range from nine to sixteen days. During this time, the follicle that just released an egg turns into a new structure called the corpus luteum, which makes a lot of progesterone and a little estrogen in case pregnancy occurs. The rise in progesterone contributes to a sluggish colon, causing constipation, bloating, and decreased cervical fluid and vaginal discharge.

If a fertilized egg implants into the uterine wall, pregnancy occurs, and progesterone and estrogen continue to rise. If pregnancy does not occur, the corpus luteum breaks down and stops producing progesterone and estrogen. These hormones then drop quickly, leading us into our bloated-and-breakout premenstrual era until our period starts. The symptoms that accompany this hormonal plunge are headaches, fatigue, breast tenderness, bloating, acne, mood changes, vaginal dryness, and low libido. After these hormones drop and you've been in your super stretchy pants until bedtime at 9:00 p.m., your period starts, and the menstrual cycle is complete.

Interestingly, studies have shown that due to the increase in estrogen and testosterone during the luteal phase, women have better pelvic floor muscle tone compared to other times in the menstrual cycle. The only other time this happens is midway through the follicular phase, when estrogen has its first peak. This important fact explains why symptoms such as urinary leakage or pelvic floor heaviness from prolapse may be less both-

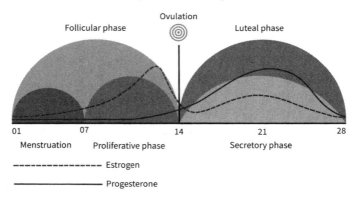

Complete menstrual cycle

Diagram of menstrual cycle with hormonal fluctuations of each phase

ersome during the midpoint of the follicular and luteal cycles (around day seven and day twenty-one of the entire menstrual cycle). Consider doing pelvic floor muscle contractions during these phases as you will get more bang for your buck.

While all you may see is period blood, behind the scenes is a well-orchestrated reproductive system set up to support a potential pregnancy and serving as a hormone machine that is the foundation of women's health.

These hormonal influences don't just affect our vaginas and pelvic floor muscles. They influence our entire body. Estrogen surges that occur during puberty, pregnancy, and both the follicular and secretory phases contribute to irritability, mood swings, and feeling super emotional. Combined with the monthly progesterone roller coaster, you may feel really annoyed at the driver who didn't use the turn signal, the partner who left a sink full of dirty dishes, or your kiddo who left a Lego on the floor that just poked the bottom of your foot. Where we are in our cycles influences our mood; my husband is happy to confirm that. And the influences aren't just emotional. Even our brain health is affected. Times of lower estrogen and low progesterone can lead to brain fog, forgetfulness, fatigue, and indecision or anxiety.

Despite the sophisticated system, like many of the other systems affecting our pelvic floor, problems with periods can arise. One in ten women experiences extremely painful menstruation, leading to pelvic and abdominal pain and muscle spasms. Many women suffer for years waiting for an accurate diagnosis. Period problems can occur when we first get our periods, after childbirth, after changing our birth control, after trauma, or when nearing menopause. Common period-related complaints I hear from women include the following:

"Every month I have such bad cramps, I have to stay home from work for a day or two."

"I cannot put a tampon in. It's just not comfortable for me. And wearing a pad limits what I am able to do."

"I get a sharp pain in the left side of my vagina a few days after my period, and it takes my breath away."

"Since I was in high school, my periods have been so painful I had to miss school."

Being well-educated about our complete menstrual cycle, including our hormonal fluctuations, helps us understand the symptoms we may experience as a result of what's happening in our reproductive system (hello, tender breasts and hard poops). That's step one. Step two is learning how to care for yourself—and what works for *your* body.

Your Pelvic Floor and Period Protocol

Your pelvic floor health is intimately tied to your menstrual cycle in a variety of ways. As you read on the previous pages, your cycle affects your bowels, vaginal lubrication, muscle tone, and more. Further, the period products you utilize have different implications for your floor. But for every menstruator, some basic practices can help you optimize your pelvic floor health during your fertile years, which can be anywhere from twenty-five to forty years of your life.

TRACK YOUR CYCLE

One of the single most empowering things you can do to take ownership of your cycle and pelvic floor is to track your cycle. You can do this on an old-school desk calendar or keep track on your smartphone and document the day your cycle starts, ends, and any symptoms you experience throughout the month. Tracking allows you to monitor and record the nature of your cycle, noting if your blood flow is heavy, light, has clots, or any other qualities about your period. All of these rhythms help you identify any patterns that may require attention, and they tell the story of your cycle. Having a sense of your normal allows you to identify when abnormalities or aberrations occur.

TRY DIFFERENT PERIOD PRODUCTS

In developed countries like the United States, we are fortunate to have a lot of options for managing our period blood flow. These include everything from traditional menstrual pads and tampons to environmentally friendly reusable menstrual cups and discs and period underwear with absorbent lining. Some folks even choose to free-bleed and use nothing. No matter if you're a middle schooler, an avid exerciser, or just want to hit the pool any day of the month, having options for period products gives women a better quality of life.

Try different period products to see what works best for you. You will likely find that some options are more comfortable than others—and that some are better during different life phases. For example, putting a tampon up your vagina is a big step for young girls. And because your floor muscles need to relax for insertion, someone who just got their period might be more comfortable using a pad until they are more in flow with their flow.

If you are opting for pads or tampons, use organic unbleached cotton products (fewer ingredients is always better) to minimize irritation to sensitive tissues and limit exposure to harsh chemicals. If you opt for a menstrual cup, you may need to try several as they vary in flexibility, capacity, shape, and material. If you use a menstrual disc, some are disposable while some are reusable, and they position differently in the vaginal canal compared to cups. And you may need a combination of these products like a menstrual cup with period underwear for your heavy days and a light tampon or liner on your light ones.

KNOW YOUR BIRTH CONTROL OPTIONS
AND HOW THEY AFFECT YOU

There are pros and cons with all birth control options—and so I always recommend talking not only with healthcare providers but also with friends to get help figuring out what might be best for you and your needs. Options include barrier methods like condoms, which prevent sperm from entering the vaginal canal, hormonal birth control options like the pill, patch, ring, and hormonal intrauterine devices (IUDs). Some of these forms of contraception alter your reproductive cycle and influence your pelvic floor health.

Hormonal birth control options are great for preventing pregnancy but can lead to unwanted side effects. A birth control ring, which is inserted into the vagina and rests around the base of the cervix for three weeks before removal, requires the ability to insert your fingers into the vaginal canal comfortably. An IUD is a plastic or metal T-shaped device implanted into the cervix and connected to a string. Some patients report experiencing severe pelvic pain after IUD insertion and removal, so painful it can trigger longer-term pelvic floor muscle tension. There is also an increased risk of dislodging an IUD with removal of a menstrual cup. Additionally, hormonal birth control options that have synthetic estrogen and progesterone alter the hormonal balance in your body and can contribute to pelvic health symptoms like vaginal dryness, painful sex, and vulvodynia (pain in the vulvar region), which I describe in Chapter 11, on pelvic pain. These hormonal changes can alter your mood and libido as well.

The pros, cons, risk factors, and side effects for every type of birth control should be explored thoroughly if and when you are choosing a birth control option. Know which device is right for you, and understand how your choice may or may not impact your pelvic floor.

I was taught to douche after my period to clean my vagina. Is this good practice?

Douching is the process of washing the inside of your vagina, and it is most often practiced to decrease odor or achieve a feeling of cleanliness after sweating, menstruation, or before or after sex. The process typically involves using a solution, anything from a scented over-the-counter wash to a homemade concoction. My two cents on the matter are simple: the practice of douching is absolutely not recommended. Not only can introducing a solution into the vagina disrupt the natural vaginal microbiome and flora, increasing the risk of infection, but it can actually introduce *new* bacteria into the vaginal canal, cervix, and uterus, leading to infection, disease, and even fertility challenges. The vagina is like a self-cleaning oven; nothing needs to be done to clean it per se. You can rinse the outside of the vagina, the vulva, between the labia, and around the clitoris by spritzing or rinsing with water in the shower or with a peri bottle or using a very gentle mild cleanser *externally* if desired. But nothing needs to be done or should be done *inside* the vagina to clean it. If you experience odor, itching, or irritation, check in with a medical provider to rule out any infection or other medical condition.

Period Problems

Bodies are complex, the pelvic floor is complex—then add the menstrual cycle and things become even more complex. Given all the factors—from hormones to muscles to organs and more—problems triggered by our cycles can arise. Addressing early signs of pelvic floor dysfunction can potentially save years of pain and struggle later on. Case in point: a number of my patients with larger-scale pelvic floor problems recall having pain with tampon insertion when they were younger. I often wonder if these women would have been able to prevent later-stage pelvic issues had they been able to talk about problems they were experiencing when they were younger.

Some menstrual and gynecological conditions like endometriosis and polycystic ovarian syndrome (PCOS) lead to severe pelvic pain. Other conditions, like premenstrual syndrome (PMS), trigger abdominal pain and pelvic floor muscle tension. Even the absence of your period, amenorrhea, can contribute to pelvic floor weakness or vaginal dryness. As embarrassing as bleeding through your shorts onto your white fabric desk chair can be (this literally happened to me while writing this book), pain and other pelvic floor problems related to your period can be traumatizing and affect your ability to attend school, go to work, have sex, and even get pregnant and carry a child. Talk to your ob-gyn, of course—and there is a lot that you can do to prevent and relieve problems that arise.

PAINFUL MENSTRUATION/DYSMENORRHEA

Painful menstruation, called dysmenorrhea, is the most common gynecological disorder that menstruating women experience. Contrary to common belief, painful periods are *not normal*. Mild cramping can occur, but severe period pain is not par for the course. Bloating? *Yes.* Fatigue? *Maybe.* Headaches? *Perhaps.* Pain? *Absolutely not.* Dysmenorrhea is due to any one, or more, of a variety of conditions, such as PCOS, fibroid tumors on your uterus, or endometriosis and adenomyosis. As a result of these conditions, a woman is likely to experience severe pelvic floor, low back, and abdominal wall muscle tension—so severe it can be quite debilitating. I go in depth into endometriosis in the next section. Follow these steps for managing discomfort during your monthly menstruation.

EXERCISE

The research is clear: mild to moderate exercise while on your period can reduce pain. Movement increases blood flow, helps tight muscles relax, and releases endorphins that can combat pain and lift your mood. While menstruating, a simple thirty-minute walk or something as intense as an hour-long power yoga class can do the trick. Remember: pelvic floor muscle strength is a bit compromised during menstruation, so opting for lower-intensity workouts is recommended.

MASSAGE

Massage is an excellent way to ease the tension that arises due to your period. Abdominal massage goes a long way in terms of relieving the cramping that arises from period pain. If a session with a professional massage therapist isn't in the budget, you can use a ball to massage tight hip muscles. Or follow the pelvic floor relaxation protocol in Chapter 2 for guidance on external and internal massage.

BUILD YOUR PERIOD CARE KIT

Have a care pack of items and tools to manage pain and discomfort during uncomfortable days. I highly recommend keeping the following in your possession.

Transcutaneous Electrical Stimulation Device (TENS) Unit. This is an electrical stimulation device with pads that can be placed over your abdominal wall or low back to relieve pain. Use the device for thirty to sixty minutes multiple times a day, as needed, but do not use it near water or when sleeping.

Heating Pad. Incredibly soothing for abdominal pain and cramping, heat softens tight muscles and soothes pain. When using a heating pad, be sure to have enough layers between the heating pad and your skin and use it for twenty to thirty minutes, then take a break to prevent burning your skin.

Medications. Anti-inflammatories or pain relievers can help manage the discomfort associated with period pain— from abdominal and low back pain, to rectal and pelvic pain, and even premenstrual headaches. Check with your medical provider about pain-relieving medication options.

ENDOMETRIOSIS

Endometriosis is a gynecological condition that occurs when tissue similar to the uterine lining grows outside of the uterus. This tissue infiltrates your pelvic cavity, sticks to your organs, and can create adhesions between the ovaries, colon, bladder, and fallopian tubes. Not only does this disease cause excruciating pelvic and abdominal pain, it's often the culprit for painful bowel movements, pain with sex, and pelvic pain that fluctuates during the menstrual cycle. And it is one of the leading causes of infertility for women in their childbearing years. Endometriosis can start at the first menstrual period and last until menopause, meaning a woman can suffer for decades and not even know the cause and cure.

I recall Leigh, a woman in her forties who called my office after 5:00 p.m. on a cold December evening in tears from pain. I picked up the line just as I was leaving my office. Leigh was desperately searching for help for her extremely painful periods when she came across pelvic floor therapy and my office number online. I shuffled things around on my schedule so I could get her in right away. When she arrived at her first appointment two days later, Leigh sat in a cozy turquoise chair in the corner of my treatment room and told me her story. I share this story as yet another example of how women's issues can get dismissed and to show how things tend to snowball when women don't get the care they need from the get-go.

Every month when Leigh had her period, she felt pain in her lower abdomen, hips, and back. She also had an overactive bladder and woke to pee two or three times at night. Her vulva burned when she peed, an issue that grew worse right before ovulation. Her bowel movements were painful, and she fluctuated between diarrhea and constipation throughout the month. Sex was excruciating, and she often avoided it because of how much it hurt, especially in the days before and after her period. These symptoms occurred every month since she started her period at twelve years old, but over the past ten years, they significantly worsened to the point of taking pain medication and missing work every month on the days of her period. She first told her primary care doctor, who referred her to a gynecologist, who prescribed her ibuprofen and birth control. That's it. Her pain persisted, and got worse. By the time I met Leigh in my office, she had seen *eleven* doctors for these problems. Pain and limitation had been her life for nearly twenty-eight years.

Recently, Leigh had started working with a fertility doctor to get pregnant. This journey was probably causing her the most anguish. She had suffered a miscarriage and had been unable to get pregnant since. After rounds of bloodwork and medications, her fertility doctor performed an abdominal surgery to investigate whether any physical challenges with her reproductive organs could prevent pregnancy. During the surgery, the doctor found adhesions that glued Leigh's bladder and bowels to her uterus and other parts of her pelvic cavity. The adhesions were so extensive the surgeon was only able to remove a small amount of them before closing her back up.

"You have endometriosis," she said. "And there is nothing more I can do." Leigh was prescribed hydrocodone, a strong pain-relieving medication, and was told she could try IVF in a few months. After five more months of this, she found pelvic floor therapy.

Leigh's story is unfortunately similar to so many other women's stories. Upon examination, Leigh had severe muscle spasms throughout her pelvic floor, abdominal wall, hips, and thighs. She was unable to relax her pelvic floor muscles for urination and bowel movements. Her posture was compromised from years of hunching over due to abdominal pain—and poor posture led to more pain. She had endured so much—all of which could have been helped from when she first got her period.

Pain is information from our bodies that something is not right. If there is anything I want you to take away from this book, it is this: if you feel pelvic pain, trust it, and keep seeking answers, until you find relief. Don't let any medical provider dismiss your pain. In many cases, pain indicates an underlying condition. And it could be endometriosis. Often I see women, young and old, for bowel or bladder issues, pelvic pain, or painful sex, and I wonder if they could have undiagnosed endometriosis, because they share these common symptoms:

- Low back or abdominal pain, typically during a period
- Pain with urination or bowel movements during a period
- Deep pain with penetrative sex
- Pain that limits one's ability to attend school, work, or daily activities
- Fluctuating constipation and diarrhea
- Fertility challenges

The diagnosis and treatment of endometriosis is complex, as the only way to diagnose it is a surgery to remove a tissue sample, which is then sent to a lab for confirmation. But from a pelvic floor therapy perspective, treating the accompanying pelvic floor tension and pelvic pain is the protocol to find relief.

FOLLOW THE PELVIC FLOOR RELAXATION PROTOCOL

Pain causes tension, and tension causes pain. Tackling pelvic floor and abdominal tension can relieve some discomfort and pain caused by endometriosis. Use stretches for pelvic floor relaxation, internal and external massage techniques to the pelvic floor, and exercise for managing the uncomfortable symptoms associated with endometriosis.

MANAGE POOPING PROBLEMS

Not all women who have endometriosis will have challenges with poops, but many will. Both diarrhea and constipation can occur. Your symptoms will determine what is most helpful. If diarrhea occurs, eat foods that help bulk up your stool (bananas, potatoes, and toast). These can also help soothe a sensitive stomach or nausea. Use a bidet or peri bottle to spritz the anal opening after bowel movements to avoid excessive wiping and skin irritation. If constipation is the issue, use over-the-counter magnesium citrate and eat high-fiber unprocessed foods to keep stool soft. Last, daily abdominal massage can promote movement of stool through the colon and improve constipation. Step-by-step instructions are in Chapter 4, on pooping.

NAVIGATE SEXUAL PAIN

Pelvic floor muscle tension resulting from endometriosis and adhesions can cause deep pelvic pain with intercourse. This pain may occur with every attempt at intercourse and even get progressively worse if endometriosis progresses. Although the adhesions and endometriosis *cannot* be addressed with therapy, the resulting pelvic floor muscle tension *can*. Use a trigger point wand to release deep levator ani and obturator interni muscle tension to relieve overactivity, explained in Chapter 2 under the pelvic floor relaxation protocol. Using an internal massage wand can get messy while on your period, so the days leading up to and after may be the ideal time to use this tool to release muscle tension. Vaginal dilators are also helpful for preparation for intercourse, especially if tension occurs with initial insertion. Follow the guidelines on painful sex in Chapter 6.

Leigh went on to have surgery from an endometriosis specialist that entailed a removal of her uterus, a portion of her colon, part of her bladder, and loads of endometrial tissue throughout her pelvic cavity. Following the surgery, she returned to pelvic floor therapy for several months to address residual pelvic floor muscle tension that contributed to painful sex and tailbone pain, which successfully resolved. Leigh's story has a good ending, but her pain and suffering went on for far too long. My hope is that this information arms and empowers all menstruators to keep advocating and searching if you sense something is wrong. And medical providers, listen to your patients, really listen to them, and help them get the relief they deserve.

I have a friend who has talked about her struggles with adenomyosis, which sounds similar to endometriosis. Are these conditions the same?

Endometriosis is when tissue similar to the uterine lining grows outside of the uterus in the pelvic and abdominal cavity. Adenomyosis is a separate yet similar condition when the tissue that lines the uterus grows *into* the muscular wall of the uterus. When shedding of the uterine lining occurs during menstruation, uterine contractions that expel the menstrual blood and lining can cause significant pain if adenomyosis is present. Typically adenomyosis can occur with endometriosis, and the symptoms of pain and discomfort can be similar to those of endometriosis.

PAIN WITH TAMPON INSERTION

Gabby, an eighteen-year-old college student, came to see me because she couldn't insert a tampon into her vagina. She had plans to go on spring break with her friends in two months, had never been able to use a tampon and only used pads, and was worried about what to do if she got her period on the beach trip. The first time she tried to use a tampon when she got her period at fourteen "felt like a sharp poker stabbing my vagina." Feeling defeated, she gave up and used pads and panty liners, which were working fine for her until she wanted the freedom to go to the beach with friends while having her period. Despite help from her mom and talking to a therapist about her anxiety about inserting the tampon, she had not yet been able to do it without experiencing pain. She wanted to just cross her legs and cry.

Gabby was experiencing a condition called vaginismus, which is tension of the outer third of her pelvic floor muscles preventing entry of anything into her vaginal canal. (I go over the symptoms and treatment for vaginismus in Chapter 6 on sex.) Using a tampon is not supposed to be painful. That said, you'd be surprised how many women struggle with it. If you have pelvic floor muscle tension or a pelvic pain condition like vaginismus, using a tampon can cause pain and further increase muscle tension. So if this is you or someone you know, I see you. Read on.

TUNE IN

The first step in addressing discomfort or pain can often be tuning in to what is happening with our pelvic floor muscles. Are you holding any beliefs that may create shame or embarrassment around this part of your body? Or is it simply just needing more instruction on how to find your vaginal opening, plunge in the tampon, and know you've done it all properly?

If it's the former, exploring some of these deeper issues can help on your healing journey while also addressing the very physical process of insertion. If it's the latter, I encourage you to unwrap a tampon and learn how to use the applicator before trying to insert it. And refer back to Chapter 2 for guidance on how to explore your floor and identify where the vaginal opening is.

RELEASE THE TENSION

Tension and guarding of the muscles at the vaginal opening contribute to pain, discomfort, and an inability to insert a tampon. Stretches from the relaxation protocol in Chapter 2 such as child's pose, happy baby pose, and a deep squat stretch assist with pelvic floor relaxation. Hold each for five to ten breaths daily. Then try inserting a tampon when you are done.

USE VAGINAL DILATORS

Using vaginal dilators, as outlined in Chapter 2, will help desensitize and relax the vaginal opening. Begin with the smallest-size dilator, and after practicing this several times with no pain, progress to the next size dilator that is closest to the size of the tampon you would like to use. Once you have used this size comfortably, try inserting a tampon applicator or tampon (if no applicator) following a dilator practice session when your muscles are already in a relaxed position.

I have a problem where I can't keep a tampon in. Ever since having kids, I feel like it just falls out of my vagina. Is this normal?

A common experience after having kids is not only a change in your periods, but also a change in what period products you need. Following birth, your periods may also have a heavier flow in the earlier days due to a larger surface area of the uterine wall after stretching during pregnancy and hormonal changes with aging and postpartum causing large clots of blood and a heavier flow. More absorbent menstrual products like super plus tampons may be necessary. But if you put a tampon in and it falls out later in the day or during peeing or pooping, your vaginal walls are likely not giving it the support it needs, and it's getting pushed out. During pregnancy, the pelvic floor muscles stretch to support a growing baby or babies. Regardless of the method of birth, vaginal birth or cesarean section, your pelvic floor muscle strength and support decrease postpartum, making the vaginal canal more lax. Pelvic floor strengthening exercises can in fact improve your ability to hold a tampon in. So if this is the scenario for you, check out the strengthening protocol in Chapter 2 to help bulk up your muscles down there to keep in your tampons.

Learn to Love Aunt Flo

Periods are more than just menstrual blood. They are signals about how our body is working and our reproductive health. During my teens, I dreaded getting my period every month and worrying about having enough tampons in my bag or whether it would hit while on vacation. In my twenties, I felt relieved when my period arrived because I was a sexually active woman, and it meant my birth control was effective. In my thirties, I felt sad every month when my period started because it meant I wasn't pregnant when my husband and I were trying to conceive. In my forties, I feel like I am watching a science experiment every month, observing my flow and mastering the algorithm of what period products I need on what days. I now tune in to what my body and pelvic floor need during my menstruation days: water, rest, nutritious foods, and gentle workouts and walks.

My perspective on my period has changed over the years, and with understanding of how the entire menstrual cycle works, my hope is that you too can tune in to these hormonal and physical fluctuations to better support your pelvic health. Whether it's pain or pooping problems, pelvic floor heaviness or period cramps, by understanding your body, and knowing what's normal and what's not, there is support available to help you navigate this regular houseguest. More than anything, I hope this information arms you to start having the conversations so many of us never had, whether it be with our daughters and sons, our sisters, our partners, our students, or our medical providers. I look forward to when we can talk to doctors about menstrual pain and it's not dismissed as normal, when maxi pads sit next to the toilet paper in every bathroom, and when we can talk about period problems as openly as we do headaches or back pain. Then we can finally change the narrative of this very natural and quite magical process of our periods.

CHAPTER 6

Let's Talk About Sex

At sixteen years old, Candace tried to have sex for the first time, but intercourse didn't work. She said it felt like every time her partner tried to enter her, he was hitting a wall. Luckily she had a very close and open relationship with her mom, whom she told. "That's *not* normal," her mom said, and she took her to the doctor. When Candace shared her experience with her gynecologist, her doctor didn't seem all that concerned. "Just relax more. Some pain is normal, and hopefully it'll get better," she instructed. From that point on, Candace felt like this was her fault. Maybe she had done something wrong. Maybe she hadn't taken care of herself in some way. She just needed to relax so sex wouldn't hurt. But with every future unsuccessful attempt, she grew more discouraged.

When I met Candace and inquired how she eventually overcame her pain to have intercourse, she stated, "Well, I was finally able to do it and lose my virginity, but only because I was super, super drunk. Basically, I just forced myself to do it." Unfortunately, Candace was not my first patient who felt the anguish of pain during sex. She was one of many.

Another of my patients who struggled with sex was a young woman named Rajani. Newly married, she had just moved to the United States with her husband and was navigating a new country in a new role as a young bride. She came to me because their long-awaited attempt to have sex on their wedding night did not go as planned. It wasn't just painful for her; it was not even possible. And she reported the same: "He is just hitting a wall and cannot get in." Six months later, after repeated attempts, nothing had changed. She felt broken, scared, and like she was failing in her marriage.

Rajani was diagnosed by her gynecologist with vaginismus, a condition in which spasms of the vaginal muscles prevent entry into the vaginal canal. With attempts to insert a finger or penis into her vagina, her muscles would tense and tighten, creating a barrier into her vaginal canal. Vaginismus is a muscle spasm of your pelvic floor muscles, and as foreign as that may feel to some, it's similar to having tension in your neck muscles leading to headaches (in this case, the ache comes from the tightening up of your vagina). And it is entirely treatable, as long as you get the right help.

Over my years of practicing, I've heard painful sex stories from women in their twenties and women in their seventies. And all of these women come into therapy believing that they've done something wrong, or that they are defective in some way. Some are able to have sex by just enduring the pain and discomfort. And some find other means of intimacy and intercourse until they find therapy.

But all of these women, including Candace and Rajani, have been able to find relief with some basic education about their pelvic floors, along with some instruction—from stretching and breathing exercises to relax their pelvic floors to more advanced techniques that include the use of vaginal dilators and more. Education and awareness about our pelvic floors and how they relate to our sexual health can not only prevent us from experiencing unnecessary pain but also decrease shame, enhance pleasure, and empower us to know and understand our bodies.

Candace came into therapy for painful sex, but with consistency and education, she was able to finally not just tolerate intercourse without pain but actually *enjoy* it. She returned to therapy years later during her first pregnancy and went on to have an unmedicated vaginal birth. Therapy helped her not just with sex, but with her pregnancy, her family, and her confidence.

Rajani completed her course of pelvic health therapy six months after her first visit. On her last day, she walked in with a huge smile on her face and said, "We did it!" She had sex with her husband for the first time without pain. She cried, and so did I. A year later, I bumped into Rajani in the freezer section of the grocery store, and she told me she was five months pregnant. I cried again. This is what pelvic floor care—care that you can do via the exercises and tips in this book—can do. This is the meaningful work I've had the honor to be a part of. And this is what's possible when we know that sex should not be painful and that pelvic floor training can help.

This book has a separate chapter about general pelvic pain. But because pelvic floor issues affecting your sex life are quite vast, I've decided a chapter on sexual health and pelvic floor conditions deserves its own space.

How the Pelvic Floor and Sex Work Together

Sex is fun. It is joyful, expressive, weird, creative. Sometimes it is a mess, sometimes it is great. But most of all, it is supposed to be pleasurable. We all deserve an excellent sex life. And I say—go get it, girl! But because a big part of sex happens in and around our pelvic floors, our pelvic floor needs to be happy for our sex life to thrive.

For the majority of women I see in my clinic, sex means inserting something (a penis, a dildo, a finger, or a toy) into the opening of the vagina. For many, sex also includes anal play, anal sex, oral sex, and even what I like to call outercourse, where nothing is inserted into the vagina but there is still sexual activity and arousal. But many argue, and I would agree, that sex starts well before any physical insertion into the vagina with

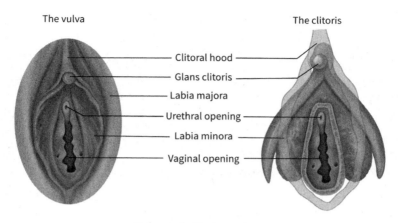

Vulva and clitoris anatomy

arousal. As arousal occurs prior to actual sex, our bodies and pelvic floor are preparing through blood flow, lubrication, and pelvic floor muscle relaxation.

There are several scientific models describing the sexual arousal cycle, the most well-known by sexual health researchers William Masters and Virginia Johnson from the 1960s. Their classic theory describes four phases of sexual response.

THE AROUSAL PHASE: WE GETTIN' READY!

This first stage occurs as a result of physical or mental stimuli like kissing, viewing or reading sexually stimulating content, or fantasizing. What we often refer to as foreplay occurs during this phase, and both physical and emotional interactions contribute to arousal.

THE PLATEAU PHASE: WAIT, I'M ALMOST THERE!

This phase follows and encompasses sexual activity and pleasure prior to orgasm. During this phase, your heart rate increases, breathing gets heavier, and you experience an increase in blood flow throughout your body, including to your pelvic floor. You can stay in this phase for a prolonged period of time.

THE ORGASM PHASE: AWWW YEAH!

This phase ends the plateau phase. An orgasm is quick and rhythmic involuntary muscular contractions of your pelvic floor muscles. Your heart rate increases; you may make loud sounds, groans, or screams; and muscles in other parts of your body—like your hips, hands, and even toes—may engage for this full-body experience.

THE RESOLUTION PHASE: WELL, THAT WAS NICE!

This final resting phase occurs when the body slows down from its excited state. Your muscles relax, and your heart rate and blood flow slow down. You may feel satiated, satisfied, tired, or snuggly, but your body and mind calm down.

SEVERAL VARIATIONS OF THIS SEXUAL RESPONSE MODEL HAVE BEEN created since then, like one from sexual health researcher Rosemary Basson, who posited that the Masters and Johnson sexual response cycle does not reflect the experience of women. She argued that the model neglects the role that closeness or attachment to a partner play in increasing the effectiveness of sexual stimulation and whether or not they orgasm in a sexual encounter. The takeaway from all of these sex researchers is that ultimately our entire body *and mind* play a role in sex, and in our pelvic floor's ability to have pain-free sex. When we look at issues of pain during sex, we need to look at the entire pelvic floor (not just the vagina)—and how the mind might be affecting pelvic floor tension. Sex is psychological and emotional as well as physical.

As you may recall from Chapter 1, the muscles of our pelvic floor are affected by our mind—and by every other single muscle in the pelvic floor. Take the clitoris, for example. The word *clitoris* is thought to be derived from Ancient Greek meaning "veiled" or "organ hidden under the skin," an appropriate description for the sensitive bulb of tissue located under a hood, or covering, of tissue. The hood of the clitoris, which serves as a protective layer from pressure and irritation, is attached directly to two of the superficial pelvic floor muscles, the bulbocavernosus and ischiocavernosus. The clitoris is deeply connected to the pelvic floor muscles, which points to how the ability to have pain-free and pleasurable orgasms is directly related to your pelvic floor function.

During the arousal phase, blood flow increases to your pelvic floor, vulvar, and vaginal tissues. Blood flow is essential to engorge the clitoris (equivalent to penile engorgement/erections), to increase lubrication of vulvar and vaginal tissues, and to increase sensitivity in all of your erogenous zones. During the plateau phase, blood flow further enhances relaxation of the pelvic floor muscles, which surround the vaginal opening, anal opening, and vaginal canal. Thus, blood flow and pelvic floor muscle function are essential for penetrative intercourse into the vagina or anus. Sex can occur without orgasm, but according to these sexual arousal models, during the orgasm phase, the engorgement of your superficial pelvic floor muscles is at its maximum until orgasm is reached and those muscles involuntarily contract and relax. Sexual arousal, intercourse, and orgasm are really quite the symphony of muscles, nerves, and tissues working harmoniously with one another. We'll cover orgasms more in depth toward the end of the chapter, but the takeaway here is that sexual pleasure is connected to pelvic floor health.

Is piercing my labia or clitoris safe?

You may find yourself wondering if some jewelry might enhance or inhibit pleasure in your genital region—and whether piercings will cause any pelvic floor issues. The most common type of genital piercing is a ring or bar placed through the hood of the clitoris, not through the actual clitoris, to increase the pressure on the clitoris during sexual activity. The second most common is a piercing through the labia. These piercings carry the same risks as do any piercings, like infection, scarring, allergic reaction to metal, tearing of the tissue, and nerve damage. Piercing in this area is as "safe" as it would be for piercings anywhere else, but (big BUT here) there are lots of nerves and sensitive tissues in this area compared to, say, your earlobe. Therefore, pierce cautiously, know you are going to a clean sterile environment, follow healing precautions that can last up to six weeks afterwards, and monitor for any signs of infection.

Having good sex is our birthright. The desire to have sex is a basic human appetite, and we should all be able to enjoy the mystery and pleasure of a good sexual life. And aside from it being a source of connection, pleasure, relaxation, and play, sex is one of the gateways to parenthood. And not being able to experience any of these benefits of sex can lead to depression and despair. One of my patients, Jennifer, had been too embarrassed to tell anyone that sex hurt. Because of her history of severe pain during intercourse with her husband, they resorted to turkey-basting his sperm into her vagina to get pregnant. Now pregnant, she was nervous that her vagina would not relax to give birth. As genius and crafty as this solution is, Jennifer deserved a better path. The distress and challenges in growing her family were largely preventable.

As with other functions that occur down south, if your pelvic floor muscles aren't working optimally, it will affect your sex. Here are just a number of challenges my patients have faced over the years:

> "My vagina feels so heavy and swollen after sex."
> "Ever since having kids, it feels like I am ripping when he tries to enter."
> "I have never been able to have an orgasm."
> "My partner has tried inserting a finger into my vagina, and I just close up like there's a wall."

"I waited until marriage to have sex, and it is so
painful I can't bear it."

"Ever since menopause, I have been bleeding during
sex."

Many of us carry extraordinary embarrassment or shame
when sex isn't working. We feel defective—and we might worry
that we are letting our partners down. There is also the question of who, if anyone, can help. Do you go to your primary
care doctor? Your gynecologist? A therapist? In movies, media,
and magazines and even during happy hour conversations, sex is
talked about only as something flirtatious and fun. But if that is
not your experience, you may feel broken. *I assure you; you are not.*

When Sex Isn't So Steamy

If your pelvic floor muscles are tense, pain can make sex frustrating and near impossible. There are countless reasons for why
your muscles may tense up: a peeing or pooping problem, a result of a birth injury, poor posture, or even trauma.

Pelvic floor tension can occur when women find themselves
delaying the urge to pee because they are unable to go when the
urge strikes, a challenge commonly experienced by teachers and
medical professionals, myself included. If you absolutely can't poop
in public, frequently holding in your bowel movements can create
pelvic floor tension, as can sitting with crossed legs for prolonged
periods, tense glutes in morning traffic, or too many virtual meetings in your office chair. After pregnancy and childbirth, we often
think pelvic floor muscle weakness is the main concern; however,
following a vaginal delivery or a cesarean section, scar tissue from
a perineal scar or abdominal scar can lead to pelvic floor tension
and painful sex as well.

Trauma can include physical or emotional trauma, sexual
trauma, childbirth trauma, medical trauma, or even conditioning from a culture or religion that sexual activity is inherently

bad. When we are in a situation that feels dangerous or scary, we might enter a state of "fight, flight, or freeze" because we feel danger (even if the situation isn't dangerous at all). When your pelvic floor muscles tense up or freeze because of past trauma, this is your body's wisdom working to protect you from further harm. Your body is doing what it is designed to do, and you need to work with your body and your mind to learn that you are safe and can relax to experience pleasure. If you feel that past trauma is related to pain or discomfort you feel during sex, working with a licensed professional who has experience in trauma or sexual trauma will be incredibly helpful in your journey toward healing and relief.

Pain with sex due to pelvic floor tension can pop up at any age, which may not be exactly what you want to hear, but debunks the myth that a "tight" pelvic floor only happens when we are young or pre-pregnancy and is a desirable state for vaginas. It is not. One morning in my clinic, a young twenty-seven-year-old woman crossed paths with a seventy-two-year-old grandmother in the waiting room, both attending pelvic floor therapy for the same problem: painful sex. I paused, took note, and thought, *This moment is such an example of how women from all ages and life stages are in need of this type of therapy. And I am so glad they found it.*

In the section that follows, I describe some of the most common sex-related challenges women experience that are related to the pelvic floor. They range from insertional pain to inability to orgasm to peeing during sex. Your pelvic floor is a factor, and the exercises and suggestions in the next pages will help.

PAINFUL SEX WITH INITIAL OR DEEPER INSERTION

In the past and even still today, many medical providers attribute pain during insertion to a phobia or anxiety around having sex. So women are told to "just relax" or "drink a glass of wine" or "consider anxiety medication." Not only does this dismiss their very real pain, but it also blames them for their experience and essentially accuses them of imagining it. More recently, the medical community re-evaluated how to best diagnose and classify painful sex and developed a term: genito-pelvic pain/penetration disorder (GPPPD). GPPPD characterizes pain with penetration as a combination of anxiety *and* a physical condition, versus anxiety alone causing the tension and pain. It's a pain–anxiety–muscle tension cycle that we need to break.

The superficial muscle layer of the pelvic floor that surrounds the vaginal opening typically relaxes to allow vaginal entry, but this layer can also tense up and *prevent* entry into the vagina. The deeper layer of pelvic floor muscle wraps around the vaginal canal, and it is this layer of muscle that is often the source of pain during deep insertion into the vagina. The first step toward relief is to release the muscle tension. Then, gradually, you can introduce touch and insertion into the vagina in a nonthreatening way.

RELAX YOUR PELVIC FLOOR

Follow the pelvic floor relaxation protocol in Chapter 2. You will start with gentle diaphragmatic breaths and external massage and add in daily stretches to relieve muscle tension. These stretches can be performed in the morning or evening, before or after workouts, but should definitely be performed prior to using vaginal dilators.

PERFORM PERINEAL MASSAGE

Perineal massage is often recommended for women during pregnancy to prepare the vagina and perineum for relaxation during vaginal birth. However, it is also an effective massage for releasing the superficial muscles of the vaginal opening to aid in pelvic floor muscle relaxation. Lie in your bed with your knees relaxed open with a pillow under them for support. Place a small amount of lubricant or oil on your thumb and gently stretch the base of your vaginal opening. Hold this stretch (it may feel slightly burny) until the sensation decreases or for 5-7 deep breaths. Release your

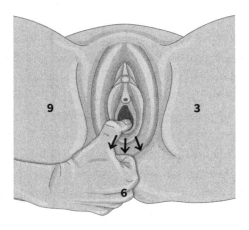

Perineal massage: thumb inserted into vaginal opening,
applying pressure toward six o'clock

pressure and rotate your thumb slightly to the left to seven o'clock
or to the right to five o'clock and repeat. Perform perineal massage for three to five minutes every other day following pelvic
floor relaxation stretches. If you are comfortable, you can also ask
a partner to massage you so that you can fully relax.

WORK WITH VAGINAL DILATORS

If touch to the vaginal opening does not result in muscle guarding and pain, progress to working on insertion into the vagina.
Start with the smallest dilator and increase to larger-size dilators
as you feel comfortable. You can work up to the dilator that is
about the same size as your partner's penis, if your partner has
one. You can also use the dilator to apply gentle pressure at different points of the opening from three to nine o'clock. Take
deep breaths and allow your muscles to soften as gentle pressure
is applied. Move the dilator in and out and practice using different positions you may be in during sexual activity.

   Progressing from inserting a dilator to having sexual intercourse is a big jump, and the following steps can help. Once the
size dilator closest to your partner is reached, practice inserting

the dilator with your partner in the room or lying next to you in bed. Progress to your partner inserting the dilator into your vaginal opening as you focus on breathing and relaxation. Use the dilator on yourself immediately prior to intercourse or have your partner insert it for you. Think of this like warming up or stretching before running a race.

Remember to work at your pace. Breathe as dilators are gradually inserted into the vagina, and pause if tension occurs. You don't have to stop the dilator session if tension occurs. Rather, focus on your breath or perform a pelvic floor contraction (Kegel), then release, to aid in releasing pelvic floor muscle tension.

USE A PELVIC FLOOR WAND

A pelvic floor wand can be used to release the deeper pelvic floor muscles if pain with deeper insertion occurs. These instructions can be found in detail in Chapter 2. Lie down on your back with your knees relaxed open and supported by pillows. Additionally, place pillows behind your back to help you easily reach the vaginal opening. Insert the wand up to the first curve and point the tip of the wand to the right and the left side of the pelvic floor muscle. Apply pressure to different spots in the muscles until you locate a tender spot or the discomfort you experience during sex is recreated. Hold for five deep breaths or until tenderness subsides. Repeat on the left and right sides until no additional tender spots in the muscles are located.

My partner and I are interested in anal play—and maybe even anal sex. What can I do to relax those muscles? Can anal sex lead to pelvic floor damage, and is it ever contraindicated? What do I need to know so we do it safely?

A lot to unpack here, so let's go. In advance, performing the pelvic floor relaxation stretches and practicing bulging or "laying an egg," both covered in Chapter 2, will help your anal sphincter (anal play entryway) to release and open when it's game time.

Go small and slowly, starting by slowly and gently inserting a pinky finger, index finger, or small anal dilator. Use a lot of lubricant here. When it comes to butt stuff, more lube is better. Try silicone- or oil-based lubricant, which can last a bit longer than water-based. Also start by trying a position that is less penetrating, like lying on your side or on your back, or for penile insertion, sitting backward on your partner's lap so that you have more control over depth. Anal fissures and hemorrhoids can occur as a result, so if pain or bleeding occur, take a pause and check Chapter 4 on pooping problems for support. And also know you may fart or have some poop bits come out, because it is, after all, your anus.

VULVAR AND VAGINAL DRYNESS

Think of a time when you've been dehydrated. Your mouth is parched. Your lips are dry and stick together. Your tongue might feel like cotton, and you yearn for a glass of water. Similar to the tissue inside your mouth, your vulva and the vaginal opening are made up of mucosal tissues that require moisture at all times, so we can even dehydrate down there. Vulvar and vaginal dryness can feel like itchiness of the labia, your underwear sticking to your vulva, or a raw sensation when wiping or touching the area. And when we are raw and dry, sex can hurt.

With arousal, fluids are released from glands surrounding the vagina to aid in moisture and lubrication. If that does not occur, touching or rubbing the tissues during sexual activity can cause perineal or vaginal tearing, burning with in/out movements, and even bleeding after sex—all of which are painful.

Vulvar and vaginal dryness can be due to a variety of factors.

One of the most common is a decrease in estrogen levels. The hormone estrogen contributes to vaginal lubrication and plumps up the vaginal and vulvar tissues. When estrogen levels decline, it can lead to thin, dry, and frail tissues and decreased pelvic floor muscle strength. Often low estrogen levels are thought to occur with aging and menopause, but we also know this can occur when women are taking hormonal birth control, are postpartum and breastfeeding, are undergoing chemotherapy or estrogen deprivation therapy, or are going through peri-menopause.

Once upon a time, petroleum jelly was pretty much a cure-all for anything skin-related.

Burn from the oven rack? *Petroleum jelly.*
Chapped lips? *Petroleum jelly.*
Cracked cuticles? *Petroleum jelly.*
Diaper rash? *Petroleum jelly.*
Dry vagina? *Petro—NO! Okay, stop right there.*

Yes, petroleum jelly can help lock in moisture, but it's actually not a moisturizing cream. It also doesn't absorb into the tissue, so it hangs out and can harbor bacteria and increase the risk of vaginal infections. Treatment for vulvar and vaginal dryness entails increasing moisture throughout the day and during sexual activity and intercourse, and through utilizing local hormone therapy for estrogen supplementation.

HYDRATE

If your skin is dry, drink water. Same for your vag. Your tissues need moisture, and they need to get it externally (moisturizers and lube) and internally (hydration). Be aware of certain medications that can contribute to dehydration like antihistamines and allergy medications, diuretics, high blood pressure or diabetes medications, and chemotherapy.

MOISTURIZE THE VULVA AND VAGINA

The easiest and most affordable option for adding moisture is to use an oil like jojoba oil or coconut oil. Start with a new jar, ideally organic, and apply after the shower, before bedtime, or throughout the day as needed. More recently, moisturizers specifically for vulvar dryness are available over the counter and can be great options. Whichever you choose, if you have any adverse reactions, itching, or infections, pause use, contact your doc, and try another brand or type of moisturizer.

Some moisturizers are specifically for the vulva, and some can also be used in the vagina. Maintaining pH balance inside the vagina is a priority to minimize the risk of bacterial growth and infection. Vaginal lotions including hyaluronic acid, which has been used for facial skin care routines, are finding their way into vulvar and vaginal care products. These are typically over-the-counter lotions or vaginal suppositories that can be inserted nightly into the vagina to increase moisture. These are great, easily accessible options.

I am three months postpartum, breastfeeding, and my vagina feels super dry during sex. Is this normal?

If you are breastfeeding or lactating, you likely have high prolactin, the milk-producing hormone. When you have high prolactin levels, you have low estrogen levels, which is why your menstrual cycle is typically delayed after childbirth. As if you needed one more reason to not want to have sex after giving birth, these low estrogen levels can cause vaginal and vulvar dryness and pain with sex. Topical estrogen, all-natural pH-balanced vulvar moisturizers, and a lubricant during intercourse can relieve dryness and increase pleasure with sex.

USE A LUBRICANT DURING SEX

Lube has interesting connotations. It can be thought of as a positive (for racy, steamy sex) or a negative (when a woman isn't aroused enough to have adequate lubrication on her own). I consider it a necessity for decreasing friction and increasing pleasure. And I highly recommend it if vaginal dryness or painful sex is something you're dealing with.

All lubes are not created equal. Gone are the days of walking down the aisle of a pharmacy and grabbing something from the shelf, because now we have many options. Lube products should be paraben-, glycerin-, petroleum-, and fragrance-free and pH-balanced, and should not cause burning or discomfort. Further, lubricants may be water-based, silicone-based, aloe-based, oil-based, cannabidiol (CBD)-based, or sperm-friendly. Let's break those down and discuss some pros and cons of each.

Water-Based Lubricants. The pro: water-based lubes are great as they are typically gentle enough for sensitive skin, and they won't break down latex condoms or silicone toys. The con: they do tend to dry up, so you may need to reapply more frequently than other options.

Silicone-Based Lubricants. The pro: silicone lube lasts the longest, so you don't have to reapply as often. It's also the slickest, so it offers a great glide with less friction. The con: silicone lubricant doesn't go with silicone toys as it can cause the material to break down. Silicone also hangs out for a bit longer and doesn't clean up as easily as a water-based lubricant. Silicone is a synthetic ingredient, so if you are trying to avoid certain ingredients keep this in mind.

Aloe-Based Lubricants. The pro: aloe-based lubes are great options as they won't break down latex condoms and silicone toys. They last longer than water-based lubes, and aloe is known to have soothing benefits for the skin.

The con: some people may have a reaction to aloe. Be aware of any redness, burning, or stinging that may occur. You can test aloe lubricant on the inside of your elbow for a few hours before putting it on your vulva and vagina.

Oil-Based Lubricants. The pros: oil-based lubes last longer than many other types and are great for daily use for hydration. The cons: some people do experience increased vaginal infections after using. Oil can also break down and rip latex condoms, so keep that in mind.

CBD-Based Lubricants. The pro: these are great if you have pelvic floor overactivity. CBD works directly with the pelvic floor muscles and tissues to help them relax while providing the moisture needed from lube. CBD suppositories are also available. The con: at this time, CBD isn't well regulated, so you will want to be sure your CBD is coming from a reputable source. The majority of CBD lubes do contain oil, so you will want to be aware if you are using latex condoms.

Sperm-Friendly Lubricants. The pro: sperm-friendly lubricants are available and have a consistency more similar to natural vaginal lubrication to optimize the ability of sperm to reach their destination. Typically, these lubricants are water-based. The con: there are no real cons except that because they are typically water-based, you will have to reapply if it's a longer sex session or there is significant vaginal dryness.

No matter which lube you choose, know you have options to find one that works best for you and your vagina. Basic rule of thumb: if it glitters, sparkles, tingles, or smells, it should not go on your vagina!

Can I use lube when trying to conceive or will this affect my chances of getting pregnant?

If you are trying to conceive, you may find yourself doing a deep dive into what will aid fertilization and what might hinder it. There are theories that lube can prevent the sperm from swimming to the egg. The more sperm that reach the egg, the more chances for fertilization. Recently, several brands have created sperm-friendly lubricants that will not affect sperm speed and style. Ultimately, a lubricant that is water-soluble, maintains pH balance, and is glycerin-free will not slow these swimmers down.

VAGINAL BURNING

Many women who experience pain with sex also have vaginal burning, which is usually due to pelvic floor nerve irritation, entrapment, or sensitivity. When we discussed muscle tension earlier, we looked at how the body learns to perceive attempts at vaginal penetration as a threat and tenses up before even being touched, thus causing more pain with touch and even more muscle tension.

This cycle leads to changes in the brain (our brains rewire to expect pain), but also changes in the *nerves*, causing tissues in the vulvar region to become highly sensitive. This can result in a burning or stinging pain with gentle touch at the opening of the vagina, so something that shouldn't be "painful" is actually quite excruciating. It's like post-traumatic stress disorder (PTSD) for your pelvic floor. This cycle becomes reinforced as a person continues to have painful experiences, meaning that the person develops increased fear, and therefore increased tension. Treatment for desensitization of your pelvic floor nerves is a three-step process.

UNDERSTAND HOW PAIN WORKS

First, acknowledge the physical component of what is happening at the tissue or muscle level of your body, and how your brain is responding. We all perceive pain differently, although the stimulus is the same. This is not to say it's all in your head. Rather, we can work with our minds in order to respond to pain in a less severe way. For example, some people can step on a tack and not even know it, while other people might step on a tack and need to lay off the walking for three days. Studies show that because the experience of pain is processed by the brain, we can work with our minds to respond to pain differently. Do what aligns with your comfort zone and values, but steps at home can include participating in outercourse, what I call sexual activity that is arousing and pleasurable that does not include vaginal penetration. Looking at photos, watching sexual activity, and participating in sexual activity that is not painful help your brain associate pleasure with sex instead of trauma, fear, or avoidance. In other words, we can train our brains to respond differently to what we think might be painful, including sex.

INTRODUCE TOUCH THAT IS NOT PAINFUL

This may start with touching externally over clothes, then over underwear, then with underwear off, then directly outside the vulva, then at the opening. Think of this like peeling layers of an onion. As you start outside and work your way inward, you can begin to welcome touch in the region as something nonpainful and neutral versus negative.

DESENSITIZE YOUR TISSUES AND MUSCLES

Follow the pelvic floor relaxation protocol in Chapter 2. Start working internally to desensitize the vulvar tissues, the opening to the vagina, and deeper pelvic floor muscles. This is typically performed using vaginal dilators. Start with the smallest size, or begin with an even smaller, but sanitary and clean, object. You can begin with something as small as a Q-tip touching inside the labia, then move to the vaginal opening, then progress to insertion. Increase to larger-size dilators as you feel comfortable.

DECREASED SENSATION DURING SEX

On occasion, patients will report that sex just feels different. "I just don't feel as much" or "I feel looser down there" are distressing reports from women who have less sensation during sex. This is reported from some postpartum women whose pelvic floor muscles are lengthened during pregnancy or vaginal birth. Similarly, many perimenopausal and menopausal women also report less sensation during sex due to lack of vaginal lubrication and decreased pelvic floor muscle strength. Decreased sensation can elicit not only feelings of nervousness or insecurity but also an avoidance of sexual activity altogether. If you suspect that you could feel more during sex, try the following steps.

STRENGTHEN YOUR PELVIC FLOOR

Follow the pelvic floor strengthening protocol in Chapter 2. The key here is to strengthen your floor to help increase blood flow to the genitals and increase the thickness of the pelvic floor muscles surrounding the vaginal canal. Increasing pelvic floor muscle strength takes time and consistency but can make a huge difference in enhancing sensation to the area. You can also perform Kegel contractions during vaginal intercourse to enhance sensation and physical contact.

USE THE RIGHT LUBRICANT

Using a lubricant can help with moisture if dryness is a factor in a lack of sensation. Keep in mind that you may need to try different lubricants to find one that decreases friction but isn't *too* slippery to prevent sensation.

USE IT, DON'T LOSE IT

When a barrier to sex presents itself, our nature is to avoid sexual activity, which can actually lead to less desire and blood flow to the genital area. If pain is not a factor, continue to engage in sexual activity that is pleasurable either on your own or with a partner. It's like riding a bicycle. You won't necessarily forget how to do it if you don't for a while, but it's definitely easier and your muscles maintain their memory when it's something you do regularly.

LEAKAGE DURING SEX OR ORGASM (AKA SQUIRTING)

Squirting, or the release of fluid during sexual stimulation or orgasm, has become a more popular topic in recent times due to how it is played up and joked about in the media. Some people describe it as a sexual superpower, and others view it as a source of shame. There's been some debate about whether the release of fluid during an orgasm is pee or female ejaculate. To set the record straight: it's typically both! Emitting just a small amount of a whitish fluid during an orgasm is possible, and in that case, it is likely ejaculate, but if there is a tablespoon or three of clear fluid, it likely has pee in it.

Some people squirt while others do not. It doesn't necessarily occur with every orgasm, and it is not a problem unless it bothers you. Squirting is more common during pregnancy, postpartum, or with aging, when your pelvic floor and bladder function tend to be compromised. If you sense any leakage during sexual activity, the following tips might help.

EMPTY YOUR BLADDER

If you do experience squirting, empty your bladder before sexual activity (in this case, it's okay to pee "just in case"). This reduces the amount of urine in your bladder, but because your bladder is never completely empty, some urine may still escape.

COVER THE SHEETS

This tip won't solve the problem, but it will save your sheets. Squirting or leaking urine can often lessen women's desire to have sex or orgasm. Placing a towel over your sheets can avoid saturating your bed with fluid and inform your partner this may happen to relieve any distress that may be associated with it.

ADDRESS YOUR PELVIC FLOOR PROBLEM

In the case of squirting, I have seen women who have pelvic floor tension leading to urinary urgency and some who have pelvic floor weakness, and they are unable to keep their urinary sphincter closed during orgasm. After reading the checklist of symptoms in Chapter 2, follow the pelvic floor protocol that aligns with the majority of your symptoms.

Ever since having kids, my vagina farts during sex. Is this normal, and what can I do about it?

Vaginal farts, also known as queefing, are a result of air getting trapped inside of the vagina, then releasing and making a loud, fart-like noise. Queefing can occur during intercourse but also during certain yoga poses or exercises like bridge pose, downward-facing dog, or headstands. When your pelvic floor muscles are weak or vaginal tissues more lax, which is the case after pregnancy and birth, air has a harder time staying in and eventually escapes. Pelvic floor muscle strengthening can help decrease the likelihood of queefing by preventing as much air from getting in and out. See my pelvic floor strengthening protocol in Chapter 2. No matter how hard you work on your pelvic floor, though, this may just happen due to the tissue changes. I know this can be frustrating and embarrassing. The only upside is that they are not smelly, just noisy.

The Big (or Not So Big) O

Orgasms are involuntary contractions of your superficial pelvic floor muscles usually preceded by sexual arousal. They can occur as a result of clitoral stimulation, vaginal sex, or a combination of both and are accompanied by a feeling of intense pleasure, euphoria, and genital sensitivity. But you don't necessarily have one with every sexual encounter, and in fact, up to 10% of women report *never* having experienced an orgasm. As with other sexual health issues, how our core and pelvic floor function plays a role in our ability to have pleasurable orgasms.

INABILITY TO ORGASM

A main complaint of women experiencing sexual health challenges is the inability to have an orgasm. The muscular contractions that occur during an orgasm are absolutely influenced by psychological, emotional, and social conditions. From a physical perspective, inability to have an orgasm or weak orgasms can be caused by hormonal fluctuation like lower estrogen level, side effects of medications like antihistamines, and weak pelvic floor muscles.

STRENGTHEN YOUR PELVIC FLOOR

Your superficial pelvic floor muscles contract during an orgasm. If those muscles are too weak, your orgasm may feel very weak or nonexistent. When performing the strengthening protocol, don't forget to do your quick Kegels, as your superficial muscles are mainly fast-twitch muscle fibers.

SELF-STIMULATE

This recommendation is not for everyone, but self-stimulation (aka masturbation) can help you discover how your body, and your unique pelvic floor configuration, work for you. You can self-stimulate with a vibrator, a dildo, or your own fingers and hands, and explore what is pleasurable for you. Do you enjoy touching the clitoris? Do you prefer internal stimulation? Do you like vibrators? Do you like lubricant? Discover what feels good to you.

Also, performance anxiety (thank you, mind–pelvic floor connection) can play a factor in why you may struggle to reach an orgasm, as there is ultimately a letting go that has to occur. Without someone else present, you may be better able to relax into the experience and focus on pleasure instead of performance.

FIND A SEX THERAPIST

Studies have shown that some women benefit from working with a therapist specializing in sexual health. If the above tips don't offer the support you need, consider finding a sex therapist to help with the emotional and mental components.

CONSTANT URGE TO ORGASM

As fun and exciting as this condition seems, constantly feeling the urge to orgasm can be quite debilitating. And believe it or not, this urge can be a pelvic floor issue. Persistent genital arousal disorder (PGAD) is a condition characterized by spontaneous and persistent sexual arousal when no sexual desire or stimuli exists. Imagine going for a walk, sitting in a meeting, playing with your grandchildren, or exercising at the gym and you feel uncontrollably warm, wet, tingly, and aroused in your genital region. Not only is it hard to focus and concentrate, it's distressing, because sexual activity and orgasm offer no relief.

There is no known cause of PGAD, although many women report that it began after a surgery, childbirth, or starting a new medication. No one treatment can cure it, but often a combination of medications (including injections or topical and oral medication to decrease nerve and hormonal activity), working with a sexual health therapist or psychotherapist to manage distressing symptoms, and decreasing pelvic floor muscle tension and pudendal nerve activity can help. The pudendal nerve is intimately involved in genital sensation; this nerve needs to be addressed and treated when managing PGAD.

RELEASE PELVIC FLOOR MUSCLE TENSION

The pudendal nerve runs from the bottom of your spine, deep under your buttock muscles, and through the pelvic floor muscles until it branches off into smaller nerves that travel to your genitalia. Tense pelvic floor muscles can irritate or entrap that nerve, which leads to increased sensitivity or activity. Follow the pelvic floor relaxation protocol in Chapter 2 and focus primarily on stretches to the glutes and pelvic floor muscles such as child's pose, figure 4 stretch, and shin-box stretch.

MASSAGE YOUR GLUTES

Outside pelvic muscle tension can contribute to inside pelvic muscle tension. Grab that massage ball and roll out your glutes and rotators. This will help minimize external tension that can contribute to pelvic floor overactivity.

USE A TRIGGER POINT WAND

Use a wand specifically on the obturator internus muscle, located on the side and front part of the pelvis. This muscle can get tense and irritate the pudendal nerve. Insert a vaginal trigger point wand and point the tip toward three or nine o'clock at the location of the obturator internus muscle. Place one hand on the outside of your knee and gently press your knee into your hand with resistance, not letting your knee move. The obturator internus muscle will contract with that motion. You will feel the muscle tighten, and perhaps feel tenderness or pain. This helps you know you are at the correct location of the obturator internus as you apply pressure to release tension.

APPLY COLD

Nerves communicate sensation between our muscles, tissues, and brain. Cold can be a great way to numb a nerve and reduce pain, warmth, and arousal. Place a cold ice pack under your pants but over your underwear for twenty minutes, then remove for twenty minutes. Repeat this process daily during times when arousal is high, if you are able, or as often as you like. Do not apply ice (or heat, for that matter) for longer than twenty minutes, as prolonged exposure to extreme temperatures can cause damage to tissue and nerves.

PAINFUL ORGASMS

Similar to painful sex, painful orgasms are often due to overactive pelvic floor muscles. Because orgasms are contractions of the superficial pelvic floor muscles, releasing those muscles is essential to relieving pain, so we can relax into the pleasure.

RELAX YOUR PELVIC FLOOR

Pause the Kegels and focus on pelvic floor muscle relaxation. Deep breathing, stretches to release tight hips and overactive pelvic floor muscles, and maintaining good posture can all help quiet your nervous system and release tension in your pelvic floor. Follow the relaxation protocol in Chapter 2.

STRETCH YOUR PERINEUM

The first layer of pelvic floor muscles fills with blood during arousal, then contracts and relaxes during an orgasm. Relieving tension or spasm in those muscles can decrease pain with orgasm.

Stretching the perineum from the vaginal opening, similarly to performing a perineal massage, can soften the superficial pelvic floor muscles that surround the base of the vaginal opening. You can perform this stretch to the vaginal opening with your finger, a perineal massage wand, or the tip of a trigger point wand.

RELEASE YOUR SUPERFICIAL PELVIC FLOOR

Roll up a hand towel to about the circumference of a tennis ball. Place the towel longways on a firm chair and sit down so the towel rests underneath your vulvar region, nestled between your two sit bones. Soften your posture and take some deep breaths to allow the towel to sink into your superficial pelvic floor muscles to release them. Hold this for five to ten deep breaths. Repeat up to three times a day and before or after sexual activity or orgasms.

From Pain to Pleasure

Sex should be fun, explorative, curious, intimate, and exciting. I'm not saying every sesh needs to be the steamiest sex of your life, but it should at least leave you feeling nourished from head to toe. But this is a tall order when a pelvic floor problem exists. In her book *Come As You Are*, American sex educator Emily Nagoski describes sexual health as a spectrum. There is no right number of times to have sex in a week or month. There is no absolute way to reach orgasm (although I do highly recommend a vibrator). Identifying the factors that influence sexual satisfaction and knowing what puts your foot on the sex-brake and what puts your foot on the sex-gas is the first step.

> A dry vagina . . . *brake.*
> Worried about wetting the bed . . . *brake.*
> Feeling self-conscious about your menopausal
> vagina . . . *brake.*
> Completely exhausted, a toddler sleeping in your bed,
> and just wanting to rack up as many hours of sleep as
> you can . . . *brake.*

The tips and tools in this chapter can help you address the factors that cause you to put your foot on the brake. You can resolve pain, get a great lube, and strengthen your pelvic floor muscles. I can't do much about the sleeping toddler in your bed except promise you that you will eventually reclaim your bed and get more sleep. And as you begin to remove your foot from the brake, you can start putting it on the gas. *You deserve it.*

It's not easy to talk about and find solutions when something in our sex lives goes awry. Just like many other pelvic health issues, embarrassment and shame accompany the very real physical symptoms we experience. The challenges above are some of the main ones I see in my patients and practice. Often women experience these for a prolonged period of time until they are either appropriately referred by a medical professional to pelvic floor therapy or find it themselves, but the sooner you seek support, the better. Start by talking to your medical provider about your symptoms. Follow my guidelines in this book. And work with a therapist in person if your symptoms don't improve or resolve.

So many women feel there is no hope or no help, but that is not the case. Candace, my patient from earlier, felt pelvic floor therapy helped her: "Even if you feel embarrassed about it—because it can be hard to talk about—it was worth it times a million. It literally changed my life."

CHAPTER 7

What to Expect from Your Expecting Pelvic Floor

I started treating pregnant women the very first week I launched my career as a pelvic floor therapist. Pelvic PT had a deep grab bag of resources to help—exercise routines to manage low back pain, stretches to relieve hip pain, and postural tips for sleeping, sitting, standing, and squatting. As the years rolled by, I took comfort in the fact that I had so many tools to draw on when my own pregnancy journey began. These simple and efficient tips and exercises were just what pregnant moms needed to stay strong during pregnancy . . . or so I thought.

Ten years into my practice and hundreds of pregnant-mom clients later, I was pregnant with my first son. And it was not at all what I had expected. I was thirty-one, and during my first trimester, I was totally exhausted every single evening. I had only enough energy to eat a bowl of Jell-O before my head hit the pillow for the night. I struggled with nausea and fatigue. I hugged the commode daily to vomit between patients. And I was absolutely *not* a straight-A student with my PT exercises. I did not have the time, nor did I have the energy. Doing thirty minutes of physical therapy exercises, which I had prescribed to so many pregnant patients in the past, was the absolute last thing on my to-do list. (Before I continue, I want to apologize to all of the moms I treated early in my career. My bad. I was an eager young PT and gave you *way* too much homework.)

Seeing how impossible it was to carve out the time and find the energy for a ton of pregnancy exercises, I became my own guinea pig. I figured out I did not need a thirty-minute-a-day routine of pelvic floor practice. I discovered a set of simple, do-able exercises and easy-to-implement habits, which I offer you in this chapter's pelvic floor pregnancy protocol. I found that I could complete this protocol in far less time to help alleviate pain and proactively help my pelvic floor through one of the biggest physical transformations of my life. The exercises and modifications are small, but their impact is huge.

Pregnancy's effects on the pelvic floor are well-known: increased urinary leakage, constipation, discomfort during sex, and core weakness. One third to one half of women will experience a pelvic floor problem during pregnancy, and these symptoms and their severity increase as a woman approaches her third trimester. Yet less than 10% of women report ever being asked about pelvic floor issues by a medical provider, and of those, very few are referred to pelvic floor PT. But the research is clear: education on pelvic floor disorders during pregnancy can actually improve pelvic floor symptoms during pregnancy and beyond.

Many women who don't receive proper pelvic floor care during pregnancy experience problems postpartum. My patient Ramina didn't find pelvic floor therapy until *after* her first pregnancy. During a postpartum massage to soothe pain in her hips, she shared that intense hip pain appeared during her second trimester. Now, every time she went for a run or exercised, her hips ached, and on top of that, she peed her pants. Her massage therapist, who was also a doula, told her about pelvic floor therapy, which led her to me. Ramina sat down in the turquoise chair in the corner of my treatment room and shared her pelvic floor woes: "My hips ache so badly that I can't sleep!" she said. "Plus, I pee my pants every single time I run, jump, cough, or even laugh and can only wear black leggings because black covers the wet spots better!"

When Ramina told her doctor about this pain while pregnant, he stated, "That's just part of pregnancy. It will get better after the baby is born." So Ramina suffered through her entire pregnancy with pain that limited her ability to exercise, an important part of her life up to that point. As a pelvic floor PT, I can tell you this with confidence: many women think the issues that arise during pregnancy will disappear once their baby is born, but that is most often not the case.

I showed Ramina postural changes and stretches to relieve her hip pain, relaxation techniques and massage to decrease pelvic floor tension, and exercises to improve her pelvic floor strength to help her leakage. Relatively quickly, her hip pain and her incontinence improved. "During my entire pregnancy, I thought I had sciatica, which it might have been, but I now understand the root of the problem was my pelvic floor," she said. Ramina and I continued to meet during her second pregnancy, which was a completely different experience for her because she was in physical therapy throughout the entire journey. She exercised throughout her pregnancy, had minimal hip pain and leakage, and had an incredibly smooth and uncomplicated birth.

In the pages that follow, I share all the tools and resources I know that support a healthy pelvic floor in preparation for and during pregnancy. But before I begin . . . If you've experienced fertility struggles, pregnancy loss, or trauma related to pregnancy, birth, or postpartum, the tools here are also for you and will help your body heal. Not every pregnancy leads to live birth. About one million women in the United States have a miscarriage every year. If you have experienced a pregnancy loss, your body has gone through an enormous transformation— and what I offer in this chapter will help you care for your body. I encourage you to approach this chapter, and the following ones on childbirth and postpartum, in a manner that is comfortable for you.

How the Pelvic Floor and Pregnancy Work Together

Pregnancy is a pretty amazing, not just in how it occurs (sperm meets egg) but also in the intense physical changes that occur to sustain the pregnancy. Your abdomen expands over forty centimeters, or fifteen inches, to accommodate a growing baby or babies. Your pelvic ligaments soften to create space in the pelvis. Your blood flow increases to facilitate growth of the placenta. Your uterus expands up to five times its normal size to house your baby until birth.

Changes in your pelvic joints, your vascular system, and your hormones all influence your pelvis and pelvic floor during pregnancy—in plenty of good ways and in some less savory ones. Pregnancy is like running a marathon for your body, and childbirth (the topic of the next chapter) is the sprint at the end.

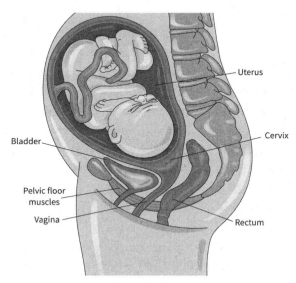

Pregnant abdomen with pressure on pelvic organs and pelvic floor muscles: a view from the side

Your body and pelvic floor are working hard day in and day out to get you to the sprint, and each trimester demands more from your pelvic floor.

FIRST TRIMESTER: YAY, BUT I'M EXHAUSTED!

The first trimester spans from the time of conception to the end of week twelve of pregnancy. During this period, an embryo, which is about the size of a grain of rice, grows into a small fetus about the size of a lime. Supporting a fetus the size of a lime is not a major strain on the pelvic floor muscles, but the hormonal changes during this early stage affect your pelvic floor.

During these twelve weeks, progesterone surges to support the implantation of an embryo into the uterine lining, the growth of the embryo, and the prevention of uterine contractions while the baby is developing. Not only does progesterone cause you to feel extremely tired, like you could take a fifteen-minute nap at any hour during the day, but it also slows down your colon motility. Constipation is hands-down one of the biggest effects of increased progesterone. You may find yourself struggling to get that baseball-sized poop out of your bottom.

Estrogen also surges during the first trimester, which, along with progesterone, leads to nausea, fatigue, anxiety, and breast tenderness. Estrogen stimulates the formation of new blood vessels to support the placenta and growing baby, but it also triggers increased urine output. Even though you might not even have a baby bump just yet, you will start making more frequent trips to pee in the first trimester. And almost one in five women experiences occasional leaks of urine early in pregnancy. Holding in pee isn't the only pelvic floor challenge that can pop up; holding in gas and stool can also get harder due to increased pressure from a growing baby and any pelvic floor weakness. While constipation is a common challenge for pregnant moms, some pregnant women will start to have anal incontinence during the first trimester as well.

Relaxin is another hormone that peaks toward the end of the first trimester; along with estrogen and progesterone, relaxin softens the ligaments of your pelvis to support your baby's growth over the coming months. This flexibility is helpful and essential for pregnancy and childbirth, because it allows your pelvis to expand and move, but it also contributes to many pregnancy-related discomforts such as low back pain, hip pain, pubic symphysis pain, and sacroiliac joint pain. Although these pregnancy aches and pains are all quite common, the effects can be extremely uncomfortable and affect your quality of life.

SECOND TRIMESTER: I'M FEELING GOLDEN— BUT WITH BACK PAIN

Once you enter into the second trimester and escape the exhaustion, nausea, bloating, and constipation of the first trimester, you may actually feel your energy return and show a cute little baby bump. Although your body will continually change as pregnancy progresses, the good news is that a lot of the rapid hormonal surges have passed. The second trimester lasts from week thirteen to the end of week twenty-seven, and by the end, the baby grows to the size of a head of cauliflower. The increased weight of the fetus and blood volume, along with your expanding uterus, place a significantly larger demand on the pelvic floor. Pelvic floor muscle fibers start to elongate to accommodate the growing pressure from above, and urinary leakage may become more frequent.

Your posture changes as you start to have an increased curve in your low back to support your growing baby bump up front. Your shoulders and upper back round forward due to the weight of your growing breasts, which are preparing to produce breast milk. Your butt tucks under to rebalance your center of gravity, preventing you from tipping forward. These pregnancy-related postural changes increase the demand on your pelvic joints, often leading to low back pain, hip pain, and even wrist and hand pain. Additionally, changes throughout the body and pelvic floor can lead to pain in your perineum (hello, achy vagina!).

During the second trimester, squeezing the equivalent of a five-pound sack of flour into your abdomen is undoubtedly going to lead to some changes. Your abdominal wall stretches and lengthens, and a greater distance between your six-pack abdominal muscles occurs. Estrogen increases at a gradual rate, reaching up to thirty times its normal level. For such an increase, there are a number of implications: besides finding yourself a bit more emotional (flashback to the time I was five months pregnant and called my husband crying on the way to work because we were out of pineapple), you will have a ton more vaginal discharge. You might find a lake in your undies, so don't forget to put on a daily panty liner. You may also have increased sexual desire due to higher estrogen levels. (Some women experience this. I for sure did not.)

THIRD TRIMESTER: GETTING OUT OF BED IS NOW AN OLYMPIC SPORT

The home stretch is here. The third trimester, starting at week twenty-eight and lasting until week forty (or until the baby arrives), is by far the most physically challenging phase for many women but also one of the most exciting. You may be setting up your nursery (make sure you exhale with exertion when pushing furniture), enjoying those front-row parking spots at grocery stores (just leave enough room to get out of the car door with your baby bump), and thinking about childbirth and creating a birth plan. For some, the joy and excitement of bringing a baby into the world grow exponentially as the days near their arrival. Other women, especially those who have suffered previous losses, have increased anxiety during the third trimester. The trimester can be a time of both enormous excitement and worry. Or both.

During the third trimester, your baby grows from the size

of a cauliflower to the size of a pumpkin—a heavy load for your pelvic floor and core. Your abdominal wall stretches even more, and finding a cozy position to sleep, stand, or sit can be a challenge. These changes can be uncomfortable, and *every single pelvic symptom gets worse*: urinary leakage, anal incontinence, perineal pain, prolapse, and low back pain. Over 50% of women experience urinary leakage in the third trimester, over 25% experience moderate pelvic organ prolapse, and over 75% experience low back pain. Despite an additional estrogen surge in this trimester, sexual activity typically declines because finding a comfortable position to play seems impossible (or you are frankly just too tired to exert the energy).

By this trimester, you have about eight additional liters of blood and fluid in your body, the equivalent of over two gallons of milk. Couple this with more relaxed tissues and blood vessels that don't pump blood as quickly through your body, and swelling occurs—meaning puffy feet, swollen ankles, sausage fingers, and also a swollen vulva. Pressure, heaviness, and achiness in your vagina are not uncommon.

Not every pregnant person experiences these issues, but you are likely to have at least one of these over the course of your pregnancy, and it is important to address whatever arises. When we neglect our symptoms and just endure pregnancy discomfort, the challenges can persist into postpartum for months or even years. Add on the effects of childbirth, lactation, and the possibility of a future pregnancy or pregnancies, and it can begin to feel like pelvic floor dysfunction is the new normal.

During my time as a pelvic PT at a local hospital, I had a conversation with the hospital director in which I suggested that information on common pregnancy-related pelvic floor disorders and tips on prevention should be part of the childbirth education classes. Childbirth preparation classes covered lots of info on how to care for a baby, from swaddling to changing a diaper and setting sleep schedules, but there was no information on how to care for the mom (and her pelvic floor) during pregnancy, birth, and beyond. Early education and intervention change women's experiences, quality of life, and pelvic floor outcomes. When I explained this to the hospital director, he said, "We don't think that is necessary. Pregnant women don't really struggle with these problems. Plus, we don't want to scare them."

We don't want to scare them.

I resigned from that job the next day. And the seed for this book grew. His mindset marginalized how much pelvic floor problems affect a woman's quality of life and put her at risk of future problems. We don't need protection from research and information that allows us to take better care of ourselves. We need education and prevention tips to help us make informed choices and care for our bodies long-term. Research supports that even a single hour of pelvic floor education can vastly improve a woman's pelvic floor symptoms.

So in the name of spreading the word, let's begin. In my practice, I commonly hear the following:

"I was throwing up in the toilet, and I totally peed my pants, soaking my shorts in urine."
"My back aches so much during this pregnancy that I can't even pick up my other child."
"My hemorrhoids are so painful, not only does it hurt to poop, but I can't even sit at work."
"I feel like something's falling out of my vagina, but my doctor said that's normal and there's nothing I can do."

Help is here, friends. Let's begin with a basic protocol for pelvic floor care during pregnancy, which I give to every single pregnant patient who comes in to see me.

Your Pelvic Floor and Pregnancy Protocol

Your body goes through massive changes during pregnancy, so undoubtedly your pelvic floor will be on the struggle bus. The tips, exercises, and modifications below are not just what I provide to all of my patients during pregnancy. They are what I used myself throughout both of mine—ask my husband, who slept on the other side of my pregnancy pillow fort every night.

MODIFY YOUR POSTURE

How you sleep, sit, and stand all affects your pelvic floor. If you find yourself turning your knees inward, crossing your legs, sleeping with one leg hiked up, or standing with your body weight on one hip (say, when carrying a heavy bag or toddler), you could use some adjustments. These postures create tension in the pelvic floor, often on one side more than the other. We looked at posture in Chapter 1, but during pregnancy, even more modifications become necessary for protecting your floor.

SITTING

When sitting in a chair, sit with an upright back versus slouching down. A firm chair or couch with a pillow behind your back or a stool under your feet can keep you from slouching. Plant your feet flat on the floor or cross at your ankles (instead of crossing your legs at your thighs).

STANDING

Your standing posture inevitably changes as your baby or babies grow and your abdomen expands. Your center of gravity shifts, leading you to arch your back, round your shoulders, and tuck your butt under (the origins of "flat mom butt" after giving birth). So you need to mindfully "right yourself" to get back into proper alignment. You can stand with your back against a wall if available, but stand upright and align your ankle bones, knees, hips, shoulders, and ears all in one straight line. Your natural pregnancy stance may be with your buttocks stuck out behind you or tucked way under. Try to avoid leaning into one hip and popping it out to the side; instead, balance your weight evenly on both feet. If you are carrying a kiddo on your hip and must lean to one side, alternate which side you carry on. Oh, and untuck your butt.

SLEEPING

As pregnancy progresses, finding a cozy position to get precious z's can feel impossible. Plan ahead because you will need all the pillows . . . and maybe a bigger bed. During my first pregnancy, my husband and I graduated from a queen bed to a king bed. We initially thought this was because a little baby would be snuggling with us in the early mornings, and more space would be welcome. Along with many of the other things I swore I would never do as a mom, like feed my kids sugar or allow video games, my toddler slept in our bed the entire night until he was three, when he transitioned to a mattress on the floor *next* to our bed.

However, during pregnancy, this additional space was welcome for all of the pillows I positioned around me every night. Seven. I used seven pillows. I know I could have gotten one of those pregnancy pillows that's a U-shaped or C-shaped, but this pillow fort around me supported every nook and cranny to help me get a decent night's sleep.

During the first trimester, you can sleep in whatever position is comfortable for you. At the beginning of the second trimester, sleep on your side to avoid compressing a super important vessel (the inferior vena cava) that brings blood flow to the baby. This becomes even more important during the third trimester, because the weight of the uterus can restrict blood flow even more. When lying on your side, place a pillow that runs lengthwise to your ankles between your bent knees to keep your pelvis aligned. As the belly grows during the second trimester, place another pillow underneath your abdomen for support. I also like a pillow under my top arm, which can be helpful if you have wrist or hand pain. If you are a back sleeper, there is good news: sleeping at a slight angle of 45 degrees by placing a pillow or two behind your back is adequate for optimizing blood flow to the baby.

EXERCISE

Despite minimal growth of your baby during the first trimester, the pelvic health changes are hard to miss. If you are already an avid exerciser when pregnancy begins, including running, yoga, swimming, or weightlifting, you can continue your typical exercise routine during the first trimester. If you want to start working out during pregnancy, but have not previously, begin with an easy activity like swimming or walking for thirty minutes, three to five times a week. Unless your medical provider advises against it, you can also absolutely perform pelvic floor exercises for strengthening and relaxation during the first trimester. This is a great time to work on pelvic floor training, before the bigger physical changes come in the second and third trimesters.

When trimester two arrives, the hormonal changes and increased uterine weight will continue to affect your comfort and performance during exercise. Don't be surprised if you feel wobbly in your ankles, knees, and hips due to ligament laxity, so avoid exercises that challenge your balance (I'm talking to my yogis here). Further, the increase in blood flow and changes in your blood pressure might lead you to feeling out of breath when you exercise. Use the "talk test" by exercising at a level of exertion where you can maintain a conversation to stay in a comfortable intensity range. Additionally, urinary leakage and pelvic pressure and heaviness can occur with higher-impact workouts like running or jumping. Exercise can still be performed (and it is recommended), but consider making modifications if leakage, exhaustion, or pain and discomfort occur.

Overall, a consistent exercise routine of thirty minutes, five times a week is recommended to keep you strong and resilient during a time of stress to your body. Exercise during pregnancy has clear benefits: decreased back pain, improved bowel movements, decreased urinary leakage, and decreased risk of gestational diabetes, high blood pressure, and postpartum depression. Exercise does not need to be avoided unless there are clear precautions or contraindications given by your medical provider. But what's safe for your pelvic floor during pregnancy? Generally safe exercises include low-impact movements like swimming, walking, cycling on spin bikes, rowing, and modified Pilates and yoga. Use caution with contact sports such as martial arts, soccer, football, or hockey. Some sports—like horseback riding, mountain biking, downhill skiing, and gymnastics—are not recommended because the potential consequences from injury are too great. Running is generally considered fine as long as you have no precautions from your medical provider.

Exercise to strengthen your body and core is just as important as straight-up movement and getting your heart rate up. But there are a lot of mixed messages online about strength training during pregnancy, so it can be hard to discern what is okay. Ultimately, when it comes to your pelvic floor during pregnancy, it's not what you do but *how* you do it. Here are the important guidelines to follow.

CO-CONTRACT YOUR PELVIC FLOOR

Contract your pelvic floor muscles with every repetition of an exercise, be it a squat, lunge, or biceps curl.

BREATHE

Exhale throughout the movement to avoid holding your breath and putting pressure on your pelvic floor or abdominal wall.

REST AS NEEDED

Take rest breaks to allow your heart rate to come down if you find yourself short of breath. For example, alternate walking and jogging intervals if you are unable to hold a conversation while running.

MODIFY YOUR WORKOUTS

Modify exercises as pregnancy progresses and you find your balance or muscle strength is affected. For example, perform push-ups and planks on the wall instead of on the ground, and decrease the amount of weight you're lifting during strength training. If you can't find any specific form of exercise that works for you, just move. Dance in the kitchen. Do a few stretches at your desk. Simply walking has been shown to benefit pelvic floor health during pregnancy. Let go of the notion of "I used to be able to do [blank]," because your body, and its needs, are different now.

The dominant narrative from pop culture magazines and fitness gurus pushes the idea that pregnant women need a "strong" pelvic floor to push your baby out. Kegel, Kegel, Kegel away during pregnancy, they say. Remember this: *your pelvic floor does not push your baby out; your uterus does.* Strong pelvic floor muscles are amazing to help with leakage, prolapse, back pain, and more, but they do not push your baby out. When the time comes to have a vaginal birth, your pelvic floor muscles need to *relax.*

During the third trimester and even prior to that, work on lengthening and relaxing your pelvic floor. Your uterine contractions open your cervix, and knowledge of how to push properly will help you lengthen your pelvic floor to help the baby come out. In the chapter that follows, I'll guide you on stretches, tips, and exercises for lengthening and relaxing your floor to get ready for birth. But just know, you don't need to Kegel your way for nine months to the delivery room. Just get regular exercise, contract your pelvic floor during workouts and activities when you exert effort, and learn how to bulge properly like you are pooping.

EXHALE WITH EXERTION

As pregnancy progresses, simple tasks can start to feel like intense workouts. When I was thirty-six weeks pregnant, I dropped a bowl of dry cereal on the floor. Instead of exerting the effort to kneel down and clean up every crumb, I said, "Oh, just leave it," and eventually had my dog Harley come eat it up. But even with a stretched-out abdominal wall and a pelvic floor that's working overtime, a simple yet important change can help care for your parts. When you are faced with a task that requires effort, and your pup is not around to help out, remember to exhale with exertion. Avoid holding your breath, which increases the pressure on your pelvic floor and abdominal wall, when exerting effort. At this point in pregnancy, exertion can include everything from lifting your toddler into their car seat to pushing a piece of furniture when you set up the nursery to simply getting off the couch. When you lift, push, or pull, exhale.

BREAK DOWN YOUR LOADS

Break down heavier loads into smaller ones to decrease the pressure on your pelvic floor. Instead of carrying three bags of groceries inside at once, just do one at a time to minimize the amount of weight you are carrying. Or consider using a wagon or stroller to help move something from one part of the house to another. In my later stages of pregnancy with my first child, my husband was traveling quite a bit. Instead of dragging heavy bags of trash from inside of the house to outside to my back alley, I would place them in a wagon on my doorstep, wheel them down the driveway to the trash cans, and then (with an exhale) lift them into the bin. These small changes may sound funny—but when you emerge from pregnancy with your pelvic floor intact, you won't regret it.

USE COMPRESSION

Increased fluid, postural changes, muscle weakness, and more relaxed blood vessels lead many expecting moms to have back

pain, swollen ankles, swollen vulvas, and varicose veins. Fortunately, not every mom will experience these, and my main
tip for prevention throughout pregnancy, and even postpartum,
is to use compression pretty much from your feet to your ribs.
And because your pelvic floor is already sustaining a lot of pressure from above during pregnancy (think hammock supporting
a pumpkin), the placement and direction of the compressions
matter. The focus is on lifting, supporting, and moving fluid
up versus squeezing in the middle, which can negatively impact
your pelvic floor muscles.

Starting from your feet: wear compression socks. Gone are
the days of the beige-colored ones that leave you with a sausage
roll overflowing the top. Some pretty cute and colorful ones are
available online with a gentle amount of compression between
15 and 20 mmHg that won't take you thirty minutes to put on.
Wear these during the daytime, when traveling, or when sitting
for prolonged periods of time. They do not need to be worn when
sleeping.

Working our way up, varicose veins can pop up in your
thighs, groin, or even your vulva. Who knew? So many amazing things are possible during pregnancy! Compression leggings or shorts can give you support in your upper thighs and
groin, but for your vulva, you need something special. Vulva
supports and compression garments help relieve discomfort
from vulvar varicose veins, pelvic organ prolapse, and vulvar
swelling. These supports pretty much look like a jock strap for
your vulva. Even a piece of lace that some brands add does not
jazz them up enough to look darling. But what they lack in
form, they make up for in function. You can wear these supports over your underwear and underneath your shorts, jeans,
dresses, or leggings to give you discreet vag support. Don't
wait for the symptoms of heaviness, pressure, or aching to ar-
rive. Put these supports on in the morning, before exercise, and
prior to activity to decrease discomfort and give your vulva a
much-needed hug.

POOP PROPERLY

I talk about pooping, and how to properly poop, a lot—and it isn't just because this is a favorite dinner table topic of my two young sons. It's important. Straining during bowel movements puts more pressure on your pelvic floor than running, jumping, coughing, or doing crunches. Because constipation is so common during pregnancy, women are far more apt to strain during pregnancy, even if they weren't strainers before. I've given you an entire chapter in this book to help with pooping problems, so revisit it as needed when you are expecting. In addition to refraining from straining, here are three additional reminders that become mission critical during pregnancy.

HYDRATE

You have a ton more blood in your body during pregnancy, and because blood is composed mainly of water, you need more water. Since constipation is already a common symptom during pregnancy, a focus on hydration can help prevent hard stools. Additionally, women are at an increased risk of a urinary tract infection (UTI) during pregnancy because urine sits in the bladder for longer or can find its way back to the kidneys. Maintaining hydration is a measure for UTI prevention.

SOFTEN YOUR STOOL

To keep your stool soft, you may need to rely on stool softeners or supplements like magnesium citrate. Always check with your medical provider first before taking any medications or supplements. The sleeve of saltine crackers and handfuls of dry pretzels that you munch on to help with nausea aren't necessarily the fiber your colon needs to soften your stool.

SUPPORT YOUR PERINEUM

Even if you use the recommended pooping position from Chapter 4 (sitting on toilet, feet on stool), you might still be squeezing out hard rabbit pellets (or giant baseballs) of poop. Applying pressure up on the perineum as you exhale and bear down provides some protection and support to your pelvic floor during bowel movements. This technique is recommended postpartum and with prolapse as well, but utilizing it during pregnancy is incredibly helpful to minimize the strain on already vulnerable pelvic floor muscles.

TAKING CARE OF YOUR PELVIC FLOOR WHEN YOU ARE EXPECTING should be as essential as setting up a nursery, packing your hospital bag, and knowing what foods to avoid. Let's turn to some of the most common conditions that can occur during pregnancy and tips and exercises on how to manage them.

Growing Pains during Pregnancy

Once pregnant, women are often treated like porcelain dolls. We are told what to eat (sushi is actually okay), what to drink (a cup of coffee a day is totally fine), and activities to avoid (running and biking are totally doable). We have weekly to monthly visits with medical providers making sure that baby and mom are healthy. But even though we are treated with such care, we aren't given the tools and resources we need when problems arise with our pelvic floors. Most doctors won't even mention the term "pelvic floor" at your pregnancy appointments. It is like it isn't even on their radar. So let's make sure all the problems, large and small, and their solutions are on *your* radar, beginning with one that is, perhaps, the most common.

URINARY LEAKAGE: OOPS, I DID IT AGAIN!

Hands-down the most common, and often the most comical, pelvic floor complaint during pregnancy is peeing your pants. What used to be an uneventful sneeze can lead to pee dripping down your pants leg in the grocery store cereal aisle. As if nausea and vomiting were not miserable enough, peeing your pants while puking in the toilet brings unwanted pregnancy effects to the next level. And while waking multiple times in the night is a nuisance to your sleep, cleaning a trail of pee from your bed to your bathroom in the middle of the night is the worst. As annoying, inconvenient, and embarrassing as urinary incontinence can be, it's also treatable.

If you're experiencing urinary incontinence, don't fret; it's never too late to address it. Pelvic floor exercises can help prevent it from getting worse as pregnancy progresses, and they give you a better chance of improving it postpartum.

STRENGTHEN YOUR PELVIC FLOOR

Whether your urinary incontinence appears in the first, second, or last trimester, you want to get that pelvic floor working. Learn to contract your pelvic floor and incorporate a very consistent pelvic floor strengthening routine if you haven't already. Follow the pelvic floor strengthening protocol in Chapter 2. Learn how to perform a proper pelvic floor contraction, then progress to performing longer holds, and eventually move into standing and upright positions when doing contractions. Pre-contract before movements like lifting, squatting, sneezing, and coughing throughout your pregnancy and into postpartum. In your second trimester, modify (use side-lying, hands-and-knees position, or support from pillows) or avoid exercises lying on your back so as not to compress blood flow to the placenta and baby. If you feel lightheaded, sweaty, or nauseous during any exercises lying on your back, simply roll to your left side.

PEE WHEN YOU HAVE TO PEE

Increased urine production, heightened bladder sensitivity, and a baby dancing on your bladder can all make you feel like you have to go . . . now . . . and quickly. So the rules of "don't pee just in case" or "wait two hours between pee trips" can be softened to accommodate the frequent and urgent calls to go. If you have the urge, by all means go ahead and pee. Responding to the urge will make incontinence less likely. If you know you will be away from the bathroom for a bit and don't feel confident you will make it to the toilet in time, a "just-in-case" pee before you start cruising the aisles of the grocery is totally fine.

SQUEEZE BEFORE YOU SNEEZE

If you haven't made this a habit prior to pregnancy, you will want to start when leakage occurs. The increased pressure on your bladder and lengthened, weaker pelvic floor muscles make it more likely for leakage to occur during coughing and sneezing. Pre-contracting your pelvic floor before a cough or sneeze, called "The Knack," can close off that urinary sphincter to prevent leakage from occurring.

I've had a lot of morning sickness, and when I throw up, I pee my pants. Can anything be done?

The increased pressure from your diaphragm onto your bladder while vomiting combined with a weaker pelvic floor during pregnancy can lead to leakage. I've had patients who told me they sit on the toilet to collect the pee drips while they heave into a garbage can. Although this can make for a more convenient cleanup, this position is not optimal for your pelvic floor. If you unfortunately find yourself throwing up and want to try to prevent pee leakage, kneel on the floor over a pail or toilet and try to keep your back flat instead of rounded while you vomit. Additionally, place a ball (like a soccer ball or soft exercise ball) between your thighs, then squeeze when you throw up. All of these can help activate your pelvic floor and reduce pressure on your bladder during vomiting. If all else fails, put a towel under your bottom while you are hugging the commode, then hop in the shower after to wash off. And start pelvic floor strengthening, stat.

DIASTASIS RECTI ABDOMINIS:
THERE'S A FOOTBALL IN MY BELLY

Diastasis recti abdominis (DRA) is a condition that occurs when the midline between your six-pack abdominal muscles stretches and creates an area of weakness in your abdomen. It is not painful but is a sign of decreased abdominal strength, and it increases the likelihood of pelvic floor dysfunction—from pelvic floor tension or weakness to prolapse. When you crunch up from a lying down position, it can literally look like a football (or alien) is coming out of the center of your belly. Between 30 and 70% of pregnant women may experience DRA, and it can persist in up to 60% of women postpartum. It can be hard to tell whether you have DRA when you are pregnant, so even if you don't see it during pregnancy, you would be wise to follow these tips.

MODIFY MOVEMENT

Inevitably, at some point in your pregnancy, you will start waking at night to pee. Your kidneys are filtering more blood, and this creates more urine. Your baby may also be sitting (or ninja-jumping) right on your bladder. To get out of bed, roll to your

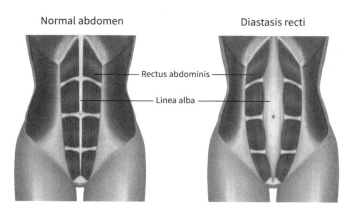

Normal abdomen

Diastasis recti

Rectus abdominis

Linea alba

Abdominal wall muscles with separation at the linea alba creating diastasis recti abdominis

side (if you aren't already there), drop your legs off the edge of the bed, and use your arms to push up to decrease strain on your ab muscles. To get back into bed, use the same process by sitting down, lying on your side, and then lifting your bent legs up onto the bed, instead of leaning back and using your abdominal muscles to lie down.

To get out of a chair, scoot your bottom to the edge of the seat, lean forward with your "nose over your toes," and push up with your hands to come to standing. This protects your abdominal wall to prevent overstraining. Proactively use these modifications during pregnancy and continue performing them in the early stages postpartum following a cesarean birth or if DRA is present.

ACTIVATE YOUR TRANSVERSE ABDOMINAL (TA) MUSCLES

Your deepest abdominal wall muscles, the transverse abdominals, wrap from either side of your low back to the front of your lower abdomen like a corset. These muscles support your spine and, when activated, create tension and increase strength in the midline of your abdominal wall (called the linea alba). To activate your TA muscles, place your fingers on the inside of your hip bones and either draw your belly button in like you are zipping up a pair of jeans or contract your pelvic floor. These muscles also contract simultaneously with your pelvic floor muscles.

Pre-contracting your TA muscles prior to any exercise or activity, including a crunch, squat, biceps curl, or any kind of weightlifting movement, increases tension between your rectus abdominal muscles. This is what ultimately helps prevent and improve DRA. I've seen some folks on social media state that crunches, planks, and push-ups are absolutely not okay for someone with DRA, when in fact that's not the case. When it comes to your core and pelvic floor strength, it's less about what you do and more about *how you do it*. If you pre-contract your TA muscles prior to the exercise, you're golden.

MANAGE YOUR INTRA-ABDOMINAL PRESSURE

Getting DRA can result from genetics, lengthening connective tissues, or poor pressure management, meaning pressure is being exerted in your abdomen, and the pressure finds its way to the weakest point in your tissues. The key to managing your intra-abdominal pressure is to pre-contract your transverse abdominal and pelvic floor muscles and, as always, exhale with exertion to decrease the pressure on your abs and pelvic floor. If you see that football pop out of your midline abdominal wall with an exercise or movement, modify that movement or avoid it.

DISCOMFORT DURING SEX: WELL, THIS IS . . . INTERESTING

Many women have an increased sexual drive during pregnancy (thanks to those high estrogen levels), while others would rather pick out nursery furniture than get busy with their partners. A wide spectrum exists with regards to sexual desire during pregnancy, and no matter where you fall on this spectrum, I assure you that you are normal and not alone. But outside of libido levels, your growing baby bump, limited ability to lie on your back, swollen vulva, and pelvic floor muscle changes all make pregnancy sex a little trickier and occasionally uncomfortable. Some of the standard positions and tricks to make sex comfortable do not apply when we are pregnant, but there are still possibilities for you so you can enjoy a healthy sex life.

FIND A COMFORTABLE POSITION

Finding a comfortable position to have vaginal sex when we are pregnant can be a challenge. During the first trimester, your baby bump isn't so big that it will get in the way, and lying on your back is still technically safe. But as pregnancy progresses and your baby bump grows, you've got to get creative to find a position that works for you and your partner. If we are talking about penis-in-vagina sex, when lying down, you can roll to your side, and your partner can be behind you in a spooning position. If you prefer to be upright, you might try being on top of your partner while they lie down or sit in a chair, which can help you control depth and speed of movement. Hands-and-knees position is also an option with a partner behind you, and you can rest on your elbows or with your head on a pillow (known as puppy pose in yoga). Standing, if you have the endurance, also works just fine.

USE PILLOWS FOR SUPPORT

For other types of sexual activities, pretty much any position you find comfortable will work except lying flat on your back. Support your head and upper back with pillows to be in a semi-reclined position. Or, lying on your back, place a few pillows or a wedge under your right hip so you are slightly rolled onto your left side to avoid compression of vessels bringing blood flow to your baby. I share these options because many women worry they will "hurt" their babies during penetrative sex, but unless you have been instructed by your physician or midwife to be on pelvic rest and avoid vaginal intercourse or you have health concerns like placenta previa or are at risk for preterm labor, sex is safe. Options are available to make it more comfortable and enjoyable during pregnancy.

MASSAGE MUSCLE PAIN

I may be stating the obvious here, but I still have so many patients who push through sex despite pain. You have permission to pause if pain occurs. More often than not during pregnancy, pain with deeper penetration occurs due to the low position of the cervix (the opening to the uterus) and potential pelvic floor muscle spasm or tension.

If deep penetration feels bruisy or tender, follow my guidelines for releasing external and internal pelvic floor muscle tension in the pelvic floor relaxation protocol in Chapter 2.

These techniques include using a ball to massage your buttock muscles, performing stretches that lengthen and relax your pelvic floor muscles prior to sex, and using an internal therapy wand (or your partner's fingers) to apply pressure on the side walls of your pelvic floor to release muscle spasm or tension. Inform your medical provider if you are experiencing pelvic pain so you can rule out other conditions, like an infection, and get the thumbs-up to insert the intravaginal wand or get a referral to a pelvic therapist who can make sure you are pressing on the proper muscles—and not your cervix—during pregnancy.

LOW BACK PAIN: I CAN'T GET COMFORTABLE

Low back pain is the most common pain that pregnant women experience and is most likely a result of changes in posture, loose ligaments of the pelvis, and lengthening muscles as your baby bump grows. Over 50% of women experience low back pain during pregnancy, and similar to other pelvic health issues, it can persist postpartum, especially if unaddressed.

SUPPORT YOUR BELLY

Proactively wear an abdominal belly support for your growing baby bump. In the second trimester it is optional, but in the third trimester, it becomes an absolute must due to significant postural changes. Most of these supports wrap around your low back and have Velcro or snaps to gently support your growing belly and take some of the pressure off your low back. But be mindful; the wrap should be supportive, not compressive. It shouldn't go around your belly and squeeze it. It should go under your bump and lift up. Wear your support during the day but not when sleeping. And follow the directions to make sure you are putting it on properly. My sister borrowed mine during her pregnancy, and I asked her how it was going. She said she could not really tell if it was making a difference, which I thought was odd. I asked her to show me how she was wearing it, and, well, she was putting it on backward.

EXERCISE

To help your low back, focus not only on strengthening your pelvic floor and core muscles, using my recommended strengthening protocol in Chapter 2, but also on upper body strengthening to manage rounded back posture, which is a result of additional breast tissue and an increased curve in your back. Planks and push-ups, which you can modify by performing them on your knees or standing with your hands on the wall, are easy and efficient ways to build upper body strength, in addition to using weight machines at the gym or dumbbells at home. Remember to pre-contract your pelvic floor with each exercise and exhale as you exert effort.

PELVIC GIRDLE PAIN: IT HURTS WHEN I . . . PRETTY MUCH DO ANYTHING

Aches and pains during pregnancy are unfortunately considered normal, but this is no reason for them to be ignored, dismissed, or untreated. Growing babies is hard work, and if anything can be done to make this experience less challenging, I say go all-in. While low back pain is the most common pregnancy pain experience, other common types of pain women experience include sacroiliac joint pain, pubic symphysis pain, and sciatic nerve pain. Although these are all separate issues affecting different body parts, following the tips and strategies below can help you get relief from these different conditions.

SOOTHE SACROILIAC JOINT PAIN

Many women often describe this as low back pain, but sacroiliac joint (SIJ) pain is something different and quite specific. This pain typically occurs on one side of the bony area between your low back and your butt cheek. Increased laxity in your pelvic joints during pregnancy allows your growing baby to have space to snuggle, but it can also lead to pain and strain on joints. Avoid activities or exercises that overstretch or strain that joint like the ones below.

- Lunge position
- Sidestepping or side squat
- Standing on one leg (tree pose in yoga)

Sleep, sit, and stand using the postural modifications I mention above, and use a sacroiliac joint stability belt (which can be easily found online) to decrease the strain on the SIJ. Additionally, pre-contracting your TA and pelvic floor muscles as instructed above helps create tension in that joint to maximize stability.

IMPROVE PUBIC SYMPHYSIS PAIN

Also referred to as your vagina bone, your pubic bone is located under the mons pubis, the fatty hair-covered tissue at the top of your vulva. Between the left and right pubic bones is a ligament that, like many other pelvic ligaments during pregnancy, softens to create space and movement of the pelvis. But an excess amount of shifting at your pubic joint can also create significant pain during pregnancy.

Use a stability belt during the day (it's not necessary at night) that wraps around your pelvis at the level of your pubic bone. Massage your adductor muscles, which attach to your pubic bones, by using a massage ball and rub from your knee to your groin, applying firm pressure to release adductor muscle tension. As with the SIJ, pre-contracting your TA and pelvic floor muscles helps create tension in the joint to maximize stability. The modifications below can avoid straining your pubic joint during pregnancy and relieve pain.

- Sit down to put on your socks, shoes, pants, and underwear
- Avoid standing on one leg (tree pose in yoga)
- Keep your knees and legs together when getting out of the car
- Squeeze a pillow between your knees when rolling over in bed

- Go up and down the stairs sideways
- Avoid butterfly/inner thigh stretch
- Sit down to shave your legs (if you are doing so at this point in pregnancy)

RELIEVE SCIATICA SYMPTOMS

Your sciatic nerve starts from the low back and upper sacral spine and travels down each side into your buttocks and down the back of your thighs. This nerve often gets compressed during pregnancy due to shifts in your pelvis and muscle tension in your buttock and hip muscles. Use a massage ball to release your buttock muscles and relieve tension in the muscles surrounding the sciatic nerve. Perform the figure 4 stretch in a sitting position to stretch the piriformis muscles, and don't forget to avoid crossing your thighs when sitting or hiking a knee up when sleeping.

Prepare for the Big Lift

While pregnancy brings with it physical challenges, especially in your pelvic floor, it is also a time when you come face-to-face with the tremendous strength of your body. A woman (and her pelvic floor) can handle a lot. I took better care of my body during pregnancy, and appreciated it more, than any other time in my life. I learned to tune in to my body and not push into pain, as I had done for so many years as a long-distance runner. I learned to love long walks with my husband on Sunday morning, which we did weekly until the day I gave birth to my oldest son. And I did my pelvic floor therapy and reaped its many benefits.

Despite the unwanted effects of pregnancy, like the nausea and pee leaks, you *do not* have to accept pain and pelvic floor problems as par for the course. Moms sacrifice a lot. Their pelvic floor health shouldn't have to be part of that. You deserve A-level care—along with that primo parking spot at the grocery store.

CHAPTER 8

Keep Calm and Birth On

I f you've ever been in labor or given birth, you know there is one thing that is certain: it is unpredictable. As much as you plan and prep and pack, you can't totally envision the course it will take. The delivery of my first son was no exception. As my due date approached, I obsessed over all the possible things that might happen to indicate I was in labor, then ruminated on what might happen next:

How painful will contractions be?
Will I know if they are contractions or just gas pains?
What if my water breaks all over my new sheets?

On a Sunday in March 2015, when I was thirty-eight weeks pregnant, my husband and I mowed the lawn and changed the lightbulbs in the garage, and he started reading chapter one in the book *The Birth Partner*, which I had given him three months earlier. I should have known those were our signs of nesting. Later that evening, I felt abdominal cramps while watching a movie. Pretty soon they were occurring regularly, around every thirty minutes, and I just knew—I was in labor. I stayed calm, told my husband, and called my doula, who said, "When your contractions are five minutes apart and last one minute for one hour, then call me." In the hours that followed, I bounced on my birth ball in front of the TV, packed my hospital bag, and ate a carton of Ben and Jerry's ice cream in the bathtub. And while I was still calm, my husband was way more worked up. He followed me from room to room with his hands cupped in front of him as if he was about to catch a ball . . . or a baby. Around midnight I made myself lie down on a heating pad in bed, where I tried to get comfortable. My contractions were now coming every six to seven minutes . . . not yet time to call my doula again.

By 2:30 a.m., I could no longer lie down comfortably; I moved into a hands-and-knees position and rocked my hips back and forth in circles while making what my husband called "very sexual moaning sounds." Following the consistent rhythms of each contraction, I moved when I needed to move, moaned when I needed to moan, swayed my hips, and breathed every time a contraction came. I was still monitoring my contractions and had not yet reached the five-minute interval. I was in considerable pain but still staying incredibly calm. But I knew it was time. "Call the doula again," I told my husband, who immediately dialed her number. We got no answer. We proceeded to call her *six more times*, and still . . . no answer. This certainly was not what we had planned.

Within the next thirty minutes, a huge and rapid shift occurred. My contractions went from every six to seven minutes to every one to two minutes and lasted thirty to forty-five seconds. The pain grew in intensity, and I could hardly form words. I shook uncontrollably between contractions, and maybe I heard my husband say, "I think we should go now"?

It was all somewhat hazy after this point. My husband packed the car while I was on our bed, still moving my hips to manage the pain. I heard a "pop" as water gushed out from between my legs. *There go my new sheets.* I felt an extreme amount of pressure at the bottom of my vagina, and I wondered whether I was about to take the biggest shit of my life or have my baby. I crawled half-naked in an intense fog on my bedroom floor all the way to the front door, letting out powerful screams with every contraction that came. My husband continued to pack the car, as he is known for his very slow, methodical movements, and this situation proved no different.

At some point, he finally scooped me off the floor and helped me into the back seat of the car. We sped through the dark streets of Dallas at 4:00 a.m. while I half heard my husband taking a call from our doula, who explained she had fallen asleep and would meet us at the hospital. Moments later our car skidded into the hospital entryway, and I slid out of the door onto my knees. I am sure I was screaming, because a group of hospital workers ran outside with a wheelchair and plopped me into it. They raced me down the hallway and practically tossed me into the hospital bed, onto my side.

"Let me check you," the nurse said. I opened my thighs, and after a quick glance, the nurse firmly stated, "You are +3 station (baby's head is in the birth canal). The baby is coming now!"

I looked up at my husband at the head of my bed and thought: *Holy moly is this happening?*

Following three strong contractions along with incredibly helpful coaching from a nurse to breathe, I pushed three times and my son was born. Three minutes passed from my arrival at the hospital to the delivery of my son. *Three minutes. Three pushes. No perineal tearing.*

My birth was chaotic, full of twists and turns—but with all the pelvic floor preparation I had done, I ultimately had the unmedicated birth I had hoped and prepared for. All of the work I did on my pelvic floor to prepare—the stretches, pushing practice, and perineal massage—resulted in zero perineal tearing. My pelvic floor showed up for me, *and* I had a very healthy baby. What more could a new mom ask for?

Delivery doesn't always go this way. Yes, I'd done my prep. And I also got lucky. Childbirth is hard on our pelvic floors— and our pelvic floors can take some twists and turns too. Just as with pregnancy, birth is complex and complicated. There are facets that are out of our control—even if you do all of the proper preparation. Knowing and accepting this is part of preparation.

In the following pages, I will share information and advice that I have found to be helpful to thousands of women prior to and after childbirth. The goal is a healthy baby and a healthy you. And the priority of this chapter, in this book, is how to manage the health of your pelvic floor in childbirth. Birth is a different experience for every single woman. The guidance I offer will help you understand labor and birth, the role your pelvic floor plays, and how to work with your body during the process so that you don't struggle with pelvic floor issues after delivery.

During my years as a pelvic floor therapist, I have heard story after story from women who felt disempowered by their births. As they unpacked their experiences, very often, tears slid down their cheeks. Some felt like less of a woman. Others felt scared to get pregnant or have another baby because of their trauma. Some felt like they failed at motherhood when it had literally just started. And time after time, I reassured them . . . this is not your fault. You did nothing wrong. Labor and birth do not conform to our agendas. Sometimes we need to pivot, often in an effort to safely deliver the baby. But also, everything you feel makes perfect sense.

My patients often tell me stories of unbearable contractions after being induced with the drug oxytocin (commonly known by its brand name as Pitocin), not being able to move freely during labor due to being hooked up to monitors, pushing on their backs while holding their breath for hours, sometimes so much so that they ended up with major hemorrhoids or prolapse. And many of those births ultimately result in a C-section, which can make postpartum recovery more difficult. Many patients express feeling like a passenger in their process instead of the driver. I know in my core that there is a better way—to birth a healthy baby *and* have a healthy mother who feels prepared, empowered, and supported—or at least not completely traumatized.

I wanted to labor at home, where I was comfortable and calm, and could move around to help my pelvis expand as the baby worked its way down the birth canal. I wanted to feel the contractions (although incredibly painful) as my cues to push and breathe. I wanted to change positions during pushing instead of having to lie on my back the entire time. I was also terrified of needles and wanted to avoid them if possible.

I knew prep didn't mean my birth would go exactly as I wanted, but it would help me feel as ready as possible. The time and thought I put in beforehand gave me confidence that I had done all I could in advance to hopefully set myself up for success in terms of how my pelvic floor would fare afterwards. And I encourage all expecting moms to do the same.

How the Pelvic Floor and Birth Work Together

We have seen moms go into labor on screens for decades. When their water breaks, they rush to the hospital, push and scream for a few minutes, and the baby is born. But the process is far more complex and lengthier than those films depict: labor starts hours, even days, prior to birth. Your pelvic floor rides a roller coaster during this entire time, and this period is called labor because— well, it's hard work. Your pelvic floor is about to perform heroics. I'm going to describe what happens to your pelvic floor and body during labor and birth without the use of interventions (medical induction, epidural anesthesia, or a cesarean section). I want you all to know how labor and birth occur independent of these (often necessary) medical procedures and understand the role your pelvic floor plays.

THE FIRST STAGE OF LABOR: THE HARD WORK BEGINS

The first stage of labor begins when uterine contractions start and lasts until your cervix is completely dilated to ten centimeters. This stage of labor is the longest and can take anywhere from eight to twenty hours, but for some women, this stage can stretch into one or two days. The uterine wall is a muscle, similar to the bladder, and the muscular contractions of the uterus help the cervix, the opening to the uterus that leads to the vaginal canal, to soften, thin, and ultimately open to allow the baby to head down your birth canal.

Because the cervix is not yet fully dilated during this stage, and the baby has not reached the vaginal canal, the pelvic floor stays relatively relaxed, and most of the action happens above. The hormone oxytocin, which increases during labor to stimulate uterine contractions, keeps the ligaments between the pelvic bones soft and stretchy. This stretchiness widens the pelvic joints so birth can progress, which is why being able to move around during labor is key . . . and why lying flat on your back in bed is not.

The first stage of labor has two phases: early phase and active phase. During the early phase, contractions are mild and tolerable, and this phase lasts from the beginning of labor until the cervix is dilated to six centimeters. The active phase of labor lasts from six centimeters of cervical dilation to ten centimeters and brings with it much more intense, painful, and frequent contractions. Toward the end of active labor, when the cervix goes from eight to ten centimeters dilated, you enter a time called transition, which is the most intense period of labor. I was likely in transition when I was in the back seat of my car screaming as my husband rushed us to the hospital at 4:00 a.m. During transition, contractions come every few minutes and last a minute or longer. You may feel significant back pain, or a sensation of needing to take a massive poop, or have the urge to start pushing. At this point your pelvic floor muscles are ready to stretch and lengthen up to three times their normal length when you are pushing.

THE SECOND STAGE OF LABOR: READY, SET, PUSH

The second stage of labor occurs from full dilation of the cervix until the baby is born, and this stage most significantly impacts your pelvic floor. The pushing stage can last up to three or four hours, which can be extremely physically taxing for the mom. During this stage, uterine contractions are frequent. Mom feels pressure on her pelvic floor and has the involuntary urge to push. This is when I felt intense pressure in my butt like I needed to poop. It's possible I actually *did* poop while giving birth, though I don't know, and I want to thank my labor and delivery nurses for sparing me those details.

Oxytocin continues to play a major role as uterine contractions help the baby descend into the vaginal canal. As the pelvic floor stretches with pressure from baby's head, more oxytocin is released, which leads to more uterine contractions. This entire cycle, called the Ferguson reflex, is a fascinating example of how the stretch of the pelvic floor muscles is essential in helping labor and birth progress. *And your pelvic floor muscles do not push your baby out. Your uterus does.* Your pelvic floor is stretching (a lot) to make way for the baby to come on down the birth canal.

The second stage ends when the baby exits through the vagina and arrives earthside. All women who have a vaginal birth will go through the first two phases of labor, but the length of time and the intensity of the experience vary. They also change if you are induced into labor, receive epidural anesthesia for pain relief, or switch to a cesarean birth during your labor.

THE THIRD STAGE OF LABOR: WAIT, THERE'S MORE

This stage is unrelated to your pelvic floor, but I share it as it's something very few pregnant women, including myself, are aware of until the time arrives. After the baby is born, there is one more step—delivering your placenta, the organ your body created that connects you to your baby via the umbilical cord. The placenta nourished your baby for the entire nine months of pregnancy. Now that the baby is born, it can retire. Most women are so focused on their new baby that they are not even aware of what's happening, but your uterus continues to contract to deliver your placenta. This stage of labor is typically very short (less than thirty minutes) and not particularly painful.

BIRTH HAS BEEN GOING ON SINCE THE START OF WOMANKIND, BUT AS medicine has progressed and innovations have been made, the process itself has changed significantly. And all of these changes have implications for the pelvic floor. One of the biggest changes we've seen over the past few decades is an increase in inductions, which are often recommended or encouraged when there is a medical risk to the mom (when, for example, she has high blood pressure), or to the baby (for example, there is low amniotic fluid), or when a number of other circumstances go down: your water breaks with no contraction, you are over thirty-five, or you have undergone fertility treatment, and more. While inductions are performed in an effort to deliver a healthy baby, what this means for your pelvic floor isn't always listed on the side effects sheet.

When you get induced, you commit to laboring in the hospital instead of at home, and you usually must consent to limiting your movements because you will be hooked up to a variety of monitors and medications. Many inductions are done with oxytocin (recall this is the hormone that promotes uterine contractions). Yay for strong contractions, but . . . this also means strong contractions *without* the ability to change positions, stand, shower, get on your hands and knees, or do movements that can help with pain management and relief. For your pelvic floor, this also means you limit your ability to widen your pelvis, and it affects the baby's ability to put pressure on your cervix to dilate. Although this process was started to try to speed labor up, labor can actually end up taking a very long time. Confusing, right? Stay with me.

What in turn happens is that your contractions get *so* strong and painful from oxytocin that you will likely need pain medication via an epidural. Yay for pain management . . . but this also means the lower half of your body will be weak and numb. Not being able to feel your contractions is likely the pain relief you are looking for, but this also blocks your ability to move around, help your pelvis expand, and feel when to push with your contractions. So the baby either does not reach your pelvic floor to activate that Ferguson reflex mentioned earlier, or you are pushing and stretching your pelvic floor really hard for so long that it goes kaput. Or you have a C-section after all this effort.

I'm not saying to do away with inductions and pain relief in an effort to spare your vagina and pelvic floor, but what I am rallying for is a way to make your delivery safe, comfortable, and pelvic floor–friendly. In my practice, I've seen hundreds of moms who question whether they could have done something differently, and why someone didn't tell them the full list of side effects and offer them additional options.

> "My baby's head was stuck. When my doctor used forceps to get him out, I ended up with a major tear in my pelvic floor."
>
> "My labor wasn't progressing after I was induced. I ended up having a C-section, and now my entire abs and pelvic floor are a mess."
>
> "I pushed for hours and felt like my eyes were going to pop out. Afterwards I had the worst hemorrhoids, not to mention bloodshot eyes."
>
> "The nurses kept telling me to hold my breath and push as hard as I could. But it didn't feel natural to me. I really think that's what caused my prolapse."

Each of these women had separate birth experiences, and all of them resulted in pelvic floor dysfunction afterwards. My goal is to arm women with tools and knowledge to decrease the risk of dysfunction, without jeopardizing the baby. Now let's go save some vaginas.

Vaginal birth sounds like it does a doozy on your pelvic floor. Would having a cesarean birth just be better for my vag?

Women who give birth vaginally often push for more prolonged periods of time, which stretches the pelvic floor muscles and nerves and increases the likelihood of a tear in the pelvic floor muscles or perineum. They also are at a higher risk for urinary incontinence and prolapse. However, cesarean birth is a major surgery, and recovery can be a bit more intensive and increases the risk of uterine rupture, hysterectomy, and hemorrhage. Ultimately it's important to know the risks and pelvic floor implications associated with both types of birth, weigh these implications for you and your baby, and discuss your concerns with your medical team so you can make an informed decision. This decision is yours. But also know that pregnancy itself is a doozy for your pelvic floor, so regardless of your birth method, there will be pelvic floor side effects.

Your Pelvic Floor and Childbirth Protocol

As I've said before, being pregnant is like running a marathon, and giving birth is the multi-hour or multi-day sprint at the end. Just as we train our bodies for running races, we need to train our bodies for giving birth. Our pelvic floor and core need preparation, but so does our mindset. Research is clear that moms who feel more educated and informed (and thus mentally prepared for the decision-making process) report less birth trauma and better outcomes—regardless of whether they had a C-section or vaginal birth. Ultimately, we all want to feel seen and heard, and have some autonomy over our bodies and our babies. There is a lot you can do to prepare for labor before labor even begins. Let's get to it.

PICK YOUR TEAM

When I moved to Dallas, I searched for a new nail salon, hair stylist, yoga studio, and of course, gynecologist. I received a recommendation from a friend who said her doc was a really warm, compassionate woman who would suit me just fine. And she did, until I was pregnant and started asking questions about my birth. I wanted a doula at my birth. (As you can recall, that didn't pan out the way I thought it would, but I knew that having a doula, or continuous support person during birth, often results in less use of pain medication, less likelihood of having a C-section, a shorter pushing stage of labor, and ultimately a higher birth satisfaction.) I saw only benefits for me and my pelvic floor in this decision.

At my twenty-one-week pregnancy appointment, I told my doctor I wanted to have a doula at my birth. She looked at me through her black-rimmed glasses and replied, "I feel like they just get in the way." Not the response I had hoped for, so I politely said thank you and left my appointment, then proceeded to call around to other obstetrician practices, looking for a doula-friendly doctor. My plan to try to give birth unmedicated was an effort to stay in touch with my body and my pelvic floor, and I knew I wanted a doctor and birth team who would support that.

Many women who desire fewer medical interventions or more holistic and hands-on care opt to work with a midwife during pregnancy. Midwives are trained medical providers who help women during labor, deliver babies, and provide postpartum care. Historically, midwives were the main medical providers for pregnant women, but as time passed and the majority of moms started birthing in hospitals instead of at home or at birthing centers, physicians gradually became the standard of care. But women who receive care from midwives often have less severe perineal tearing, a shorter pushing stage of labor, fewer C-sections, and reduced use of forceps or vacuum-assisted births, which are risk factors for pelvic floor muscle injuries. Midwifery care is a great option for low-risk births and has benefits for your pelvic floor health and healing.

Ultimately, the team you choose should support how *you* want to give birth. They should make your priorities their priorities. Talk to your friends and family members who have given birth and ask about their experiences and their teams. Seek a recommendation from someone who had the type of birth that sounds desirable to you. Meet that doctor or midwife. Ask your questions. Share what you know about the pelvic floor, and make sure they can work with you to prioritize the health of your floor and body, no matter how your birth story plays out. If you want a doula, I recommend finding one in your first trimester, because they can book up faster than daycare spots. Ask yourself as you meet these care providers, "Do I feel calm, supported, and comfortable taking a poop in front of this person?" That is the level of intimacy you will have with them.

PREP YOUR PERINEUM

Perineal massage is mission critical when preparing for vaginal birth. As you may recall, your perineum is the area between your vaginal and anal openings where all of your pelvic floor muscles come together. This area is also commonly the site of tearing during a vaginal birth. Historically, physicians would perform an episiotomy by surgically cutting into these pelvic floor muscles with a scalpel to help the baby exit the vaginal opening. Now that the medical community has realized tearing spontaneously has better outcomes, episiotomies are no longer a routine practice and are only done when it's medically necessary (for example, if the baby is stuck in the birth canal or needs to be born with immediacy).

At thirty-four weeks of pregnancy, start perineal massage. There are a number of possible positions if you are practicing self-massage, but if these positions are too difficult for you, there are perineal stretch devices (they look like shoe horns) to make it a bit easier to reach this body part. To practice solo:

1. Lie in bed, sit on the toilet, or place one foot on a stool (use something for balance if needed) and insert your right thumb into your vaginal opening (short fingernails recommended here).
2. With the pad of your thumb facing down and inserted up to the first knuckle, apply firm pressure down toward six o'clock like you are stamping your thumb firmly to get a fingerprint. If it feels like you are just pushing on soft tissue, you likely aren't deep enough and need to insert the thumb deeper into the opening. You should feel a slight to intense burning sensation when you press and hold on the muscles at the vaginal opening.
3. Hold pressure for five deep breaths. Then rotate your thumb to the right toward nine o'clock and repeat, and then left toward three o'clock and repeat.
4. You will press on each point on the clock from three to nine o'clock and hold until the burning decreases, which may take about thirty to sixty seconds.

The whole process should take just three to five minutes and be repeated daily or every other day in the weeks leading up to birth. If doing it yourself is not the most comfortable or accessible, try standing with one foot on a step stool, sitting on the toilet or the edge of a bathtub, or recruiting your partner for help (they would use their forefinger instead of their thumb). Lube is optional. Handwashing before and after is not.

Remember to take deep breaths while performing perineal massage. When you are giving birth, perineal massage from a nurse or doctor can be helpful but is not shown to have the same benefits as massaging prior to birth. However, placing a warm washcloth over your perineum to soften the area just as the baby's head is crowning can also help prevent severe tearing.

When I delivered my son, I felt a strong urge to push during a contraction just as his head was exiting my vagina. Between my last two contractions, the nurses instructed me to breathe but not to push because they wanted his head to stretch me. On the next contraction, he came out. I truly think my perineal preparation saved me from perineal tearing, as I did not have to shoot him out with force.

STRETCH IT OUT

Your pelvic floor acts like a hammock that supports your pelvic organs, including your growing baby inside your uterus throughout pregnancy. Strengthening your pelvic floor muscles during pregnancy helps prevent that hammock from getting super stretched down there. But as your due date approaches, stretching your pelvic floor and releasing tension in your hips and thighs help you prepare. The best position to relax the pelvic floor muscles is the squatting position. When women give birth, they often squat or lie on their backs with their knees up. (Recall that the best position for pooping is also squatting because it relaxes your pelvic floor.) To get ready for labor and birth by releasing tension in your hips, I recommend a morning and evening routine of the following stretches. Descriptions for these stretches can be found in Chapter 2 under the pelvic floor relaxation protocol.

- Child's pose
- Cat–cow pose
- Knee to chest stretch in side-lying
- Figure 4 stretch in sitting
- Deep squat stretch

GET MOVING

In the pelvic PT playbook, motion is lotion. Having regular movement during labor can help with pain relief, widen and expand your pelvis, and facilitate the baby coming on down the birth canal. Movement can also help your labor progress, and certain movements will help the necessary pelvic floor muscles lengthen and relax. Whether you are giving birth at home or in a hospital or anywhere in between, I recommend talking to your medical provider in advance about your options for movement and what will be available to you during your labor.

All of the stretches you have been practicing during pregnancy and mentioned above are all excellent to do during labor and will support your birthing. In addition, you can walk, lunge, gently bounce on a ball, crawl in the hands-and-knees position, or sway your hips in a circle or side to side.

If you receive an epidural for pain relief or you are confined to a hospital bed, you will likely be hooked up to a variety of monitors, which limit your ability to walk around or change positions. If you are in this situation, try to change positions every thirty minutes. A peanut ball, a birth ball the shape of a peanut, can be very helpful and is often available at a hospital (or you can bring your own). Place it under your knees while lying on your back, or between your knees while lying on your side, with one leg straight to support the other. This can help widen your pelvis during the labor process.

PREPARE TO PUSH

Recently a patient showed me a video from her hospital childbirth education class in which a nurse gave a presentation of what to expect during birth. The nurse stated, "You need to have really strong pelvic floor muscles to push really hard to get your baby out. So, practice your Kegels now."

This is 100% incorrect. To start (and I've mentioned it more than once in this book), *your pelvic floor muscles do not push your baby out.* Your uterus does. Although strong pelvic floor muscles are beneficial during pregnancy, your pelvic floor muscles need to be flexible and able to relax for vaginal birth. We don't need them to push your baby out; we need them to get out of the way.

Before going into the big game, you need to practice. For

childbirth, that means learning how to push *before* you give birth (when you might be in a brightly lit room, uncomfortable, possibly medicated, and surrounded by medical professionals staring at your nether regions). Learning how to push will help you prepare for the big day, and you will also be able to find out how you like to push. Practicing in advance allows you to try on different positions to figure out what might be most comfortable for you, so you have your pushing strategies when it is game time.

A lot of controversy and discrepancy exist between medical professionals on the best ways to push. Pelvic floor therapists, including myself, may coach you on how to exhale and breathe during your uterine contractions, while labor and delivery nurses may coach you to hold your breath and push as hard as you can for ten seconds. Do what feels most natural and effective for you during birth, which may in fact vary and change as the minutes, even hours, pass. You may start one way and then want to try another. Practice in advance by grabbing a mirror and watching your perineum relax and bulge as you push your perineum out. You can literally see what might be most effective for you. And just like with movement, *talk* to your medical provider in advance about your pushing options and preferences.

LABORING DOWN

Once your cervix reaches ten centimeters, the second phase of labor officially begins, and you will be encouraged to start pushing. Laboring down is the process of not actively pushing right away but waiting for a period of time, usually between one and two hours, to allow you to rest while the baby moves down the birth canal. The benefit of laboring down is you spend less time pushing, which in turn means less pressure on your pelvic floor. This can decrease the chance of perineal tearing and a need for instruments like forceps or vacuums that can lead to pelvic floor trauma.

However, recent studies have shown that a longer second stage of labor can change blood oxygen levels in babies and increase their risk for infection. After these findings, laboring down is no longer recommended by the American College of Obstetricians and Gynecologists. As a PT, I land at neutral on laboring down. If your provider is recommending it, and you have a lot of trust in your provider and it feels right, or you need a rest, waiting thirty minutes to an hour to start pushing can give you some time to rest. But if you are being encouraged to push at full dilation, go ahead and start when your uterine contractions are occurring.

Talk with your medical provider before your birth so you know what to expect and what your options are. If you have an epidural for anesthesia, you'll likely be encouraged to start pushing right away.

SPONTANEOUS PUSHING

When you are pushing, oftentimes your labor and delivery team will "coach" you on how to push. The typical pattern is to tell you to hold your breath and push as hard as you can for ten seconds. The alternative to this is "uncoached" or spontaneous pushing, which means you push when you feel the urge and in whatever way feels most natural and comfortable for you. You can breathe or hold your breath. Research shows that the second stage of labor is slightly shorter (by thirteen minutes) with coached pushing, but typically there are no additional advantages to you, your floor, or your baby. However, when the provider is not in tune with the mother, there can sometimes be side effects of coached pushing, such as problems with bladder function, increased incontinence, and decreased pelvic floor support postpartum.

For this reason, I am not a fan. I absolutely understand the desire for your birth team to want to coach you so the baby can be born, but because there are no proven advantages to you or your baby while there are plenty of potential negative effects on your pelvic floor, I'm on team spontaneous pushing. Breathe and push when you feel the urge to push or have visible uterine contractions on your monitor. One thing to note: if you've had an epidural, the sensation of contractions may be minimal, and you may not even have strong contractions or urges to push. In this case, a monitor that shows when your uterine contractions are occurring can function as a guide for when to push. If you decide to have an epidural, I suggest keeping it at a lower level of intensity so you can still feel pressure in your vagina (or butt, like in my case) during contractions.

AVOID PURPLE PUSHING

A very common belief is that holding your breath gives you more power to push, and so it is not uncommon for providers in the delivery room to instruct women to do what we call purple pushing, or holding your breath when you push. As a result, some women's skin might turn purple or blue. Another term for this is a Valsalva or closed-glottis pushing.

Holding your breath while pushing puts excessive force on your pelvic floor. Some moms can push up to three hours. Purple pushing will not only exhaust you but may also stretch and weaken your pelvic floor, leading to a higher risk of incontinence and prolapse after birth. Also, breath holding can cause the pelvic floor to contract when you want it to be lengthening and relaxing. And studies have shown no benefit to this practice for babies or moms. As a pelvic PT, I am not a fan.

There are many ways to breathe on your big day. I encourage you to choose which breathing method works best for you, and that may vary over the course of the pushing stage. For example, many moms breathe forcefully or make sounds while pushing, but when the baby is crowning, they find that holding their breath to push at the end is most helpful. The takeaway is, you have options.

TRADITIONAL PUSHING POSITION

During the pushing phase, most moms are positioned lying on their back with their feet in stirrups or their knees hugged to their chest. While this position does help lengthen the pelvic floor and provide clear and visible access to the vaginal opening during birth, your pelvis is limited in its ability to open and widen. Whether you've had an epidural or not, you can also lie on your side, which can help the baby adjust positions within the pelvis, relieve back pain, and offer a different option for pushing if the baby isn't coming out. In some situations, with support from another person, you may even be able to get into a hands-and-knees position, offering another option for pelvic mobility and movement.

Prior to birth, I encourage you to take a mirror or place your hand over your perineum (the area between your vaginal and anal opening) and practice pushing in different positions. Lie on your back with your knees relaxed, open wide. Lie on your side with one knee hugged to your chest. Get into a hands-and-knees position or squat over the floor. With the mirror positioned so you can see your perineum, practice bearing down to push in each of these positions and see if one position feels more comfortable or will help you lengthen your pelvic floor and push your perineum out better. Then practice this with holding your breath or breathing out and see if one of those feels better in each of these positions. This information helps you know what pushing options work best for you.

If you must lie on a bed in a fairly traditional birthing position, I suggest lying on your side. This is by far my favorite position for moms to birth in. It's easy to assume with an epidural, it allows the pelvis to widen during crowning, and it minimizes the severity of perineal tearing because the pelvic floor muscles don't reach their maximum stretch. A stirrup, a partner, a doula, or a nurse can hold your top leg bent and hugged toward your chest while you are lying on your side.

Does getting into a bathtub with warm water during labor help my pelvic floor?

Many expecting moms consider strategies to help them stay relaxed and manage pain during labor, and soaking in a tub or birthing tub can be one of those options. Warmth in a tub can not only be an effective way to manage pain during labor but also helps with pelvic floor muscle relaxation. Studies show labor shortened by about thirty minutes and less use of epidural anesthesia in moms who labor in water. You can lie on your back or side, or even get into hands and knees or child's pose depending on the size of the tub. However, the American College of Obstetricians and Gynecology recommends this practice only during the first stage of labor for moms delivering between thirty-seven and forty-two weeks of pregnancy with no complications. Water immersion during the second pushing stage of labor and birthing in a tub are not recommended due to increased risk of infection or inhaling water into the lungs or umbilical cord trauma while lifting the baby out of the water. Talk to your medical provider about this as an option for the first stage of labor. Additional options like dim lighting in the room, having calming music, aromatherapy or use of essential oils, and limiting visitors while in labor can all add to a calm and relaxing environment to optimize the relaxation of you and your pelvic floor.

MY TOP PUSHING TIPS

To sum all of this up, ideally you do not get induced unless medically necessary to give you the freedom to move around at least during the early phase of labor when you are still dilating up to six centimeters. After that, most women will opt for pain relief via epidural anesthesia, when you will then likely be lying in a bed for the remainder of labor. Should this be the case, here is your pelvic floor plan summing up everything above for labor and birth:

- Change positions every thirty minutes. A peanut ball, birth ball, and pillows can all be used to change your position to keep the pelvis mobile and allow room for widening. If you aren't progressing or aren't comfortable while on your back, roll to your side. Again, the most effective position for pushing is often the one that feels right for you.
- Wait to push until you are ten centimeters. You can request to labor down if you'd like or you need some additional rest.
- Push during your uterine contractions. In a hospital setting, you will likely be getting coached, but pushing when you feel a contraction, feel pressure in your bottom, or see the contractions on your monitor will make your pushes more effective.
- Breathe out and exhale during pushing *if* you want to breathe out. You don't have to hold your breath if that does not feel effective for you.
- Feel free to make sounds while pushing. You can moan, growl, grunt, or hum, all of which can allow opening of the throat instead of completely holding the breath.
- Using a warm compress on the perineum and birthing while lying on your side have been shown to decrease the risk of severe perineal tearing.
- When a baby's head is crowning, allow the head to stretch the vaginal opening between contractions until you start pushing again with the next contraction.

PREPARE YOUR MIND

As I've mentioned before, your mind is connected with your body, your pelvic floor, and birth. I recall a friend telling me she was having a home birth and was dilated to eight centimeters. Then her husband's phone rang, and he picked it up. When she heard her mother-in-law's voice on the other end of the line, her cervix closed back to four centimeters. I also knew heading into birth that I wanted as calm and quiet an environment as possible, which is why my husband didn't call any of my family members until after my son was born. I knew my mind needed to be in the right place, focused on my body, breath, and contractions. As your expected due date approaches, take some time in advance to prepare your mind. This can range from listening to relaxation or meditation tracks to journaling, doing gentle yoga, or even working with a therapist. The connection between mind and body is strong and undeniable, and we must address one to influence the other.

PACK YOUR POSTPARTUM CARE KIT BEFORE BIRTH

There's nothing like making a Target run at 2:00 a.m. when you need some maxi pads and stool softeners after having a baby. One of the most proactive things you can do before childbirth is to prepare for after childbirth, just like you prepare for baby care by ordering baby wipes and butt paste. Getting what you will need for your care is just as important.

Maxi Pads and Panty Liners. Your uterus continues to contract in the weeks following birth, causing you to bleed for the first four to six weeks, maybe even longer, following a vaginal delivery or cesarean section. Select organic, unbleached pads and liners and plan to change them out frequently postpartum. You can place the pad or liner inside the stretchy disposable underwear (or diaper) that you will get from the hospital (and you can order them for home). Transition to using some big, stretchy underwear as blood flow gradually decreases.

Compression Briefs. I mentioned these for use during pregnancy, and I am a fan of these for postpartum care as well. Compression briefs lift from the bottom up to support your groin, vulva, and tummy when your pelvic floor and core are exhausted after birth. Some women use "waist trainers" that squeeze the middle of the waist, but these put pressure *down* on your vulnerable and weakened pelvic floor, which isn't good. I recommend wearing compression briefs immediately after birth over your maxi pads and underwear (they are also great for holding in ice packs over a C-section scar or vulva), but they don't need to be worn at nighttime while sleeping. Continue daily for four to six weeks as swelling decreases, as you walk and move around more and regain some pelvic floor strength.

Ice Packs. Ice is your friend immediately postpartum. Ice decreases swelling and inflammation, which occurs whether you tear or not, and it helps with pain relief. You can get ice packs in advance that are specific for the perineum or lower abdominal cesarean incision. These can be placed directly on your skin or over a pad or pair of underwear. Place over your vulva following a vaginal birth or over your scar if you've had a C-section. Use the first three to five days after giving birth for twenty minutes three to five times a day.

Pee and Poop Support. Take stool softeners on day one postpartum to keep your poop soft and easy to pass when you are healing down south. Also, a peri bottle to cleanse yourself after pees and poops will be a relief so you don't have to aggressively wipe. You can also use witch hazel pads to wipe or soothe healing tissues and hemorrhoids, and don't forget a squatty potty (hopefully you know why by now).

Cesarean Birth Preparation Protocol

Over 30% of the births in the United States are via cesarean section (C-section), and it's the most common surgery performed in the United States. This percentage rate has steadily increased since the 1990s in some part because the majority of C-sections are first-time births, and many moms have a repeat C-section for a future birth, thus further bumping up that percentage.

If you know for sure you are going to have a C-section, follow all the parts of the main protocol on the previous pages, but here are some special considerations to include. This preparation won't include pushing practice as it does with vaginal delivery preparation, but incorporates exercises to release hip tension, stretches to improve posture and scar mobility, and preparing for postpartum recovery.

LENGTHEN AND STRENGTHEN

Although there is less focus on lengthening the pelvic floor during cesarean preparation, carrying tension in your hips, thighs, and back during pregnancy and into birth can make recovery a challenge. Focus on lengthening the sides of your abdominal wall and releasing tension in your neck and back, which will allow for optimal posture and mobility postpartum. Specifics for performing these exercises can be found in the strengthening and relaxation protocols in Chapter 2.

- Thread the needle
- Cat–cow pose
- Modified downward-facing dog
- Modified bird dog

CHANGE UP YOUR POSTURE

Sleep with a pillow underneath your waist and your tummy to help stretch the side abdominal wall and prevent one side of the abdomen from getting tense and tight. Alternate which side you cross your legs on while sitting. These modifications prevent your pelvic floor and core muscles from getting overly tense, tight, or asymmetric. Avoid tucking your butt under when standing to maintain optimal core and booty activation, essential for cesarean recovery. Pregnant moms are notorious for this posture due to trying to balance the weight of the baby up front, but this crunches your lower abdomen, which needs to stretch and lengthen to help you stand upright after surgery.

ADDITIONAL ITEMS FOR CESAREAN POSTPARTUM CARE

Everything listed above in the vaginal birth care kit is needed for a C-section with the addition of a few more items.

Small Pillow. In the first few weeks following surgery, the incision from your scar will be tender, and activities as simple as riding in a car, pushing to poop, and feeding your baby can cause pain and discomfort. Keep a small pillow handy, one about the size of a twelve- to sixteen-inch couch pillow or even a stuffed animal from your kiddo's collection. While riding in a car wearing your seat belt or while breastfeeding your baby, place the pillow over your clothes where your abdominal incision is located to provide additional protection to the healing incision. If you have a coughing or sneezing spell, place the pillow over that same area and apply gentle pressure against it during each cough or sneeze to avoid increased intra-abdominal pressure causing injury or popping open the incision.

Soft Underwear. Again, your incision will be tender, and scratchy old pregnancy undies may not be what your body needs or tolerates. Plus, you'll need something to hold in the ice packs and maxi pads. Have a pair of soft underwear. There are many made specifically for cesarean recovery that cover your incision and can offer a layer of gentle protection under scratchy clothes.

Abdominal Support. Following any abdominal surgery, your abs are going to feel weak and struggle to support you. This is normal, albeit challenging for a mom who still has to care for a newborn baby. You will need a soft abdominal binder to wrap around your low hips and tummy for a little extra support. Some hospitals provide one of these, but you can also purchase one in advance to have on hand. This should not have clips or fasteners of any kind but should secure with a strip of Velcro and be soft enough to wear throughout the day. It is not needed at night while sleeping.

The Rebirth of Birth

Whether you are a thinker and planner and want to prep as much as possible as you head into the unknown experience that is childbirth or you have had a challenging, or even traumatic, birth experience and aim for it to be different the next time, we all have common goals: a healthy baby *and* a healthy you, both physically and emotionally, after birth. You have every right to feel comfortable, confident, and supported in your birth experience and look forward to a new season afterwards without pain, leaking, or even regret.

When my patient Angelina was pregnant with her first child, she figured she would follow her doctor's lead on what to do. She was thirty-eight years old, and her doctor recommended labor induction at thirty-nine weeks of pregnancy. (Once you are thirty-five years old, the medical community is more likely to consider your pregnancy "high-risk" and recommend interventions.)

She went through a typical sequence of events with induction, then an epidural, then oxytocin because labor was not progressing quickly enough. Then she was finally dilated to ten centimeters. At this point, she was coached to push for hours while holding her breath and lying on her back. Exhausted and defeated, she was then told by her doctor they would wait thirty more minutes before performing a C-section. Angelina was determined to get that baby out. So she pushed as hard as she possibly could. And he eventually did come out. But the experience had been so hard and aggressive that she tore from her vagina to her anus. She said she was relieved she didn't end up having a C-section after laboring and pushing, but also said her recovery was traumatic. She couldn't sit for weeks afterwards and had pain with bowel movements and sex for months. As you can imagine, she wanted a different birth experience with her second pregnancy.

Angelina came into my clinic at thirty-seven weeks pregnant

with her second and said she wanted to prepare for childbirth. She and I both knew we likely had two weeks at best to get her body ready, so we went to work. I worked with her to address some hip pain she'd had since her first birth. Then I taught her perineal massage, how to bulge and bear down in different positions, and a routine of daily stretches to perform heading into her last few weeks of pregnancy. I saw Angelina for three visits prior to her birth.

She spontaneously went into labor a day before she was scheduled to be induced, and said she had an incredibly smooth delivery. She pushed for thirty minutes and had no perineal tearing. This is the type of birth I wish people heard more about, because I know it is possible. When I saw Angelina at her postpartum pelvic floor therapy visit, she expressed how grateful she was that she prepared in advance this time. And how empowered she felt during labor and pushing. This was a dramatically different and incredibly healing experience for her.

Our medical system of childbirth needs a rebirth. It needs to center the needs of the mother, and her body, along with the needs of the baby. Here is how I see it: childbirth is about birthing a baby for sure. But it is also about birthing a mom—one who deserves to feel strong and capable instead of broken and confused. And with the methods and tips above, along with a solid and supportive medical team, my hope is that we can move the needle toward that, one mom at a time.

CHAPTER 9

The Postpartum After-Party

I stood in the shower and let warm water run over my body. I had just passed through the most transformative physical experience of my life: the birth of my son. I had prepared for months, listening to hypnobirthing recordings in warm baths, performing pelvic floor relaxation stretches every morning and evening, and setting aside time for my husband to do perineal massage. And after nine months of pregnancy, hours of labor, and an intense and rapid vaginal birth, I leaned against the shower wall of my labor and delivery room and sighed.

A few minutes earlier, a nurse had come into the bathroom and informed me they were ready to transfer me to my postpartum room on another floor, but first I had to pee. I took some big, deep breaths as I leaned against the shower wall, trying to coach my pelvic floor muscles to relax so my pee stream would start. All of my years of instructing other women on how to pee were coming in handy: *take big, deep breaths, don't push, be patient, allow your pelvic floor to let go to start your stream.* Moments after birth, I was already coaching my pelvic floor to perform.

It worked. Finally, my stream started. And after that sweet relief, I was rolled in a wheelchair to my hospital room, where my baby, husband, and I would camp out. Over the days that followed, I implemented more of the techniques and strategies that, as a pelvic floor therapist, I knew would help me in the early days of postpartum recovery:

- Ice my vulva to help with swelling and pain
- Exhale when lifting my baby out of the bassinet
- Walk the halls of the hospital to promote blood flow
- Roll over and use my arms (instead of my abs) to get out of bed
- And take the stool softeners!

I felt grateful for my education and expertise during that vulnerable time for my pelvic floor. And as I stroked my sweet newborn's head, I thought many times about how every woman needs these same strategies after giving birth. Postpartum can, of course, be a very joyous time—but it can also be quite painful.

At any given moment, millions of women are in the postpartum haze. Over 3.5 million babies are born in the United States every year, and up to 90% of moms who birth vaginally have a perineal tear, a laceration that can extend into pelvic floor muscles all the way to the rectum. All of these women need postpartum support. And yet the only instruction regarding my vagina that I received in the hospital, voted the best place to birth in the city of Dallas, was, "Let me know if you have a blood clot bigger than a golf ball." No one guided me on how to move, lift, heal, pee, poop, or manage my pain. And I received zero in terms of a pelvic floor care plan upon returning home.

As I sat on the toilet, attempting my first postpartum bowel movement (I used a hospital garbage can on its side to support my feet as a makeshift stool), I thought there has to be a better way. Every postpartum mom deserves to know how to care for her body and pelvic floor after birth. They need education on how to perform the simple everyday functions such as peeing, pooping, and lifting after their pelvic floor and abdominal wall have been put through the wringer. They deserve longer-term recovery support, guidance to strengthen their bodies, a protocol to return to sex and exercise, and care *after* the baby is born that is more in alignment with the consistent and frequent check-ins that occur *before* the baby is born.

If you get anything out of this chapter, I want you to know that pelvic health changes that commonly occur postpartum, such as leaking urine, constipation, hemorrhoids, pain with sex, cesarean scar sensitivity, or pelvic organ prolapse, *are not normal.* Your body is not broken; the medical system is fractured. And everything in this chapter (and in this book) is offered in an effort to show you what you *can* do. You can improve and even prevent these common pelvic floor changes that occur after birth for years and decades to follow. The two billion moms worldwide need to know how to care for their postpartum pelvic floors.

Historically, women lived in closer communities with their families, and after giving birth, parents, female relatives, and other women helped care for a mom and her new baby. It is the norm in many other countries for family and community members to help with household chores, cooking, and childcare in order to give a new mom an opportunity for rest and recovery. In Chinese culture, new moms participate in "sitting the month," where a new mother receives care from family members to allow her "loose bones" to return to normal. In Mexican culture, women rest for forty days during a time period called *la cuarentena.* Muslim women also observe a rest period for forty days. And in Japanese culture, a woman is cared for by her mother until approximately eight weeks postpartum. Many countries and cultures support caring for a new mom between three and five months after birth.

And there's more: in some countries, women are encouraged to abstain from sex to allow for appropriate healing up to one hundred days. In the US, women are advised to take a break for a standard of six weeks. Despite these variations and differences in other cultures, the common thread is that *the mother is mothered.* The focus is not solely on caring for, protecting, and feeding the newborn baby, but also restoring the mother's health, which in turn gives her body and pelvic floor time to heal.

Women in the United States are not guaranteed a single day

of paid maternity leave and, likely living far from family who can lend support, are forced to return to household duties or work well before their bodies are healed. While postpartum doula care can help fill this need in the United States, that care is paid for by the mother and is not accessible to many people. With unpaid parental leave, the high cost of childcare, and lack of family and community support, the heavy lifting of caring for a newborn falls on the mother who is recovering from ten months of pregnancy and then childbirth.

Standard medical care in the United States consists only of a six-week postpartum visit with an obstetrician (perhaps a few more from a midwife) that usually entails a brief physical examination, a psychological screening, a conversation about birth control, and clearance to return to sex and exercise. Other than this six-week checkup, a mom does not have any other planned medical care after leaving the hospital or birthing center. *Mind blown.* Studies show that at six weeks after a vaginal birth, pelvic floor strength is reduced by 54% and pelvic floor endurance by 53%. In other words, when a postpartum woman is "cleared" to return to intense physical activity, her pelvic floor is functioning at less than 50%.

There are other aspects of postpartum care that need to change too: from breastfeeding and lactation support, to the cost of childcare, to the lack of paid and unpaid leave from work (one out of every four postpartum women returns to work within two weeks of giving birth, citing financial reasons). Each of these things deserves attention, but my focus is on your pelvic floor and core rehabilitation. If you are reading this, you may have been sent back into the world to care for your newborn baby, and perhaps older children as well, or you are returning to the workforce, but you have received very little guidance, if any, on how to care for your body. These circumstances place your long-term pelvic floor health at risk.

Postpartum pelvic floor therapy needs to be the standard of care for women because pregnancy, childbirth, and modern-day mom life can do a doozy down south. Until that day comes, follow the guidelines in this chapter. Let's begin with some postpartum pelvic floor education 101.

How the Pelvic Floor and Postpartum Work Together

Immediately after a vaginal or cesarean birth, the hormones estrogen and progesterone (which were super high during pregnancy) take a nosedive as the hormones oxytocin and prolactin both increase dramatically. Oxytocin causes your uterus to contract, heal, and shrink back down to its pre-pregnancy size. These uterine contractions, also known as "after-pains," can be triggered by breastfeeding or lactation and cause postpartum vaginal bleeding, called lochia, following birth. So regardless of whether you had a vaginal or cesarean birth, you will have vaginal bleeding for about four to six weeks. These after-pains can be incredibly intense, so much so that after a completely unmedicated birth, it was these contractions that had me begging for pain relief medication.

Prolactin also surges in the early days following birth in an effort to boost breast milk supply, which also causes estrogen levels to decrease. Over time, low estrogen levels contribute to vaginal dryness, vulvar itching, decreased vaginal lubrication, low libido, and decreased pelvic floor muscle tone. So your pelvic floor stays in a vulnerable state well after birth when you continue making breast milk. This estrogen decline is in no way a reason to stop lactating unless you are ready, but it does shed light on how the healing and recovery process of your pelvic floor persists well beyond the six-week mark.

Most birthing women will experience a perineal tear during vaginal birth, which can range from as small as a paper cut on the labia to a significant tear into your pelvic floor muscles extending to the anal sphincter and rectum. *Ouch!* Additionally, moms who have a cesarean section will have a lower abdominal incision, typically horizontal just above their pubic bone. These wounds will go through a phase of healing that can last anywhere between three weeks and a year. So even though "postpartum" medical care halts at six weeks postpartum (and most working women are expected to return to the workforce by twelve weeks postpartum), our bodies are still very much healing until one entire year after giving birth. One of the most tricky but critical matters when it comes to your pelvic floor and core is wound healing.

A cesarean or perineal wound takes a while to heal. The first phase of healing, hemostasis, includes the formation of a blood clot to halt bleeding. The second phase, the inflammatory phase, takes place for three to five days and brings warmth and redness to the area as healing cells make their way to the wound. After this inflammatory phase, and depending on the extent of the wound, the proliferative phase begins, when new blood vessels form to bring blood flow to the area, lay down new collagen, and assist with wound closure. This is a crucial time that spans three to fourteen days after birth. Because the wound is not yet closed, the majority of wound infections occur during these first two weeks after birth. A good and competent care team will advise you to look out for signs of infection such as prolonged redness, swelling, increased pain, an odor, or oozing of the wound and immediately report to your medical provider if any of these signs occur.

After ten to fourteen days, the wound enters the last phase of healing, the remodeling phase. Now the new tissue gets stronger, and collagen continues to build to create scar tissue at the site. This last phase starts around week three and lasts . . . up to a year. A laceration in your pelvic floor following a vaginal birth or an incision in your abdominal wall after a cesarean birth needs up to a year of care and attention to prevent further pelvic floor problems down the line.

At best, your pelvic floor and abdominals may be ready for

very gentle activity after two weeks, but even at six weeks, scars are still forming. And even after a wound is completely healed, scar tissue at the site of the wound forms, and this tissue is 20% weaker and less elastic than previous tissue. Because most of us don't know this, many of us are lifting and going about our business as usual three months in, which makes healing more difficult. Our bodies are not the same, yet we attempt to return to the same pre-pregnancy activities but with weaker tissues. And we might not get the signal right away that we are causing harm to our bodies.

After birth, our nerves also need a vacation. The pudendal nerve, which courses through the pelvic floor and supplies nerve function to the muscles that hold in pee and poop and maintain pelvic organ support, can get super stretched during vaginal birth. So although there is no longer a several-pound baby sitting on your bladder, injury to this nerve leads to urinary leakage, fecal leakage, and decreased pelvic organ support. And because the pelvic floor connects with the spine for core support, injury to the nerve can even cause low back pain. Function of this nerve can gradually return after two months, but by then, many women have already returned to work.

I met a mom of twins whose husband broke his finger, and he was prescribed twelve weeks of physical therapy. Three sessions of hand therapy a week for three months. Meanwhile, after the birth of her twins, which was an emergency cesarean section, she was sent home with an ice pack, some ibuprofen, and two newborn babies, and told to follow up with her doctor in six weeks. While pelvic rehabilitation and physical therapy are not (yet) the standard of care after giving birth, I think every mom who has had a C-section will tell you how challenging the recovery was and how confused and lost she may have felt.

A cesarean section requires cutting through seven layers of skin, tissue, muscle, and organ. After slicing outer layers of skin, fat, and fascia, the abdominal wall muscles are separated in the middle to reach the peritoneum (the inner lining of the pelvic cavity) and ultimately the uterus, where the baby resides. After the baby or babies and placenta are delivered, the uterus is stitched closed, most often with a vertical up-and-down incision, followed by the abdominal wall closure, most often with a horizontal incision called a "bikini-cut" above the pubic bone. For an uncomplicated incision, skin and muscle healing takes three months, while uterine incision healing can take a full six months. Healing takes time.

FROM WOUND HEALING TO NERVE HEALING TO MUSCLE FATIGUE AND more, your pelvic floor is needy after giving birth. Neediness is normal! But if you don't attend to those needs, you will likely run into issues. Over the years, either in my clinical practice or even just at a cocktail hour, I've heard dozens of postpartum struggles, all of which relate to the pelvic floor.

> "I was just lifting a laundry basket full of clothes and felt something drop in my vagina."
> "My daughter pressed on my stomach and touched my C-section scar. The pain made me want to jump out of my skin."
> "Every time I have sex, my vagina feels like it's tearing open."
> "When I sit up after lying down, it looks like a football is coming out the middle of my belly."
> "I tried to go for a short run in my neighborhood. I turned around before the end of the block because pee was streaming down my leg."
> "Something doesn't feel right down there. It's like ever since I gave birth, things just feel out of place."

These are a small sampling of the stories I've heard over the years. But here's the good news: whether you've had a postpartum issue for six months or a few years or many decades, there are ways to address the problem. These pelvic floor PT tools and techniques can make a big impact.

How long should I wait to get pregnant again so my pelvic floor has enough time to heal?

Some moms express concern about how soon to get pregnant again after a previous birth (called interdelivery interval) to optimize pelvic floor health. While some studies show a return to pelvic floor strength as early as two months postpartum, others state that waiting until thirty-six months after birth can decrease the risk of urinary incontinence. Many factors including whether you had a vaginal or cesarean birth, length of pushing stage of labor, body mass index, and whether you are breastfeeding or lactating all play a factor. If you are wrestling with this question, I encourage you to speak with your medical provider to determine medically if there is a recommendation on waiting a certain period of time based on your uterine healing or other medical conditions, and then consider the goals for your family.

Being over the age of thirty-five increases the risk of pelvic floor challenges. So does breastfeeding or lactating. But your fertility also changes as time passes, and depending on the goals you have for your family, waiting an extended period of time can pose a risk in that capacity. It's safe to say about a year can be a good time to wait. Most folks have significantly decreased breastfeeding or lactating by this point, hormone levels have somewhat normalized, and you are getting a little bit of rest and a smidge of exercise. If you get pregnant sooner than this, which many of my patients have, you can still optimize your pelvic floor health with the tips and guidance in this book.

Your Down-There Care Plan

Often my postpartum recovery advice to new moms is to take it slow and listen to your body. While these may feel like loose guidelines when you want hard rules on how to heal and protect your body, listening to your own needs for rest is important. I've never met a mom whose recovery took *too long* because she waited to get back to exercise and activity, but I have worked with many moms who went back *way too soon* to high-intensity exercise and activity, and their pelvic floors suffered long-term damage. As you proceed through my tips below, taking you from day one post-birth until the weeks and months afterwards, tune in to your body. If pain or bleeding increases, slow down and contact your medical provider.

HOW TO POOP

You got pregnant. You grew a baby. You went through birth. Now . . . you need to have a bowel movement. Many women tell me that taking their first poop after childbirth was even more painful than giving birth. Some very simple strategies can make this event much less traumatizing.

> **Hydrate and Take Stool Softeners.** Following blood loss, not having food or fluids for hours or even days, and the side effects of pain medication, your stool can get very hard and uncomfortable to pass. Hydration is key, especially if breastfeeding or pumping. Drink enough water to make sure your urine is almost clear. Take stool softeners as directed for the first several days to weeks after birth. Other options for softening your stool include magnesium citrate or glycinate supplements, prunes or prune juice, and a diet rich in fruits and veggies. If you are taking stool softeners, wean off them slowly instead of stopping cold turkey to give your body time to adjust so your colon doesn't get backed up again. (But keep drinking that water.)

Support Your Floor and Core. Place your feet on a squatty potty or stool (head to Chapter 4 for more pooping posture details). Following a vaginal birth, you can place the pads of your fingers covered in toilet paper on your perineum (area between the vaginal and anal opening) and apply gentle pressure upwards toward your head. If you had a cesarean birth, place a folded towel or small pillow at least twelve inches long over your abdominal area where your incision is located. Exhale as you bear down to empty your bowels, maintaining firm pressure against your perineum or abdomen. If your stools are hard or large, you may have to exhale and bear down several times to effectively empty your rectum.

Don't Delay the Urge. When my first son was born, my husband worked from home in our bedroom, so I ended up wearing my baby on my chest a lot. It was the only way I could get him to nap and not cry. One afternoon when wearing him, I had the urge to poop. Never ever in my life had I taken a bowel movement with another human in the bathroom. I knew delaying the urge was not ideal, but I also did not want to start a tear-fest. So I went into the bathroom, pulled down my pajama pants, and pooped while wearing my baby. Afterwards, I called my best friend and told her about my bathroom trip. She said, "Oh, I've done that tons of times. Sometimes I pee wearing him too." *Excuse me, what?* Is taking a bowel movement while holding or wearing your baby really a normal part of motherhood?

I can't speak for everyone, but after this first memorable experience, it was normal for me. And it will likely be for you if you follow my guideline not to delay the urge. When the urge hits, it's because the stool is ringing the doorbell in your rectum. Delaying the urge will make that stool get harder and more painful to empty, which is not great for healing your perineum and pelvic floor. So when the urge calls, head to the bathroom to have your BM, baby-wearing and all.

Keep It Clean. When your perineum is healing or your abs are so sore you can't lean forward to reach your bum, wiping after a bowel movement can be messy or almost impossible. Enter a peri bottle, which is usually provided by hospitals, or you can order one online. Fill the bottle with warm water (some folks add a few drops of witch hazel), then spritz over your bum and anal opening after a bowel movement to cleanse the area. Follow with a pat dry with toilet paper. Avoid using any wipes with alcohol as that can burn sensitive tissues.

HOW TO PEE

One of two things is going to happen with your bladder immediately after giving birth. You are either going to struggle to get your pee stream started, or you are going to stand up and all of the urine from your bladder is going to pour out. Don't stress; this will improve.

If you can't get your pee stream to start, and the threat of inserting a catheter into your urethra is on the line, sit on the toilet and take some big, deep breaths to help your pelvic floor muscles relax. Use a stool under your feet to further relax your pelvic floor and a peri bottle to spray warm water over the urethral opening to further relax your urinary sphincter. Putting peppermint oil drops in toilet water can also be helpful to relax your sphincter to start your stream. I like to tell moms to pack this in their hospital bags or keep it in the bathroom at home. Put five to ten drops in toilet water, sit on the toilet, and take some big, deep breaths to help your pelvic floor relax.

If this doesn't work, stand in the shower, place one hand against the wall to support your body weight, and take some deep breaths as the sound and warmth of the water assist in relaxing your pelvic floor. This is obviously not the most practical or long-term solution, but it is effective until the practice returns to normal.

If it burns when your urine streams out against sensitive tissues or a wound, lidocaine sprays, which you can apply before peeing, can "numb" the area to provide relief. You can also try sitting backwards on the toilet, facing the wall, and leaning forward to direct your urine stream backward. This can help direct your urine stream away from a sensitive perineal wound. After you finish peeing, spritz the area with warm water from a peri bottle and pat yourself dry with toilet paper.

HOW TO EXERCISE

The benefits of postpartum exercise are clear: improved heart health and bone health, better sleep, reduced anxiety and depression, and weight loss, which can decrease pelvic floor dysfunction. It also provides a temporary escape from the overwhelming demands of feedings, nap schedules, and endless laundry. When it comes to exercise, follow this axiom: build the foundation of your home before you put up the roof and walls. First rehabilitate your core and pelvic floor, the muscles and structures that support your organs, before you return to your pre-pregnancy exercise regime. You need to make sure you can keep in urine and stool and that your spine is supported before you take on Pilates, running, pickleball, and weightlifting.

The question I get most often after birth is, "When can I return to exercise?" I am a huge fan of movement and activity, so I get how hard it is to hold back. Even I went back to running too soon. New research has come out suggesting waiting a full twelve weeks after birth to resume one's pre-pregnancy exercise routine. That said, many medical professionals will give us the thumbs-up to return to exercise at six weeks. As a PT, I know that our physical bodies are not ready to return to our pre-birth or pre-pregnancy workouts that early. So where does one start? I often tell my patients to begin with a habit of walking. Walking is an excellent substitute for the first few months. It is also a fantastic first baby step to feel out how your body is doing before adding weights, speed, or complex movements to your exercise gig. Put on some tunes, or a good podcast, and enjoy. In addition, there are other exercises you can do to build yourself back up.

MODIFY YOUR MOVEMENT

How you move matters. Many of the same strategies you implemented during your pregnancy carry over into the postpartum period. When getting in and out of bed, roll to your side and use your hands to push up instead of crunching up or having someone pull you. When getting out of a chair, scoot your bottom to the edge of the seat, lean forward, and again push up on the armrests or seat with your hands to come to standing. These techniques minimize the strain on your pelvic floor and abdominal wall.

GO FOR A WALK

As challenging as it may feel, and as many times as you may have cursed me during your pregnancy for this exact same advice, you need to walk. Get out of bed and walk around your home or the hospital, even if it's just around the bed, especially following a cesarean section surgery. Upright movement helps your posture, blood flow, and healing, and decreases the risk of blood clots. A protocol on how much you should move or walk following birth varies; some guidelines suggest to stay in bed for the first five days to a week, and others say you can start running by three weeks. I believe practical and safe guidelines are somewhere in the middle. I love walking because it's easy and free, and if the weather is nice outside, you can get beyond the walls of your home (especially if guests from out of town are overstaying their welcome). Here are some general recommendations for walking, which can be modified based on your pain levels and recovery.

1. Days 0 to 6 (Week 1): Walk five minutes a day in hallways and around the house.

2. Days 7 to 13 (Week 2): Walk ten minutes a day; can be broken into two five-minute walks.
3. Days 14 to 20 (Week 3): Walk fifteen minutes a day; can be broken into two eight-minute walks.
4. Days 21 to 28 (Week 4): Walk twenty minutes a day without interruption if possible; can be broken into two ten-minute walks if needed.

MONITOR HOW YOU LIFT

Don't forget to exhale while lifting, which you will likely be doing a lot of during motherhood. Holding your breath when you load your body—say, when lifting a stroller into the trunk, a car seat with a seven- to ten-pound baby, or even a toddler into and out of the tub—puts pressure *down* on your pelvic floor and *out* onto your abdominal wall. This increased pressure without adequate muscle and tissue support (due to a healing pelvic floor and abdominal wall) can lead to increased risk of a hernia, pelvic organ prolapse, diastasis recti, and urinary leakage. With every lift, it's one, two, three, exhale.

STRENGTHEN YOUR PELVIC FLOOR

After giving birth while lying in my hospital bed, I thought: I kind of just want to do a Kegel to see how it feels. So I did, and this followed: radio silence. No contraction. Zero. My mind told my body, my pelvic floor specifically, to do one thing, and the message wasn't connecting. I had zero ability to contract my pelvic floor. Why? My pelvic floor was exhausted!

You may not necessarily feel a strong contraction initially, but performing gentle Kegels in the first three to five days after giving birth can help promote blood flow to the pelvic floor and aid in healing a perineal laceration. Then move through the following progression for pelvic floor connection and core activation postpartum.

1. Days 0 to 6 (Week 1): Perform ten quick pelvic floor contractions, drawing in deep core muscles simultaneously, two or three times a day while lying down.

2. Days 7 to 13 (Week 2): Perform ten long-hold three- to five-second pelvic floor contractions, drawing in deep core muscles simultaneously, two or three times a day in a sitting position.

3. Days 14 to 20 (Week 3): Perform ten quick contractions and ten long-hold three- to five-second pelvic floor contractions in a standing position. Initiate bridge exercises, one to three sets of ten repetitions.

4. Days 21 to 28 (Week 4): Perform ten long-hold five- to ten-second pelvic floor contractions in a standing position. Initiate ball squeezes lying down and bird dogs in hands-and-knees position. One to three sets of ten repetitions. Descriptions can be found in the pelvic floor strengthening protocol in Chapter 2.

5. Weeks 5 and 6: Perform upper-body exercises (performing pelvic floor and core contraction with each repetition) while sitting such as biceps curl, overhead press, and overhead triceps extension with less than ten-pound weights for one to three sets of ten repetitions. Incorporate pelvic floor contractions into day-to-day movements such as going from sit to stand, squatting down, lifting your car seat, or picking up your baby.

Now stop and assess. Before taking on additional pelvic floor exercises, take the pelvic floor questionnaire in Chapter 2 to determine the appropriate protocol that aligns with your symptoms. We all heal differently. Some women might need to strengthen their floor after birth; other women would benefit from relaxation. Make sure you follow the protocol that's right for your condition.

If you fall into the relaxation category, return to Chapter 2 to practice the relaxation protocol. If you fall into the strengthening category, follow these steps:

6. Weeks 6 to 8: Perform the following lower-body exercises in the standing position: squats, lunges, marching in place, side squat, step-ups, and calf raises with no weight. One to three sets of ten repetitions.
7. Weeks 8 to 10: Perform the exercises above with less than ten-pound weights. Add in single-leg bridges, single-leg calf raises, single-leg sit to stand, and wall sits with no weight for one to three sets of ten repetitions.
8. Weeks 10 to 12: Add less than ten-pound weights to single-leg bridges, leg calf raises, wall sits, and sit to stand for one to three sets of ten repetitions. Add in exercises with impact such as single-leg hops, jumping in place, jogging in place, and jumping jacks for thirty to sixty seconds.

All of the above activities should be performed without pain, leakage, pressure in the vagina, or a feeling of heaviness or something falling out. If you experience these or any other pelvic floor symptoms, stop the exercises, retake the pelvic floor questionnaire in Chapter 2, and follow the protocol that aligns with your symptoms. If more individualized guidance is needed, check in with a specialist. If you are able to reach twelve weeks for strengthening without any pelvic floor symptoms, you can confidently return to jogging and higher-impact activities, gradually building up intensity and endurance.

Another option for pelvic floor strengthening is using pelvic floor weights. Yes, your pelvic floor can actually lift weights! These can be beneficial for many postpartum moms, as they gradually add "resistance" to pelvic floor exercises and offer something to "squeeze around" when performing Kegels. If you do want to incorporate these, wait until six weeks after birth and get clearance from your medical provider that insertion into the vagina is safe. Detailed use and progression with vaginal weights is in the Chapter 2 strengthening protocol.

I've heard vaginal steaming can help with postpartum healing. Is this legit?

Reportedly linked back to ancient times, vaginal steaming, also known as V-steaming or yoni-steaming, involves sitting or squatting over a pot of hot water infused with herbs and wrapping your lower body in a blanket (to keep the steam from escaping) for twenty to thirty minutes. The steam is said to help cleanse your vagina, increase vaginal moisture, and even balance your hormones and increase energy after birth. But the steam only reaches the external vulva and vaginal opening, so deeper experiences of cervical or uterine cleansing can't physically be achieved with this practice.

Also, I have a major vulva warning here. Placing hot water and steam so close to vulvar and vaginal tissues can cause damage. A study reported a woman getting second-degree burns on her labia and vulva from V-steaming because the excessive heat burned her delicate skin and tissues. I don't recommend vaginal steaming. If you do decide to steam, proceed with caution and know it's giving your vulva and vagina a tiny facial, but it isn't creating any real positive change down there.

Reclaim Your Floor and Core

Even if you follow all of the recommendations for prevention and recovery, problems down south may still occur as birth can be unpredictable and our bodies undoubtedly experience physical change. Many common pelvic floor challenges related to peeing, pooping, and sex are in those respective chapters in this book. Below are some postpartum-specific problems (and their solutions) that may arise.

PERINEAL TEAR SCAR TISSUE RESTRICTION

Scar tissue is a collection of cells and collagen that covers the site of an injury; it is dense and thick, and it does not move as smoothly as its pre-injury skin. It can be tight, sensitive, or lead to symptoms ranging from a minor itch to severe pain that last for years.

Over half of the women who return to sex after childbirth have pain, especially in the first three to six months after childbirth. Perineal scar tissue forms, and even after it's considered "healed," it can still feel incredibly tight and painful, leading not only to pain with sex but also to problems with urination, bowel movements, and even back pain. Tissue healing occurs during the first several months to a year, so the remodeling phase is the best opportunity for change.

In the initial weeks after birth, ice, pain medication or anti-inflammatories, lidocaine spray, and a sitz bath (a soak for your sensitive bottom) will help you manage pain and promote healing. And after your six-week postpartum check, when you get confirmation that your wound has healed and sutures have dissolved, begin perineal massage. The details on performing perineal scar massage are in the relaxation protocol in Chapter 2.

I had a perineal tear, and my doctor stitched me up super tight, saying this will be better for sex. Is this standard after a perineal tear or episiotomy?

Historically called "the husband stitch," the practice of adding additional stitches is an effort to "tighten" the vaginal opening following a perineal tear or episiotomy. It is medically unnecessary, not standard practice, and is in fact considered medical malpractice as it can be harmful for the patient. Yet it still happens and causes significant pain and discomfort with attempts to insert something into the vagina. While little evidence is available as to how often this process occurs, I myself have heard a physician say, "I'm going to stitch you up tight to make your husband happy." There are also instances when this can occur unintentionally, and stitches at the vaginal opening can heal and cause significant restriction. You may feel like your vagina is tearing or ripping as a result. If either of these is you, check in with a medical provider to discuss your symptoms as it can be revised surgically if necessary.

CESAREAN SCAR TISSUE RESTRICTION

My patient Julianne, a fifty-four-year-old labor and delivery nurse, was referred to pelvic floor therapy by a urologist (a doctor who specializes in peeing problems) for incomplete bladder emptying and frequent urination. She tried a bladder medication for a while to no effect; it only caused constipation. She underwent a battery of tests confirming her bladder, urethra, and urinary sphincter were in good working order, and an ultrasound showed she retained one hundred fifty milliliters of urine in her bladder after she peed, over triple the normal amount that should remain. Not sure of the culprit, her physician encouraged her to try pelvic floor therapy.

In my office, Julianne shared that she was the proud mom of three boys, all of whom were now in their twenties, and all of whom she delivered via cesarean section. During the physical evaluation, Julianne lay down on my exam table with a sheet draped over the lower half of her body. I lowered the sheet just above her pubic bone to examine her cesarean scars. As I pressed above, below, and all along the scar, Julianne winced in pain. "I had no idea it was so sensitive down there," she stated. "I guess I never really touched it, so I wouldn't know."

Julianne's scar was similar to many of the cesarean scars I had seen over the years. It was a "cesarean shelf," which is when the scar is sandwiched between two bulges of the abdominal tissue above and below. Her three scars (one from each cesarean) were squished together and tight to her skin. They looked stuck. I knew immediately that her scar tissue restriction might be the culprit behind some of her issues.

Over the course of five therapy sessions, I performed massage to Julianne's scar and instructed her on how to do the same at home along with proper peeing and urge suppression techniques. After her five sessions, we measured the urine in her bladder, and it was back to normal. She had been urinating every hour for years, had increasing urinary tract infections, and was unable to empty her bladder, all because of the scar tissue from her C-sections.

Scar tissue can have a negative impact on your pelvic health, including pain with sex, constipation, abdominal pain, and skin sensitivity, because it often goes unrecognized and unaddressed as a source of pelvic health problems. Even if the pelvic floor problems you are experiencing now are from a birth or surgery decades ago, they can still be helped. It's never too late to care for your pelvic floor.

Although a C-section may "spare" the pelvic floor in some capacity, the effects of cesarean scar restriction go beyond the abdominal wall. Cesarean scar restriction can not only cause itching, numbness, hypersensitivity, burning, or pain with everyday activities like wearing pants or leaning against a countertop but also contribute to constipation, painful menstruation or ovulation, incomplete bladder emptying, back pain, infertility, and even painful sex. Over 30% of first-time moms who gave birth via a cesarean section reported pain with sex at three months

postpartum. Up to 40% had painful menstruation. Proper rehabilitation of a cesarean scar is essential for improving postpartum
pelvic health.

PERFORM SCAR DESENSITIZATION

Similar to the initial healing phase of a perineal scar, in the
early days after a cesarean section, ice, pain medication, anti-
inflammatories, and a heating pad can help soothe pain. Prior to
scar massage, many pelvic health therapists encourage patients
to do what we call "scar desensitization" to help decrease scar
sensitivity and build up skin tolerance to different textures and
forces. Begin this process one to two inches above and below the
scar as soon as day one after surgery, but do not work directly
over the scar until it is completely healed. Start with softer textures like a soft makeup brush or a piece of felt, silk, or satin.
Follow with a soft washcloth or piece of denim or burlap, brushing the area for three to five minutes daily. Once the scar has
healed, you can perform this directly over the scar and continue
for three to four months.

START SCAR MASSAGE

I have treated many moms after a C-section, and as I perform
scar massage on their healed incisions, tears have streamed down
their cheeks. Not because of pain necessarily, but because they
were disconnected from this part of their body since giving
birth. Depending on your birth experience and recovery, perhaps fear, anxiety, or trauma leaves you not wanting to look at
or touch your scar. Massage might seem out of the question. But
performing scar massage will help with the long-term health of
your scar and pelvic floor, and can help with the healing of your
heart.

If you are performing scar desensitization as above, you may
already be somewhat comfortable touching your scar. If not, a
great way to start connecting is to place your hand over your
clothing that covers the scar and take some big, deep breaths.

After a shower or bath, simply brush a towel over your scar. Eventually you can place your hand directly onto the scar and take some big, deep breaths. As you grow more comfortable touching your scar, begin the scar massage practice below, which can be started as early as two weeks after a C-section to months or years later. It's never too late, but in the first year is ideal as tissue is still in the remodeling phase.

Using an all-natural oil like almond oil, coconut oil, or vitamin E oil or an unscented lotion, start with firm pressure one to two centimeters in depth and gently rub across your abdominal wall two inches above and below your incision site. Move side to side and up and down while maintaining firm pressure massaging around your scar. You may feel sensitivity or tenderness, working within your comfort level. If your scar is less than six months old, you want to use less pressure and perform this massage daily for five minutes, up to two or three times per day. If your scar is older than six months, you can use more intense pressure and perform it three or four days a week.

Once your scar is completely healed and free of scabbing, which can take anywhere between four and six weeks, and with clearance from your medical provider, you can work directly on your scar. Start by following the guidelines, rubbing parallel to the scar. If the scar is less than six months old, use light to moderate pressure. If the scar is older than six months, use more intense pressure. After four to six weeks, as discomfort decreases, you can start moving perpendicular to the scar with your fingers and moving them in circular or crisscross motions to work the tissue in different directions. Consistently massaging your scar not only will improve tissue mobility and pelvic floor function but also can improve the appearance by reducing redness and puffiness.

USE SILICONE

Once the wound is completely healed, dry, and free of scabs, use silicone scar gel or tape over your scar. Silicone is believed to hydrate the scar, slow the overgrowth of collagen, cosmetically flatten the scar, and decrease redness. The recommendation is to apply a silicone strip or silicone gel over a clean, dry scar and leave on for twelve to twenty-three hours per day. Remove the tape or silicone when bathing and reapply afterwards, and continue use for six months. Many of my patients have used silicone and found it to be a total game-changer for scar healing.

It's worth noting that some women will develop what's called a keloid scar, when the body overproduces collagen in the scar healing process and results in a puffy, inflamed, and often red or brown raised scar. The cause or contributing factors in keloid scars is mostly unknown, but should you start to notice this, pause the scar massage and treatments and check in with a dermatologist.

I had a cesarean birth but have had pain with sex since giving birth. Can cesarean scar restriction cause pain with sex too?

Yes. Vaginal delivery and cesarean sections are equally as likely to result in pain with sex, and it can take on average six months to return to pre-pregnancy sexual function. Cesarean section surgeries cut through layers of muscle, tissue, and fascia, which creates scar tissue after healing. This scar tissue can lead to fascial restriction from the abdominal wall all the way to the pelvic floor. In addition, pelvic floor muscle tension along with vaginal dryness can occur in all postpartum moms. So unfortunately, C-sections don't completely spare your pelvic floor. If you experience pain with sex after a cesarean, try the tips for scar tissue restriction and cesarean scar massage above.

DIASTASIS RECTI ABDOMINIS

Diastasis recti abdominis (DRA), which I discussed in depth in the pregnancy chapter, can persist in up to 60% of women postpartum. Whether or not you implemented DRA prevention exercises during pregnancy, you will want to start on the exercises below as soon as you can after birth. They help improve DRA from progressing as you rebuild your core strength.

FOLLOW THE STRENGTHENING PROTOCOL

Your deep abdominal wall muscles, or your transverse abdominals, co-contract with your pelvic floor muscles. So when you properly do a Kegel, your transverse abs turn on. And when you are trying to activate your transverse abs, your pelvic floor contracts as well. The reason this is important is that activating your TA increases the tissue tension between your six-pack muscles and improves your DRA. Following the pelvic floor strengthening protocol in Chapter 2 will simultaneously help you improve your DRA over time.

MANAGE YOUR INTRA-ABDOMINAL PRESSURE

We are so busy after the baby's arrival, always rushing to take care of another human's needs, that we ignore our own. Whether it's jumping out of bed quickly or straining on the toilet to pee because the baby is crying and you need to hurry, very often we aren't paying attention to *how* we move. These activities can put increased strain on your abdomen and pelvic floor, which are still weak, healing, and vulnerable. In an effort to decrease that extra unwanted pressure, follow these tips for movement, some of which are similar to the recommendations provided for pregnancy.

- Roll to your side to get out of bed instead of using a crunch-up maneuver.
- To get in and out of a chair, avoid using your abs to lean up and instead use your hands to scoot your bottom forward to the edge of the seat.

- Exhale with exertion to decrease the pressure on your abs when lifting weights and baby.
- Avoid a waist trainer (which can put pressure down on your pelvic floor) but consider compression underwear that goes over your tummy so you get support below and at your core.
- When possible, modify movements that cause that football to pop out of the midline of your belly as you work to strengthen your core.

PAINFUL SEX

The cervix, the opening to the uterus, takes about six weeks to close after giving birth. In an effort to prevent bacteria from entering, which could lead to a uterine infection, the standard recommendation is to wait six weeks before returning to intercourse or insertion of anything into the vagina (e.g., a tampon or sex toy). This is the guidance for a vaginal or cesarean birth.

If you had an episiotomy or perineal tear, check in with your medical provider to ensure your wound is healed and stitches are dissolved. This is typically done at your six-week postpartum visit. Once the sex restriction is lifted, if you don't feel ready to return to vaginal intercourse, trust yourself. Despite your cervix being ready, you may not be. Nine out of ten women have pain the first time they have sex after birth. Your body is still very much healing, you are likely sleep-deprived with a small human in your bedroom, and getting it on may be low on your list of priorities. I waited twelve weeks after my second son was born to return to sex. When you are ready to give it a go, the guidelines below will help make it more comfortable.

Decreased estrogen levels following birth cause the skin of the vulva and vagina to be dry and sensitive, making any rubbing or friction during sex very uncomfortable. Proactively plan to use a lubricant for this first romp and afterwards as long as dryness occurs (more on lube options in Chapter 6 on sex).

Sexual positions that were comfortable prior to birth may no longer work after birth, at least for a little while. If you sustained a severe perineal tear or had an episiotomy, pressure or rubbing on the lower part of your vagina may be sensitive. Try lying on your back or side. If you had a cesarean birth, any pressure on your abdomen or scar may be too much. You may want to try being on top, in hands-and-knees position, or lying on your side. Explore different positions to find what works best for you during these early stages.

Set reasonable expectations. Your first time back to intercourse after birth may be more like a creative session of information-gathering rather than the steamiest sex of your life. Take some relaxing deep breaths before initiating sexual activity. Communicate with your partner about using a lubricant, trying a particular position, and going slowly. And more than anything else, don't push through pain. You may still be healing. Your pelvic floor muscles may be tense. Your tissues may be dry. If you experience pain, take a pause and return at a later time. If you experience bleeding, let your medical provider know, and check any incisions that may need additional medical attention. In Chapter 6, I have an entire section on painful sex to walk you step-by-step through getting relief.

A More Powerful Postpartum

I've never met a mom who doesn't recall some traumatic aspect of her postpartum pelvic floor experience. It may have been intense pain at her perineum and being unable to sit down for days, a cesarean scar so restricting that hunching over was the only way to walk, lifting a laundry basket and feeling a drop in her vagina, such severe back pain she couldn't pick up her other children, a bowel movement so painful she passed out on the toilet, or such severe burning when she peed that she held her bladder and needed to get catheterized. These experiences stick to your soul; even decades later, a lump still forms in your throat or your eyes water when you recount these awkward and painful moments.

When I meet these women and hear their stories, I feel saddened by their experiences, but I also feel empowered, because I know there are solutions. And I've witnessed hundreds of moms benefit from them. Pain and pelvic floor problems are *not* the inevitables of becoming a mother. These are *not* the sacrifices we should have to make. These are *not* the prices we have to pay to birth babies. Because *there is a better way.*

I am so incredibly hopeful that the tools and tips throughout this chapter help you recover from one of the most transformative times in your life. So that not only will your baby be cared for after birth, but also you.

CHAPTER 10

Your Pelvic Floor on (Meno)Pause

With every passing decade, I'm surprised not at what I lose with aging, but at what I gain. Looking back, my twenties were a bit of a shit show. Yes, I graduated college, earned a doctorate degree, and met my husband, but I was also riddled with self-doubt, insecurity, and indecision about my path in life. In my thirties, I became a mother, which has been not only the most rewarding role thus far but also the most demanding. Picking tiny Lego pieces out of my carpet is hard work. My pregnancies and births changed the trajectory of my career. I experienced firsthand the challenges women face in healthcare and launched my social media account, The Vagina Whisperer, and my online pelvic floor workout platform as a result.

Since entering my forties, I've found confidence in my career (pelvic health or bust!), my sense of self (trusting my own intuition more), and my body (embrace the side boob). I worry a lot less about being skinny and much more about being healthy. I care much less about people's opinions of me as I feel solid in my values. I also prioritize the importance of a good sunscreen, a great workout, and a solid night's sleep. Midlife is a great opportunity to shed all the BS that held us back in the past—and it is ripe for reinvention.

But the dominant paradigm tells us otherwise. Since entering my forties, I am also bombarded with an onslaught of ads for supplements, skin care serums, foods, injectables for both my face and vagina, and even shampoos to combat aging. You'd have to be living under a rock to not get the memo: the inevitable process of aging is something we need to fight for as long as possible. Don't get me wrong; I tweeze my gray hairs and have a solid nighttime skin care regimen, but discerning between aging "fixes" and what truly supports health in middle-age and our elder years is challenging.

Despite the joys of growing older, aging brings with it a set of concerns that require our attention. As we move into our forties and fifties when perimenopause and menopause hit, taking care of our pelvic floors becomes a nonnegotiable if we want to avoid pain, disability, or diapers down the line. The time we set aside to care for the strength, flexibility, and functioning of our pelvic floor needs to come before we color our hair and Botox our frown lines. If you don't, you'll end up with the forehead of a thirty-year-old, but you may be leaking urine when you laugh.

Perimenopause through menopause is a time of enormous hormonal transition. And because our hormones have a huge impact on our floor, we will all experience a moderate to severe number of changes to our pelvic floor during this time. You might wake up a few extra times a night to pee or have Mojave-level vaginal dryness during sex. You might leak a bit of urine when coughing or sneezing. You might even have a heavier flow during your now irregular periods. And many of us are having babies in our late thirties and into our forties, so the transition from pregnancy to postpartum to perimenopause blurs together, and we are unsure where one season stops and another starts. The result can be pelvic floor problems that are inconvenient, uncomfortable, and confusing—but which we still might think are par for the course.

Menopause does bring with it some good news. For example, you no longer have to worry about period blood staining your white pants. But just as your hormones decline, so do your muscle strength and collagen production, which contribute to the pelvic floor issues women experience in midlife. Although it feels like women never get a break when it comes to our pelvic floors, there is a lot we can do to ease these transitions and improve our symptoms when they arise.

How the Pelvic Floor and Menopause Work Together

Menopause, by definition, occurs on the day when you have not had a period for twelve consecutive months. On average, women reach this monumental day at the age of fifty-one, and it's something we should commemorate—just as we should commemorate the day we get our periods as young women. This day is a turning of the page into a new season of life, and a mighty good reason to get together for mahjong or margaritas with friends!

Menopause is the natural biological process when your ovaries stop releasing eggs and halt production of estrogen, testosterone, and progesterone. After this point, you will no longer have a period (so you can officially toss the tampons or period underwear), and you can no longer get pregnant (peace out, birth control!). But because estrogen and other hormone levels basically take a cliff dive, there are some not-so-fun symptoms like hair loss, weight gain, and low libido.

Perimenopause can start ten to fifteen years *before* menopause and is a time when your hormones are more unpredictable than hurricane season in New Orleans. Think of perimenopause as the equivalent of getting a notification that some bad weather is headed your way. Prepare for the hormonal shifts of menopause, just like you prepare for a hurricane by gathering flashlights and extra gallons of water. With proper prep, you might end up with something as benign as a lawn chair blown over in the wind. But with no prep it all, menopause might feel like the roof is getting ripped off your house.

If you are in your thirties and have irregular periods, need more lube during sex, or feel low-energy no matter how much you sleep, you may already be in perimenopause. For those who reach menopause later in life (say, fifty-five and beyond), you may feel like you are oh-so-ready to transition to your next season, but Aunt Flo just keeps popping up. Either way, your hormones spend over a decade in roller-coaster mode. In addition to irregular periods, you'll likely experience other physical changes that may include hot flashes, night sweats, chills, headaches, muscle aches, dry skin, mood changes, anxiety, depression, irritability, decreased libido, difficulty sleeping, heart palpitations . . . and a more vulnerable pelvic floor. *Awesome.* Many of us tend to overlook these pelvic health changes because we are managing a lot of the other day-to-day struggles (not to mention work or child-rearing or aging parents). And further, if we do mention bladder or sexual health changes to our health-care providers, they chalk them up to "a normal part of aging."

If by now you are completely overwhelmed and dreading this life stage, take a few deep breaths, return to the first paragraph of this chapter, and remember that aging also comes bearing gifts. Not all age-related changes are bad. The day I hit menopause, I am taking all of the money my future self will save on period products and treating myself to a spa day. Because yet again, I have entered another season as a woman, have lived another year, and I want to celebrate that. But I get it. Change is hard. While the culture might tell us to reject or resist aging, when it comes to your pelvic floor, you can't totally stop the shift in hormones and the shifts in collagen production—so instead, I encourage you to own it. Own these pelvic floor changes, seek to understand them, and then follow the protocols in this chapter—and you will for sure struggle far less.

Consider Denise, a fifty-two-year-old woman who came to see me because she noticed bright red blood when wiping with toilet paper after having sex with her husband. Blood when wiping is not uncommon if you are around or on your period, but Denise had not had a period in over a year. She reported feeling raw during sex and became concerned when she noticed pink stains in her underwear afterwards. While these changes were subtle, she did the right thing by coming to pelvic floor therapy to get things checked out. When I inquired about other pelvic health symptoms, Denise told me she was waking a lot at night to pee and had been getting one to two urinary tract infections a year for the past several years.

Denise thought all these issues were odd, but not too problematic. Unbeknownst to her, these nighttime bathroom trips and bleeding during sex were menopause-related. Decreased estrogen levels due to menopause caused her vaginal tissues to become thin, fragile, and more prone to tearing during sex. Changes in her hormones were also behind her frequent urination and irritation to her bladder. I informed her that these pelvic floor changes were related to menopause and that they could, in fact, improve. She asked why no one had told her this sooner. *This is a common refrain.* Time and time again, I hear that women just haven't been informed that although these changes are common, help is available.

After pregnancy and childbirth, menopause is the next biggest risk factor for a woman to develop pelvic floor problems. We women will live an average of eighty years, meaning we might spend up to half of our lives in a perimenopausal and postmenopausal state with hormones that are going haywire. Our pelvic floors *will* change. Our tissues, muscles, and organs will change. But you can accomplish so much by educating yourself early in your life, accepting the changes, and then incorporating new routines and exercises so the changes don't take total control.

Recently I saw on the news a seventy-one-year-old woman who had previously been suffering from arthritis and joint pain and could barely walk up stairs. Her daughter was a personal trainer, and convinced her mom to start lifting weights, work out daily, and make dietary changes to combat her chronic health issues. As a result, her mom lost seventy pounds and felt she was in the best shape of her life—at seventy-one. She is an example of what we can accomplish in our later years. We know to wear sunscreen to protect our skin. We remember to get our mammo-grams to screen for breast cancer. We are told to strength-train to prevent osteoporosis. Likewise, we can take time to support our pelvic floor when we approach and enter menopause.

Let's go through each of the hormones and consider what happens when they decline.

ESTROGEN:
YOUR KEEPS-THIS-SHIP-SAILING HORMONE

During perimenopause, your ovarian production of estrogen gradually declines until you reach menopause, when your ova-ries completely stop producing estrogen altogether. When your estrogen plummets, it affects your musculoskeletal system, your cardiovascular system, and even your nervous system and brain (hello, brain fog!). Your pelvic floor function—from the urinary system to your reproductive system—will also shift. As men-tioned in Chapter 5 on periods, estrogen is largely responsible for regulating our periods, increasing vaginal lubrication, keep-ing our vaginal walls plump and strong, and enhancing sexual desire. And because your pelvic floor contains a zillion estro-gen receptors, when estrogen isn't there to latch on and do its job, our vaginal walls and pelvic floor muscles become less sup-portive, less heroic, and more prone to injury. Before and after menopause, you will experience some (or, unfortunately, all) of the following:

- Vulvar and vaginal dryness
- Painful sex
- Urinary incontinence
- Pelvic organ prolapse
- Increased urgency of urination
- Increased frequency of urination
- Frequent urinary tract infections
- Waking at night to pee
- Decreased libido

But wait, there's more. Estrogen also contributes to the production of collagen, a protein that our bodies produce to help tighten skin, strengthen bones, and aid in muscle strength and performance. If you walk down the aisle at Whole Foods, you'll at some point come across an entire section of collagen powders, pills, and supplements promising thicker hair and nails, stronger bones, and tighter skin. As estrogen, and thus collagen, decrease with aging, we are met with more wrinkles in our skin, weaker bones, and less muscle mass. Women lose about one third of their skin's collagen in the first five years after menopause and roughly 2% each year for the next twenty years. So we can thank our estrogen and collagen decline not only for our crow's feet but also for our thinning vaginal tissues and bladder walls.

While these pelvic health changes are a "normal part of aging," menopause should not mean we are all doomed to experience urinary leakage and discomfort during sex. It does mean, however, it's high time to commit to pelvic floor strengthening and flexibility exercises (which you can easily do while binge-watching your favorite show on Netflix at night).

PROGESTERONE: YOUR PERIOD-AND-POOP HORMONE

Progesterone is a hormone that prepares the uterine lining for pregnancy with each menstrual cycle and, along with estrogen, takes a nosedive during perimenopause. Often the very first symptom of perimenopause is when you get ghosted by your always regular monthly period due to decreased progesterone levels. You may experience irregular periods, and your cycles may be much longer than the average twenty-three to thirty-five days and become less frequent.

The imbalance of estrogen to progesterone can also lead to really heavy periods. I'm talking about a crime scene bathroom situation when you've soaked through a super plus tampon in an hour and stained your undies. If you are on hormonal birth control, your periods will be lighter and more consistent, and you will be fortunate enough to skip out on this monthly messy situation. If you have a hormonal IUD for birth control, you may not get a period at all. But for the rest of us, our period may become irregular and heavy as perimenopause is in full swing.

Progesterone levels also affect how well poop moves through your colon, which is why a few days out of every menstrual cycle you may experience bloating, abdominal discomfort, and constipation. You also may experience hard stools and constipation, leading to excess straining with bowel movements.

TESTOSTERONE:
YOUR SEXY-TIME-AND-STRENGTH HORMONE

We often think of testosterone as a male hormone, but women produce testosterone too. Testosterone falls under a group of hormones called androgens, which are sex hormones that stimulate puberty and increase blood flow to the vulva. Testosterone is made in our ovaries, adrenal glands, and fatty tissues—and you can thank big T for its role in mood support, energy, muscle mass, and sex drive. As testosterone and other androgens decrease with aging and menopause, so does your muscle strength, mood, memory, energy levels, and sexual function.

Different from the rapid decline of estrogen and progesterone, testosterone levels peak in our thirties but then decline at a gradual pace through the menopausal transition. Low testosterone levels are likely the biggest contributor to a declining sex drive and a major factor in decreased overall muscle mass in your body.

Will hormone replacement therapy (HRT) fix my pelvic floor changes during perimenopause and menopause?

Tackling the pelvic floor changes related to menopause is not an *or*, it's an *and*. HRT is supported in the research as an effective treatment for hormonal supplementation during perimenopause and menopause and to aid in decreasing the negative changes in pelvic floor health. But a few caveats exist.

HRT comes in many forms ranging from oral pills to patches on the skin, pellets, gels, injections or creams, and suppositories to be used locally on the vulva and vagina. Typically a combination of these is used under the guidance of a physician who is well-versed in hormone therapy.

Additionally, HRT is not for everyone. It is not always recommended for some folks due to their medical history, like a history of breast cancer and other estrogen-driven cancers. Doing your research, working with your physician, and going with what feels right for you are essential when making the decision whether to use HRT and what types.

Last, HRT in isolation will not fix your pelvic floor problems. Regardless of whether you use hormone supplementation, you also *must* perform pelvic floor exercises to manage pelvic floor problems related to menopause. Start these exercises proactively during perimenopause and maintain healthy pelvic floor habits through menopause and beyond.

If you haven't gathered by now, menopause is a time when pelvic floor complaints run rampant. Women are hot and they have to pee. Sit at a table with women between the ages of forty and sixty and you will likely hear the following.

"Everything feels really dry, like my underwear sticks to my parts."

"Something is literally falling out of my vagina."

"Sex! What's that?!"

"I feel like I have to constantly pee."

"The shop is closed."

I only wish I could attend every forty- to sixty-something book club and women's group to address these common complaints that come up.

So what can *you* do? If menopause is far off in the distance, make yourself aware of the changes you should expect. If menopause looms on your doorstep, now is the time to begin the exercises and protocols offered in this chapter. And if menopause is years or even decades behind you, it's not too late. The goal is to implement pelvic floor tips and exercises to minimize the severity of your pelvic floor symptoms. You can have great sex well into your seventies. You don't need to resign yourself to buying incontinence diapers in bulk. And you *deserve* to live a life without constant pelvic discomfort.

I had my ovaries removed, and I am not yet menopausal. Can I expect the same changes in my pelvic floor during menopause?

Having your ovaries removed by a procedure called an oophorectomy can happen for a variety of reasons (typically cancer or disease). When these organs are removed, you will go through what is known as "surgical menopause," which will trigger an abrupt and rapid decline in estrogen, progesterone, and testosterone. Without ovaries, you will no longer have a period or be able to get pregnant.

All of the symptoms that occur in the time frame leading up to menopause occur all at once: hot flashes, night sweats, vaginal dryness, and low libido. Hormone replacement therapy can be a helpful treatment, unless your doctor advises otherwise based on certain preconditions. So ultimately, yes, you will experience the same changes one would with menopause.

But there are other things you can do to support your body after such an abrupt change. Follow the pelvic floor recommendations in this chapter, and consider using supplements like ashwagandha for stress relief, calcium and vitamin D for bone density, and fish oil for inflammation. And optimal sleep hygiene, regular weight-bearing and resistance exercise, proper nutrition, and hydration will be your friends.

Your Pelvic Floor and Menopause Protocol

Imagine me coming to your next girls-only weekend with you and all your BFFs. As your friend, after talking about my favorite lubes and whether sex gets better as we age (the answer is, it can!), I'd tell you a story about how I was initiated into perimenopause when I woke myself in the middle of the night thinking I'd peed the bed. Turns out my heavy period had completely soaked through my tampon and period underwear and seeped onto my favorite Egyptian cotton sheets. A new era had begun.

Then I would lay out my top six tips for pelvic floor preventative care during the hormone rodeo of this life phase. Yes, we've gone over some of these tips in previous chapters—but here I talk about the importance of these practices when our fertile years start to fade.

HYDRATE

If you're suffering from hot flashes and night sweats, you are losing water. And many of us might end up decreasing our water intake in an effort to minimize how often we pee . . . or leak. In addition, some medications we might take during the perimenopausal and menopausal years contribute to skin dryness and constipation, or have a diuretic effect, which pushes fluid through our bodies more quickly. So when we age, we actually need to work a little bit to stay hydrated. Water supports natural vaginal lubrication, dilutes your urine to decrease risk of urinary tract infections, and gets absorbed into our colon to aid in digestion and pooping. Your urine should be almost clear to a light yellow as an indicator you are adequately hydrated. So go get the giant water bottle and drink up, Buttercup. It's good for your skin too!

MOISTURIZE

Along with many of you, my facial skin care routine includes roughly six to eight steps on any given night. Fortunately, my vulva skin care routine has just one or two steps. During perimenopause and menopause, your vulvar and vaginal tissues lose elasticity, get super dry, and can feel itchy and burn. In Chapter 6 on sex, I cover a lot of options for vulvar moisturizers and lubricants. When perimenopause arrives, it becomes even more important to regularly and consistently apply a moisturizer to your vulva and vagina. To keep it simple: apply a pH-balanced, paraben-free moisturizer to the vulva at the same time every day. Lots of vulva balm and moisturizer options are out there. Try several to find one that works best for your tissues.

MOVE

Muscle mass and bone density decrease with aging, which leads to general muscle weakness and fragile bones. The easiest and most accessible exercise you can do at any age is walk. When walking, the impact on your bones increases your bone density and strengthens the muscles in your core, hips, and pelvis. Walking can also improve balance, which we tend to lose as we grow into our older years (hence the likelihood of falls as we age), and it brings blood flow to our pelvic floor. Whether it's parking toward the back of the parking lot, a nightly loop around the neighborhood, or a morning mall walk with your best bud, get your steps in. Weighted vests for walking are an option for additional benefits of bone health and muscle-building. Regular exercise also aids in sleep, which suffers during the peri years, and it increases production of endorphins, which are feel-good hormones that can boost libido—a bonus side effect!

STRENGTH-TRAIN

With aging, we experience a decrease in bone density, bone strength, and pelvic floor muscle strength. These bone changes also increase your risk of a rounded spine, which can further impair how well the pelvic floor muscles function and provide support for pelvic organs. A strength-training regimen using hand weights, resistance bands, or weight machines at the gym is critical. Strength training combats bone loss, helps new bone regeneration, strengthens weakened muscles, and improves posture. If you don't already strength-train, begin as early as thirty-five when testosterone levels start to decline. If you haven't started yet, it is never too late.

Current recommendations for strength training include two to four sessions a week, lifting free weights (preferred to using weight machines) for three sets of eight to twelve repetitions until muscle fatigue, which is a complex way of saying your muscles should be tired by that last repetition. Common exercises like biceps curls, overhead press, squats, and lunges can all be done at home, at the gym, and in a workout class and are a simple and effective way to start building muscle mass.

CO-CONTRACT

A co-contraction is a Kegel while doing something else at the same time. You can do them during your strength-training workouts, before a cough or a sneeze, or when lifting something heavy. To target the pelvic floor, you must also perform pelvic floor strengthening exercises to combat the gradual and inevitable increase in muscle and tissue strength. Your *Golden Girl* routine can include the pelvic floor strengthening regimen offered in Chapter 2, but you can also get more bang for your buck when you add in a Kegel co-contraction to your daily activities.

Try incorporating co-contractions into one regular activity you do every day. With time, it will become a habit.

ADDRESS THE FEMALE BRAIN

Last, but certainly not least, when it comes to your menopausal years, you need to address your mood and your mind. The way our brains function is a matter of chemistry, and when that chemistry changes due to hormonal fluctuations, higher cortisol levels, and the stress of navigating a major shift in our lives, our moods will shift. Many women report feeling like a different person in their menopausal years because of these brain shifts. Anxiety, depression, irritability, and anger will frequently rear their heads. You may feel down and depressed about an onset of urinary leakage preventing you from running or traveling. You may feel distance from your partner with whom you have decreased sexual activity. You may feel grief about no longer being able to get pregnant. Not only will you find yourself next-level frustrated when your home thermostat is two degrees above your liking, but you might find yourself far more irritable over details that you used to shrug off.

I mention all this because taking care of our emotions and moods will impact our ability to weather the changes to our pelvic floor. Recall in Chapter 1 how stress and distress can lead to tension in the pelvic floor? We need to be proactive about our moods. If you are more irritable, and spending time in nature is the secret sauce to ease your triggered mind, then make time for that twice-a-week hike. If sessions with your therapist help you navigate the changes in midlife, make some appointments. Even something as simple as cozying up with a pet can be an important and necessary calming force. Support for your mind is support for your body.

The Misadventures of Menopause

Okay, you probably get it now. Menopausal changes are inevitable. But they are especially hard if they go unaddressed for a prolonged period of time. The consequences can go from mild to severe. Little leaks can lead to full-blown bladder emptying when you stand up. Skid marks in your undies can lead to complete loss of your bowels when you can't make it to the bathroom. A slight bulge in your vagina can lead to significant pelvic organ prolapse requiring surgery. These examples are not to scare you, but rather to encourage you to take prevention seriously and proactively address pelvic floor issues now.

Throughout my career, there have been some landmark moments that propelled me to be outspoken about women's need for better pelvic healthcare, which ultimately led me to writing this book. One of those times was during my own pregnancy and preparation for birth, when I discovered firsthand the profound benefits of pelvic floor therapy. And the second, equally as impactful, was when I treated postmenopausal women who had undergone surgery to repair pelvic organ prolapse. As I mentioned previously, many of these women had synthetic mesh surgically inserted into their vaginal walls to provide support but grave pelvic floor complications emerged when the mesh started eroding.

One patient stood out. Martha, a fifty-five-year-old woman and mom of three "big babies," was postmenopausal when she came to see me. Her first pelvic floor struggles started in her forties, when she began having occasional urine leaks on her morning jogs. Her leakage got worse over the next few years, which forced her to stop running altogether. At an annual visit with her gynecologist, she was diagnosed with a bladder prolapse. A simple surgery using a small piece of mesh to tack her bladder up would do the trick. She had the surgery, and an easy recovery followed. But months later she felt a sharp shooting pain in her vagina. Thinking and hoping it would go away with time, she brushed it off.

The tipping point came when she was having sex with her husband, and said he felt something scratching his penis. After her vaginal pain increased and another attempt at sex resulted in a scraped penis, she checked in with her surgeon, who discovered that the mesh from her surgery was not only piercing through her vaginal wall but also infected (and it was indeed scraping her husband's penis). The mesh was shredded into little pieces, all of which had become embedded throughout her vaginal walls. Not easy to remove. Now in severe pain, Martha underwent three additional surgeries to remove as much of the mesh as possible. And if that wasn't enough, the remaining scar tissue from the mesh continued to cause pain. And then her bladder prolapse returned. Martha was miserable.

Our healthcare system failed Martha. What started as small pelvic floor issues, which are quite common with age, spiraled into major long-term dysfunction and a surgery that went awry. I've seen a number of midlife women who have been traumatized from these complications. And during the course of treatment, I always lamented the fact that there was so much that could have helped these women's conditions, which would have avoided surgical intervention altogether.

Many of the conditions below can occur at any point in life, but due to the hormonal declines and decreased tissue and muscle support, they are more likely to happen or get worse during menopause. The following tips can not only improve these situations but perhaps even prevent them from occurring. Here we go.

PEEING YOUR PANTS

Both stress incontinence (leaks with coughs and sneezes) and urge incontinence (leaks with the urge to pee) are far more likely during menopause. Decreased muscle strength and less closure of the urethral sphincter lead to more leaks during activities like walking to the bathroom and even simply getting up from a chair. If urinary leakage is an issue during your menopausal journey, go to the leakage guidelines on bladder health in Chapter 3. Memorize them. Practice them daily. But in addition to those general guidelines, try incorporating the following practices into your daily routine for this extra-special phase.

FOLLOW THE PELVIC FLOOR STRENGTHENING PROTOCOL

Your pelvic organs need support from your pelvic floor muscles. Your urinary and anal sphincters need to hold in pee and poop. Strong Kegel contractions can help suppress the constant urge to pee. Follow the pelvic floor strengthening protocol in Chapter 2 to increase pelvic floor muscle strength and connective tissue support. You might be asking yourself, "Will I have to do my pelvic floor exercises forever?" And my answer is yes, just like you have to brush your teeth every day. Just five minutes a day of strengthening exercises go a long way. Your muscles get progressively weaker with aging. You have to continue to strengthen your pelvic floor muscles to combat that.

Perform three sets of ten quick contractions daily, relaxing fully between repetitions. It is important to perform them in the standing position, as standing and walking are common positions where leakage occurs. Also perform three sets of ten long hold contractions daily, holding each contraction for ten to twenty seconds, with five to ten seconds of rest between contractions.

KEGEL BEFORE YOU COUGH OR SNEEZE

Not only do your pelvic floor muscles get weaker with aging, but they activate more slowly as well. Imagine how you get out of a chair when you're young. You can just jump up. With aging, we tend to move more slowly, which is also true with our pelvic floor muscles, leading to an increased risk of leakage. Try performing "The Knack," a pelvic floor contraction/Kegel before you cough or sneeze, to help close your sphincters to prevent urinary leakage. Occasional leaks may still occur, but "The Knack" will enhance your pelvic floor strength and improve the activation of your pelvic floor muscles. This is another "must perform forever" tip.

MANAGE NIGHTTIME PEES

Frequent peeing before bedtime or waking multiple times at night to pee are common experiences during perimenopause and after menopause. Not only are they stealing precious z's, but walking in the dark or when you are tired can be dangerous. This, coupled with weaker bones during menopause, increases your risk of falls and fractures. Do yourself a favor and clear a pathway from your bed to the bathroom, removing all rugs, clothing, wires, or anything that can be a tripping hazard. Drink the majority of your fluids in the first half of the day, and cut off fluids two hours before bedtime. If an urge presents, use the urge suppression techniques in Chapter 3 to help with frequent urination. Over time, these techniques will train your body to go before your bedtime, rather than three to five times in the night.

POOPING YOUR PANTS

Unfortunately, pooping your pants as you age is a common occurrence as well. Fecal incontinence, or the loss of the stool, is discussed in Chapter 4 on bowel function, but commonly occurs with menopause due to decreased strength of the external anal sphincter along with loose stools. Fecal incontinence can start as skid marks or streaks in your underwear or feel like you can't clean your bottom well enough. If unaddressed, it can progress to complete loss of bowel contents with the urge to poop. This is debilitating and highly impactful for women, often leading to fear of leaving home, avoiding travel and socialization, and increased risk of skin irritation in the tush area. Good news is, there are a number of preventative PT tricks—and things you can do to improve the situation.

FIRM UP YOUR POOP

Loose stools are more likely to leak. And because of hormonal fluctuations, dietary changes, and side effects of medication, loose stools can be a common occurrence during menopause. Review the fecal incontinence section in Chapter 4. You may find long-term dietary changes are necessary. Decreasing dairy, fatty foods, and fried foods can lower the likelihood of loose stools. And regularly eat a piece of white toast, a potato, or a bowl of rice to keep your poop solid and easier to hold.

PROTECT YOUR PRECIOUS TISSUES

If you experience any fecal staining (aka skid marks in your undies), it is important to protect your skin and tissues so other problems don't arise. Moisture and fecal matter next to your skin can lead to irritation and infection. If you notice staining, change your underwear as soon as possible. Or use a liner inside your underwear. You can easily change out the liner when the staining occurs. I recommend using organic cotton incontinence and menstrual hygiene products. And remember to bring a spare change of undergarments when you are traveling. When you are home, you can use a bidet to clean your bottom, then pat yourself dry with toilet paper, or use a hair dryer on a cold setting to dry.

STRENGTHEN YOUR BACKSIDE

Your external anal sphincter is skeletal muscle that can be strengthened. Performing the pelvic floor strengthening protocol in Chapter 2, with a focus on some specific exercises, will significantly help you "hold it" if the urge arises, so you can get to the bathroom in time.

- Bridges with a Kegel. Lie on your back with knees bent and feet planted firmly on the ground. Place a pillow or ball (about the size of a soccer ball) between your knees. Perform a Kegel contraction and squeeze your knees together gently. Maintaining the Kegel and knee squeeze, lift your hips off the floor until they line up with your knees and shoulder. Hold for five seconds and return to the starting position. Repeat for three sets of ten repetitions.
- Squats with a Kegel. In a standing position, contract your pelvic floor and focus on squeezing the anal sphincter

as you lower down into the squat and as you return to upright standing. Perform three sets of ten repetitions.
- Endurance Kegels. Hold your Kegel for up to thirty seconds with thirty seconds of rest between repetitions. If a thirty-second hold is a challenge, start with a five-second hold and five seconds of rest, increasing to ten-second holds and ten seconds of rest, then twenty-second holds and twenty seconds of rest. Perform ten contractions daily in the standing position. Bonus: place more of the weight in your heels when doing standing Kegels to activate your external anal sphincter (your butthole). You can hold on to a countertop for balance.

PELVIC ORGAN PROLAPSE

Together, estrogen, progesterone, and testosterone support the strength of our floors, so it can feel like three strikes and you're out when all three begin to subside. As you recall from Chapter 1, one of the primary functions of the pelvic floor is to support your organs held in the bowl, which it does with the help of ligaments that suspend your organs in your pelvic cavity.

Think of a boat in a dock: your pelvic organs (uterus, bladder, and rectum) are the boat. Ropes are attached from the side of the boat to the dock; the ropes are your ligaments. The boat is floating and supported by the water underneath; the water is your pelvic floor muscles. If the water level (your pelvic floor) drops or decreases, the boat (the organs) will rely more on the ropes (ligaments) to support it, and those ropes will stretch, fray, or even break if they are unable to support the weight of the boat. When this happens, the boat will fall down (your pelvic organs will prolapse).

Pelvic organ prolapse (POP) occurs when your organs descend in your pelvic cavity and push into your vaginal walls due to decreased tissue support from above. POP can happen with chronic straining, decreased muscle support that occurs with menopause or after childbirth, and decreased ligament support (which becomes more likely during menopause due to decreased collagen). Half of all women over the age of fifty have some degree of POP.

POP can be surgically fixed by pulling the organs back up using your internal ligaments and/or muscles, which is the equivalent of replacing the ropes supporting the boat. The challenge with this remedy is that it does not raise the water level supporting the boat (the pelvic floor muscles have not been strengthened to support the organs), and the boat will continue to hang on the ropes, making it likely they will break again. Chronic straining or not breathing properly with exercise are the equivalent of jumping on the boat and can increase the risk of POP. This along with not properly strengthening the pelvic floor muscles is why POP surgeries often fail after ten years and must be repeated. In order to give your organs optimal and longer-lasting support, you have to strengthen the pelvic floor (raise the water level) *and* scale back on activities that increase your risk of prolapse occurring (stop jumping on the boat).

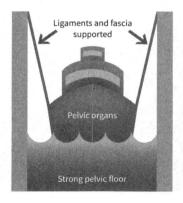 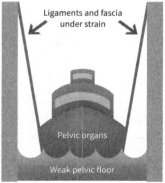

Boat supported by ropes and water as an analogy for pelvic organs supported by ligaments and pelvic floor muscles

My top three tips for prolapse are to decrease straining (stop jumping on the boat), get support (take the pressure off the ropes, or ligaments), and strengthen your pelvic floor (raise the water). All of these must be done to effectively prevent prolapse and prevent it from getting worse.

STOP JUMPING ON THE BOAT

High-pressure activities like coughing and sneezing are often unavoidable, so using "The Knack" mentioned earlier by contracting your pelvic floor before a cough or sneeze will help support your organs with the increased pressure from above. But the biggest pressures on your pelvic organs will likely come from straining: straining to poop, pushing when you pee, and holding your breath when lifting or exercising. Those activities place significantly increased pressure on your pelvic floor muscles and ligaments, and over time weaken those structures and contribute to prolapse.

POOP PROPERLY

Support your perineum and exhale when you poop. Constipation puts more strain on your pelvic floor compared to coughing, running, or even jumping. Keep your poops soft and easy to pass (refer back to Chapter 4 for guidance on optimal pooping habits). Proactively place a piece of toilet paper on your perineum and press up as you bear down and exhale to poop.

PEE PROPERLY

Sit down and lean forward or back when you pee if you feel like you don't empty your bladder well. Play around with this a bit to see if leaning forward or backward helps you to empty. After peeing, shake your hips side to side, stand up and sit down again, and see if any additional urine empties. This maneuver, called double-voiding, helps empty any additional urine. Don't push when you pee, which places unnecessary pressure on your bladder and pelvic floor (more jumping on the boat). Sit, breathe, and relax your pelvic floor muscles, and your bladder can push pee out for you.

EXHALE WITH EXERTION

Holding your breath leads to increased pressure on your pelvic floor muscles and ligaments, which are already vulnerable and under duress during the perimenopause and menopause periods. Exhalation prevents an excess of pressure on your organs and muscles and is a necessary lifelong habit, but particularly during menopause, when tissues, muscles, and ligaments tend to be weaker and more prone to injury when lifting a bag of groceries, lifting a child, pushing out a hard poop, or even lifting dumbbells in your fitness classes.

USE AN INTERNAL SUPPORT DEVICE

Depending on the extent of your prolapse and the cause (weak ligaments versus weak muscles), using an internal device can offer support to your vaginal walls and pelvic organs. A pessary is a silicone medical device that is inserted into the vaginal canal to lift your organs and support your vaginal walls if weakness and prolapse occur. Due to the varying types of prolapse and its causes, a medical provider such as a nurse practitioner, urologist, urogynecologist, gynecologist, or even a pelvic floor therapist in some states can fit you for a pessary to find the right one for your needs.

There are over-the-counter options that can be used as internal bladder or pelvic floor support. Using a lubricant may be necessary when inserting to combat vaginal dryness. If your vulvar and vaginal tissues are frail and thin around menopause, topical estrogen (prescribed by a medical provider) and a daily vulvar and vaginal moisturizer can help.

These devices can be worn throughout the day or only during time when you may experience more pressure, leakage, or symptoms, such as in the afternoons or later in the day, when exercising, jogging, or hiking, during times of prolonged standing or walking (think walking the aisles of Target), or while performing your pelvic floor exercises.

STRENGTHEN YOUR PELVIC FLOOR

You have to raise the water. I mentioned the importance of strengthening as part of your menopause protocol. Holding Kegels for a longer amount of time can improve the endurance of your pelvic floor muscles and offer more muscular support for your prolapse. The majority of the pelvic floor muscles are endurance muscle fibers, and you will work more of the muscle and help support your pelvic organs better with endurance exercises. If your muscles fatigue easily when you perform endurance contractions, try them while lying down or lying on your side, and then progress to standing. Performing these exercises in the morning before your muscles get fatigued will help.

GETTING IT ON . . . MENOPAUSE-STYLE

Sex may feel like it isn't worth the effort during menopause due to discomfort and bodily changes. Fortunately there are lots of ways to help you enjoy sex into your later years.

GET CREATIVE

Because decreased estrogen and testosterone levels contribute to a lower libido, you will need to get creative about integrating physical connection into your life if you are wanting to get the mojo going again. Planning ahead for a weekly romp, having a morning session before afternoon fatigue hits, or even bringing in different sex toys to spice things up in the bedroom can be helpful. If we are talking about penetrative sex and your partner is also experiencing sexual challenges, like difficulty maintaining an erection, using toys and outercourse (sexual activity not including insertion of anything into the vagina) can also continue to promote connection, intimacy, and satisfaction.

CHANGE POSITIONS

Because your pelvic floor muscles get increasingly fatigued, trying different positions for intercourse may help you find one that is more comfortable for your prolapse. Try these modifications. If you have a bladder or urethra prolapse, try hands-and-knees position on all fours (known as doggy style). If you have a rectocele or rectal prolapse, try lying on your back or on your side. With a uterine prolapse or apical prolapse (top of the vagina coming down), opt for lying on your back, side, or on all fours to avoid being on top.

LUBE IT UP

Without question, proactively use a lubricant during intercourse. Your vulvar and vaginal tissues are prone to dryness, tearing, and increased risk of infection, and using a lubricant on your partner and/or at the vaginal opening will decrease friction and promote pleasure. See how to choose the right lube in Chapter 6, on sex.

USE IT OR LOSE IT

If you decide your sex life is a thing of the past, good on you and skip ahead. But many women grieve the decline in sexual activity due to the changes in their bodies and those of their partners. Blood flow to the pelvic region from arousal, orgasm, and exercise all help maintain healthy tissues and pelvic floor muscles to keep your vagina ready to rumble. Not having sexual activity or intercourse for prolonged periods of time is like not watering a garden for months or years. Then you go back for vegetables, only to realize the soil is dried up and all your plants have died. You must tend the garden to keep it lively.

Check out Chapter 6 on sexual health to not only understand the relationship between our pelvic floors and sex but also gain tips and insights to start having pain-free and pleasurable sex.

MASTERING MENOPAUSE

When we reach our menopausal years, we are entering what you might call our wisdom years. We have the opportunity to take all of our life experience and self-knowledge to manage our health and well-being from a wiser and more empowered place. Menopause brings with it pelvic floor changes and challenges, but with education and taking ownership over those changes, we can make them far more manageable. Denise, who I mentioned earlier, came to therapy and learned how to use vaginal dilators to relax her pelvic floor muscles and prepare for intercourse. She used a vulvar moisturizer and requested a topical estrogen cream for her vulva and vagina to plump her tissues. She incorporated Kegels into her Silver Sneakers workouts at the gym. She cut off her fluids a few hours before bedtime and used urge suppression techniques to cut down her frequent nighttime pees. Denise got better, as do so many women who get the support they deserve.

I am just now entering my perimenopausal years, as are many of my friends. On a girls' night out, the conversation often weaves its way back to the pelvic floor. One friend talks about how heavy her periods are. Another shares that she has occasional leaks when playing tennis. Another discloses she is choosing sleep over sex even though her kids are entering middle school. I am thrilled I can sit with friends and have these conversations, share that The Vagina Whisperer's vagina is also changing, and talk through the many things we can do to support our floors.

We have fumbled our entire lives as vagina owners, from when we had our first period to our first pelvic exam, from our first sexual experience to navigating pregnancy and birth. We are entering a stage in life when we are wiser, when we know we need to be the drivers in our health. We can be proactive, we can be informed, and we can talk to each other and learn from one another. We don't need to suffer. In fact, we can enjoy our bodies and pelvic floors well into our golden years.

CHAPTER 11

When Your Pelvic Floor Is a Pain

When my son was five, he and I spent Mother's Day weekend planting flowers in our garden. After a trip to the store to pick out some of his favorites, we got on our knees to pack in new soil and give our front yard a glow up while soaking in the perfect eighty-degree weather before the sticky New Orleans summer heat rolled in. As far as Mother's Day goes, it was pretty much ideal.

But the next day, little itchy spots popped up on my knees. And when something itches, I scratch it. And scratch it some more. And suddenly, I had an intensely painful reaction complete with pea-sized bumps all over my ankles, shins, and thighs. The pain and itching were so bad that I could not sleep, sit, or hold a conversation. I just wanted to crawl out of my skin.

The day after that, I was forced to cancel my patients because I could not bear to wear my work pants or have anything on my legs. I was completely incapable of taking my mind off my suffering to care for others. Instead, I made an emergency appointment with a dermatologist who said, "Looks like a skin reaction. Just take Benadryl and use over-the-counter anti-itch cream." I followed these instructions as the bumps continued to spread over my legs, back, neck, and chest like in a horror movie. I packed ice packs around my body to numb my skin. After the cold wore off, I got into a warm oatmeal bath to soothe the pain and itching. And I applied every anti-itch cream to every nook and cranny of my body to get some relief.

After a few weeks and a whole lot of medication, patience, and extreme restraint from scratching, the pain *finally* let up. It turns out I had an allergic reaction to the soil that led to dermatographia, a condition causing welts on my skin in response to the scratching. The point of the story is, being in distress for several weeks controlled my life. It was physically uncomfortable, but mentally and emotionally taxing as well. I was a wreck. My discomfort got in the way of my ability to work, think, exercise, sleep, and be present for my family.

This is what pain and discomfort does to us. It has the potential to bring your life to a screeching halt. I always thought I could handle pain relatively well. Many of us do. I had two unmedicated births, which were *very* painful, but that kind of ache was temporary, and I knew the end result would be something wonderful—a child. The difference with my skin reaction was that it was constant and relentless, and it wasn't producing a cute newborn baby. The unknown of it alone was psychologically taxing.

The suffering from my skin reaction was the closest I've come to what my patients experience when they have pelvic pain. And in my case, I could see the evidence of my pain on my skin! Pelvic pain is not an itchy bump on skin, a burn on a finger, or a broken bone on an X-ray. It cannot always be seen, but it is just as real and often even more debilitating. It can arise from an unknown cause, be difficult to diagnose, and be even more challenging to cure. Pelvic pain can make it difficult to sit down, get up from a chair, drive to work, pee, have a bowel movement, or wear pants.

We've looked at different forms of pain and discomfort throughout the book—from constipation pain to pain with sex—but here at the end of the book, I want to address pain in general. Many women experience more amorphous and general pelvic pain. And they can't identify the cause. Pelvic pain can be sharp and shooting, dull and achy, throbbing, itchy, burning, searing, or ringing. It can vary in intensity, duration, and location. But overall, pelvic pain is often unbearable, and it drains our life force.

One in four women experiences some mysterious pelvic pain in their lifetime. If you are hurting now, this chapter is for you. And if you don't have pelvic pain of any kind, this chapter is also for you—because understanding the workings of pelvic pain can be handy for prevention, dealing with it if you face it later in life, or even supporting someone struggling with it. But what is pain, anyway? A basic understanding of pain and how it works is an important first step in addressing how to relieve it, particularly when it is in your pelvic region.

Pain is sensory information sent from our nerves or tissues to our brain to let us know something is not quite right in our bodies, and we need support or protection. Depending on how long it lasts, pain can be either acute or chronic. Acute pain comes on suddenly, typically as a result of an injury from an event like breaking a bone or birthing a child. But if pain persists for weeks or months on end, even after the injury has healed, it becomes chronic. Chronic pain often happens because of how we respond to the original acute injury. Perhaps we have tense muscles, limited mobility, or nerve damage. Chronic pain is much more mysterious and harder to treat—given how it can lead to a slew of additional challenges like depression, anxiety, insomnia, fatigue, and muscle tension. A lot of the pelvic pain patients I see in my clinic suffer from chronic pain. Very often they don't know the source of the pain, and almost always they have no clue how to address it.

Pain can also be characterized by where it originates and what it feels like. Nociceptive pain, the most common type, is the result of pain receptors in your tissues, skin, or internal organs from episodes like stubbing your toe, tearing a ligament in your knee, or bladder pain with a urinary tract infection. Neuropathic pain results from damage to our nerves or nervous system, often without a specific injury occurring. Neuropathic pain can feel tingling, sharp, shooting, or searing, like that feeling after you've sat on the toilet and scrolled on your phone for too long and then stood up to tingling in your feet like you are walking on pins and needles. That sensation can be attributed to a posture you hold for too long. But true neuropathic pain results from a touch that should not be painful, like clothing rubbing your skin or a simple loving tap from your partner, but causes extreme pain due to misfiring nerves or a dysfunctional nervous system.

Entire books on pelvic pain are available, some of which are listed in the back of this book, with deep dives into the causes of pain and tips for treatment. But ultimately, here's what you need to know: pelvic pain can't be seen, making it difficult to pinpoint what is going on within the pelvic bowl of nerves, muscles, and organs, and often leads to women suffering unnecessarily for very long periods of time. Pelvic pain is not a sling you wear on your arm where people may kindly offer you support or give you space to avoid further injuring you. On the outside, you look perfectly fine, but underneath, you are struggling. And those struggles affect your ability to do everything from sitting or wearing underwear to being able to work or have sex. In fact, on average, it can take up to *seven years* for a woman to get an accurate diagnosis of her pelvic pain.

By the time women with pelvic pain get to pelvic floor therapy, they've already suffered for years, seen multiple physicians, and even been told nothing is wrong with them. Some have even had parts of their body like their uterus or ovaries removed! At this point, the pain is likely chronic, requiring treatment that addresses not only the physical issue and limitation but also the mental and emotional components of what hurts. Physical pain can lead to changes in the brain and nervous system, requiring a more mind–body approach and multidisciplinary treatment for long-lasting healing.

One patient, Nancy, traveled over seven hundred miles from

Oklahoma City to New Orleans to see me for therapy. She had been experiencing severe vaginal and vulvar pain for almost ten years. The pain started one Saturday after riding bicycles with her husband. She and her husband loved to go for hour-long rides on the weekends. Over time, she began to feel a burning sensation on her labia every time she rode her bike, and she wasn't able to sit for the rest of the day after a ride. But who wants to give up a romantic bicycle voyage with their partner? She kept going. And after a while, Nancy's labia hurt all the time, and her vulva burned every time she peed. She stopped wearing underwear and wore skirts during the day and T-shirts at night to sleep. She could not sit at work, so she stood all day. And then came the foot and back pain. She stopped having sex because the thought of touching the area made her tense. She stopped going on bike rides with her husband because any pressure on her labia caused searing pain. I only wish I could have helped her sooner.

Nancy's pain journey continued. She had multiple treatments including antibiotics for possible infections (although the tests were always negative), creams to numb her labia, nerve blocks to decrease sensation to the area, and Botox to relax her pelvic floor muscles, which worked a tiny bit but wore off after several months. Finally she met with a surgeon who recommended she have her labia removed. Desperate, she went through with the surgery. Afterwards, she still could not sit, the sutures itched, and wiping after peeing and pooping was excruciating, so she spritzed the area with water as best she could. Worst of all, after the initial recovery period passed, her labia pain was still there. Upon returning to see her surgeon and reporting her lack of relief, he said, "I just didn't get enough tissue. We need to go back and trim more." Nancy agreed to do one more surgery and had more of her labia tissue removed, but her pain, yet again, did not improve.

It was only then that she made it to pelvic floor therapy, still in search of relief. And it helped. Nancy was able to decrease the tension of her pelvic floor muscles with internal trigger point massage in therapy and using an internal pelvic wand at home for self-treatment. She performed daily stretches and breathing techniques at the start and end of each day and when her pain started to increase after prolonged sitting. She worked with vaginal dilators, focusing less on insertion into her vagina and more on gentle touch of the vulva and vaginal opening, retraining her brain that touch does not necessarily equal threat. She started wearing loose-fitting underwear again. She took big, deep breaths to start her urine stream, which helped her pelvic floor stay relaxed, and she had less burning when she peed. She was able to sit at work for longer periods of time using a seat cushion. Her back and foot pain decreased as a result. She didn't go back to bike riding with her husband, and she didn't return to sex. But she got pieces of her life back after an incredibly long journey of pain and recovery.

Early diagnosis and treatment of pelvic floor muscle dysfunction are super important steps for preventing and managing pelvic floor discomfort. You can see a pelvic therapist in person or simply turn to the tools in this chapter. You do not have to suffer. Relief is possible.

How the Pelvic Floor and Pain Go Together

Pelvic pain is complex and multifactorial. It can be like chasing a ghost. Sometimes it begins after slipping on steps and landing on your tailbone. It could be residual from a urinary tract or yeast infection. It may be suffering from childbirth or a surgery. It can be from riding a mechanical bull or leapfrogging an entire 10K. But for many people with pelvic pain, the pain starts when no danger is in sight. And complicating it even more, the origin of the pain isn't always where it's felt. No matter the origin or cause, pelvic pain almost always involves the nerves and muscles of the pelvic floor. And when we learn how the nerves and muscles work together, we can begin to understand the pain we might be experiencing—both the why of the pain and how to help the pain.

When you remember the sheer complexity of the pelvic floor anatomy, it can begin to make sense that pelvic pain can be so mysterious. Thirty-six muscles attach to the bones in your pelvis. And dozens of nerve branches extend from your spinal cord to your pelvic floor that control sensation and muscle contraction and relaxation. Of these branches, sensory nerves carry signals to the brain that help you experience touch, taste, smell, and sight. If you touch a hot stove with your hand, sensory nerves in your hand send a signal to your brain to let you know that stimulus is painful. When your brain receives the signal of danger or pain from the hot stove, motor nerves, which help with movement, carry signals from your brain to your muscles to move your hand so that it doesn't get burned. One of the primary motor and sensory pelvic nerves in the pelvic floor is our friend the pudendal nerve.

The pudendal nerve is an infamous nerve in the pelvic floor region that signals to the pelvic floor to contract the urinary and anal sphincters, and it is also responsible for sensation to the clitoris, vulva, and perineal body (the skin and tissue over the perineum). The Latin origin of the word *pudenda* means "to be ashamed," which unfortunately sheds light on perhaps why this part of our body, our genitals, was and still is poorly addressed in our medical system. Because of its pathway, this nerve can get injured easily. From prolonged sitting on a saddle (like on a bicycle or motorcycle) to the intensity of vaginal childbirth and even the movement of deep squats during workout routines, this nerve can get squished or irritated. And when this nerve gets injured, all sorts of issues can show up, including hypersensitivity with touch to the genitals, difficulty holding in urine or bowel movements, pain with urination or bowel movements, pain with orgasm or sex, and pain in the clitoris, anus, rectum, vulva, and vagina.

A similar experience exists in the widely known condition carpal tunnel syndrome. An impaired movement pattern in the shoulder can lead to muscle tension in the forearm, compressing a nerve in the wrist and resulting in pain in the hand. Similarly, when the pudendal nerve gets impinged, pain may be felt in the clitoris, or labia in Nancy's case, far from where the nerve originates. We wouldn't cut off a hand that's in pain, just like Nancy's labia should not have been removed. We need to take a step back and think about all of the systems involved before drastic measures such as these are taken. And if we can somehow find a way to relax the muscles and free the impingement of this nerve, very often many of the issues will begin to go away.

Trauma, compression, and stretch to the pudendal nerve contribute to pelvic pain. When pain occurs, all our muscles tense up in that region, which further irritates the pudendal nerve and leads to more pain and long-lasting, chronic symptoms. A cycle of pain and muscle tension occurs, and to break this cycle, you need to address all the components to give yourself sweet and long-lasting relief. Women with distress downstairs due to

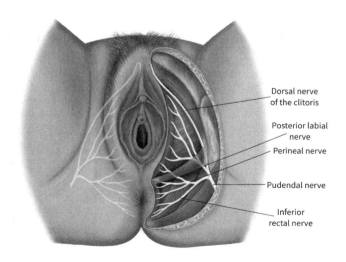

Pudendal nerve branches to the female genitalia
and pelvic floor muscles

pelvic floor muscle dysfunction deal with a variety of symptoms, and often ones you couldn't even imagine are related to muscles.

> "When I wear tight pants, my vagina feels like something is poking it."
> "Every time I sit for longer than five minutes, my tailbone hurts."
> "It feels like hot acid is being poured on my vulva."
> "After every ride on my spin bike, I have these sharp shooting pains to my clitoris."
> "When I have the urge to poop, I feel like an ice pick is stabbing me in my butthole."

Whenever women come into my office with any sort of pelvic pain complaint, one of the first things I do (after a good listen) is walk them through a four-step pain protocol to give them some tools to manage their pain and hopefully some relief. As providers, we can never promise or guarantee that we can help your pain go away. The goal is to make your pain less intense and less frequent so that you can hopefully return to the things you love to do.

Managing Your Pain Protocol

Before we get to specific pelvic pain situations, it is good to develop some more general habits around managing your pain. It is easy to go through life being faintly aware of vague pain—but when we lean into it, and pay closer attention to it, we can learn more about the source of the pain and how to alleviate it. When pain knocks at the door of your floor, try the following.

TRACK YOUR PAIN
Grab a notebook. Your pain has a story. To address the physical aspect of your pain, identifying the triggers is the first step. Keep a pain diary where you write down the time of day your

pain occurs, its intensity level, what activity or movement you were doing prior to or during the pain, and how long it lasts. Anything that helps relieve it can be extremely helpful to note. Try to tune in to when and how severely you experience the pain. Are you constipated, stressed, exercising, wearing a certain pair of pants, eating a certain food, or sitting a certain way? Very likely a pattern will emerge. And patterns can often help us identify the source or trigger of the pain.

PAUSE THE TRIGGERING ACTIVITY

Once you determine what might be causing or exacerbating the pain, you might need to get off the horse for a while. Maybe you need to sleep with more pillow support, use a standing desk to avoid sitting, or take a break from pickleball. Listen to your body. Sometimes our triggers are not always avoidable, but the goal is to decrease exposure to the triggers to give your muscles and nerves some rest. You may not be able to completely avoid these activities, but making an adjustment to avoid a clear trigger is key.

RELAX THE PELVIC FLOOR MUSCLES

Muscle tension contributes to pain, and pain contributes to muscle tension. No matter whether your pelvic floor muscle tension is the chicken or the egg, it needs to be treated to help you get relief. The relaxation protocol in Chapter 2 is the pathway to ease pelvic floor muscle tension, spasm, and overactivity for pelvic pain conditions. Manual techniques like ball massage or cupping can release external tissues, while internal pelvic floor massage with a finger or wand can release pelvic floor muscle tension and relieve pudendal nerve irritation. Stretching and breathing exercises help quiet your nervous system and restore relaxation to tense muscles. Throughout this chapter, we will go through different issues, and I will offer various pelvic floor support therapies that you can do to help yourself. Commit to them.

GRADUALLY RETURN TO ACTIVITY

As your pain improves, gradually add back movement or an activity that was previously challenging or triggering. Think baby steps. For example, in the case of clitoral pain, if wearing jeans was problematic, start wearing a pair at home for a short interval, like for one hour. If symptoms do not increase, in the following days, progress to wearing the jeans for a longer period, like three hours. Then progress to wearing them for an entire day. If that goes well, wear them for activities outside of the house. Just as with other pelvic health issues, stay under the threshold of what your body can tolerate. If pain occurs, do not push through pain but pause, breathe, and utilize the tools below to help manage your symptoms.

Common Culprits of Pain in Your Pelvis

There are probably hundreds or even thousands of things that can create pain in the pelvis, and we can all fall victim to them. In the months leading up to my wedding, I did a workout program five days a week to "get into shape." I had always been a regular exerciser, but like many other brides-to-be, I was on a mission to get into my best shape ever. My pre-wedding workout program involved a lot of squats and lunges to firm up my legs and core. After several weeks, I felt a slight pain in my tailbone. Then I noticed that every time I sat down, I had pain in my butt crack. When I got up from sitting any longer than ten minutes, my body creaked because my tailbone would ache. I remember driving to taste our wedding cake, and I had to roll onto my side and recline my car seat because my tailbone was at a five out of ten on a pain scale of one to ten. Wedding planning is stressful, so I admit I was also probably guilty of butt-clenching. When I walked myself through the protocol, it was clear my tailbone was talking to me: easy on the squats. Unclench your butt. Stop stressing about what color toenail polish you should wear. Luckily, I knew what to do, so I was pain-free when I walked down the aisle. But every woman, and person with a pelvic floor for that matter, should be privy to this same insight.

Tailbone pain is just one type of pelvic pain that can occur involving the muscles, tissues, and nerves in your pelvic region. Below are some of the most common pelvic floor culprits women experience. Remember: your goal here is management and function. And, hopefully, some relief. You might not get the pain to go away entirely, but the tips below will help. In addition to these strategies, consider including a pelvic floor therapist and a physician who have experience with pain management in your care.

PUDENDAL NEURALGIA: YOUR PELVIC FLOOR IS ON FIRE

Recall my patient Nancy who had her labia removed? Nancy had pudendal neuralgia. A neuralgia refers to pain that is felt in one or more nerves and that can follow the path of that nerve—which will create pain elsewhere in the body. In Nancy's case, her pudendal nerve was irritated or damaged, and her labia hurt. Removing her labia did not help. She got relief only when we treated her pudendal nerve and the muscles and tissues surrounding it.

Most people with pudendal neuralgia report minimal or no pain upon waking in the morning, and it increases as the day progresses or following a certain activity, like sitting or riding a bicycle. Because the pudendal nerve travels to many different parts of the vulva and pelvic floor muscles, pudendal neuralgia symptoms can range from feeling like you are sitting on a golf ball to feeling like a hot poker is in your vagina or rectum. How this pain starts also varies as it can be caused by compression of the pudendal nerve from something like sitting or bike riding, a stretching injury from something like a deep squat during a workout, or injury during an event like childbirth or vaginal surgery.

Women with pudendal nerve pain can experience a variety

of different symptoms from discomfort during pelvic examinations, tampon insertion, or sex to pain while sitting or even rectal pain during bowel movements. The treatments for these will be similarly focused on pelvic floor relaxation.

AVOID SADDLE SITTING

Pudendal neuralgia was once known as cyclist syndrome as so many cyclists experienced this sharp, shooting pain or fullness in their rectum because of compression and irritation to this nerve. Because the pudendal nerve runs right between your sit bones, sitting on a saddle, like a bicycle seat, horseback, or motorcycle seat can compress that nerve. To resolve pudendal pain, avoid saddle sitting.

USE A CUSHION WITH A CENTER CUTOUT

Women with pudendal neuralgia often report pain with sitting except when sitting on a toilet seat, because there is no pressure on the nerve. Specialty cushions with a center cut out can be used every time you sit or as often as possible. Seat cushions or adaptive bike seats can also be used for cycling in order to prevent exacerbation of symptoms on a saddle.

RELEASE EXTERNAL MUSCLES AND TISSUES

Releasing the muscles and tissues along the course of the pudendal nerve is key to pain relief. Cupping or using a massage ball along your sacrum around the midline of your butt cheeks (aka your butt crack) and along your glutes, inner thighs, and abdominal wall will release external muscle tension and restriction.

PERFORM INTERNAL PELVIC FLOOR RELEASES

The pudendal nerve runs right through your pelvic floor and alongside your obturator internus muscle. Use a pelvic floor massage wand to release the pelvic floor and obturator internus muscles internally on both sides of your pelvis. Place the tip of the wand internally on the muscles at two to five and seven to eleven on the pelvic clock and hold for five to ten deep breaths as muscle tenderness decreases.

ADDRESS THE CENTRAL SENSITIZATION

In addition to working on the physical contributors to your pain, it is important to address the mental component. This is true not only for pudendal neuralgia but also any pain that is chronic in nature. Learning how pain works and how it changes the brain over time can influence how your brain and body respond. Many books on how to "decentralize" pain are offered in the resources section in the back of this book. And if accessible, working with a therapist who specializes in chronic pain can be beneficial as well.

VULVAR PAIN: YOUR VULVA AND/OR VAGINA HURTS

Vulvar pain includes the entire region of the vulva including the clitoris, labia, vestibule located inside the labia minora, and vaginal opening. Vulvar pain, called vulvodynia, can be provoked with pressure or touch to the area—for example, during vaginal intercourse or direct touch to the vulvar area. The pain can also be unprovoked and occurs at spontaneous times. The specific cause of vulvar pain is not easily identified and often exists alongside other pain syndromes like irritable bowel syndrome, fibromyalgia, or painful bladder syndrome.

Vulvar pain can be localized, occurring at a specific spot on the vulva, or generalized, and the entire vulvar area is involved. With vulvar pain, the pelvic floor muscles are short, tight, and hypersensitive. Pelvic floor therapy aimed to release tight muscles and to decrease irritation to nerves in the area is effective in alleviating pain. As rare as this condition may seem, roughly 8% of the female population experiences vulvodynia, yet it takes an average of seeing five healthcare providers for a woman to receive an accurate diagnosis, let alone appropriate treatment. Unfortunately, this has led to many women suffering for a long time, making a huge impact on their quality of life.

My clitoris is super sensitive, and every time something touches or rubs against it, I want to jump off the table. Would these tips help?

Clitoral pain is a subset of localized vulvar pain, often due to hypersensitivity or irritation to a branch of the pudendal nerve that provides sensation to the clitoris and clitoral hood. The same strategies to treat vulvar pain below are beneficial and can be found in Chapter 2 under the pelvic floor relaxation protocol. Strategies include massaging trigger points in your abdominal wall with your fingertip pressure or using a massage ball to relieve glute tension. When showering, use your index and middle finger to gently pull back the clitoral hood and rinse with water. This area can collect a whitish discharge or substance called smegma that can cause clitoral irritation.

PAUSE THE KEGELS AND RELAX
YOUR PELVIC FLOOR

Kegels will likely make vulvar pain significantly worse. Instead, follow the pelvic floor relaxation protocol in Chapter 2 to help release tense pelvic floor muscles. A number of relaxation stretches will help bring relief. Stretches performed with deep breathing can not only ease pelvic floor muscle tension but also quiet your nervous system. Since sitting can often be an uncomfortable position for women with vulvar pain, focus on the following stretches and hold each stretch for ten deep breaths, really allowing your muscles to soften and relax. Breathe deeply in the posture. These stretches can be performed daily in the morning and evening or anytime an increase in symptoms occurs.

- Single knee to chest stretch
- Butterfly stretch

- Happy baby pose or modified happy baby
- Child's pose
- Standing hip flexor stretch
- Modified downward-facing dog stretch

USE VAGINAL DILATORS

Vaginal dilator training is outlined in Chapter 2 and is an effective method to relax pelvic floor muscles, desensitize nerves in the vulvar region and vaginal opening, and help progress toward pain-free life. Perform the relaxation stretches above prior to dilator insertion. Use a lubricant and start with a small-size dilator, gradually progressing toward a larger size that feels comfortable and pain-free.

PERFORM INTERNAL TRIGGER POINT RELEASE

Use a pelvic floor wand to help release the muscles. Ensure you can insert a vaginal dilator that's the same diameter as the wand without pain prior to using the internal pelvic wand. Use the tip of the wand to release tension or tender points on both sides of the pelvic floor and on the underside of pubic bones next to the urethra at eleven and one o'clock.

AVOID SKIN IRRITANTS

Because the causes and triggers of vulvar pain are largely unknown, utilizing precautionary vulvar hygiene practices is important to prevent irritation to sensitive tissues and nerves. As a first step, make sure to rinse the vulva with water only. The sensitive tissues of the vulva can be easily irritated with chemicals, especially for those who experience vulvar pain. To properly cleanse the area, rinse the tissues between the labia and around the clitoris with warm water. This will minimize any further irritation. Always remember to pat yourself dry when you are done washing. Also, after a shower, rinsing, or peeing, avoid aggressively wiping your vulva. Use a bidet, peri bottle, or shower head to cleanse the area and reduce excessive wiping. Then pat the area dry with an organic cotton towel if available or toilet paper. To thoroughly dry the area, use a hair dryer on the cool setting. (Pro mom tip: this is also how I dried my son's bottom when he had a diaper rash, and it worked like a charm.)

Avoid irritating creams, lotions, bubble baths, and shower gels. Your vulvar tissues are *hyper*sensitive when vulvar pain is present, and many of the washes and moisturizers can cause additional irritation and pain. Again, only rinse with warm water. If you take a bath, soak in warm water. Epsom salt can be added if that does not irritate your vulva, but avoid bubble baths. Use vulva moisturizers (even organic coconut oil or jojoba oil works) that are pH-balanced and paraben-free.

You can also try going commando (when possible and as much as possible) or wear loose shorts, pants, or skirts. Your vulva is easily irritated by underwear and materials touching the sensitive tissues. When you do wear underwear, wear all-cotton (organic if possible) underwear. Limit wearing synthetic pants or leggings. Your vulva and vag need to breathe, and wearing synthetic pants and leggings can trap warm air in the area, leading to an increased risk of infections. Wear loose cotton clothing that can absorb sweat and moisture away from tissues and help reduce irritation to the area.

In terms of pads and tampons, use organic and unbleached products. So many chemicals are in menstrual care products, and placing those next to sensitive tissues is not recommended.

USE LUBRICANTS THAT ARE OIL-BASED OR WATER-BASED

Because vulvar pain often contributes to sex that hurts, using a lubricant may be essential when attempting intercourse. All-natural oil-based lubricants like coconut oil can be a great place to start, but please remember oil-based lubricants cannot be used with latex condoms as oil will cause the condom to break. Water-based lubricants that are not warming or scented and are paraben-free are also a great option for intercourse and using vaginal trainers and dilators.

My labia feel itchy and painful. Could it be my pelvic floor causing this?

Your pelvic floor muscles can be a component, but other dermatological or autoimmune conditions can affect your vulva as well. If you notice a gradual change in the labia getting thinner, almost like they are disappearing, along with chronic itching, irritation, or sensitivity of the labia, contact a dermatologist or gynecologist for additional examination. It can be a sign of lower estrogen levels (common during postpartum, lactating, or perimenopause) or autoimmune and dermatological conditions that require treatment from a physician. To soothe the tissues, get relief, and manage the itching, use a moisturizing balm specifically for the vulva (check out Chapter 6 on painful sex for tips on vulvar moisturizers), take Epsom salt baths or soaks, and wear all-cotton underwear and clothing to avoid excessive heat or sweating in the area.

COCCYX PAIN: YOUR TAILBONE HURTS

Your coccyx, commonly known as your tailbone, is a triangular-shaped bone located at the very tip of your sacrum. This bone has attachments to muscles and ligaments in your pelvic floor and buttock muscles, moves when you go from sit to stand, and helps support you when sitting upright. *Coccyx* in Latin means "cuckoo," referring to the curved shape of the bone, similar to a cuckoo's beak. *Dynia* means pain, which you will see in many of the pain diagnoses we talk about. The formal name for tailbone pain is coccydynia.

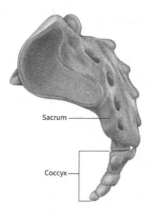

Sacrum and coccyx bones: a view from the side

Tailbone pain can feel like tenderness or an ache in the region of the tailbone or surrounding muscles and tissues. It typically gets worse with prolonged sitting, getting up from sitting, and during sex, exercise, or bowel movements. Tailbone pain more commonly presents in women than men and can result from a sudden injury during childbirth or a fall (like that time I tried to snowboard, fell directly on my bottom, and could barely sit for days). It can also occur gradually with prolonged sitting on hard surfaces, a lot of glute-strengthening exercises without adequate relaxation or stretching, pelvic floor tension, or increased movement of the coccyx. If you experience tailbone pain, try any or all of the following tips, and it should gradually subside with time.

RELAX YOUR PELVIC FLOOR

Kegels or any pelvic floor–strengthening exercises are not the answer. Follow the pelvic floor relaxation protocol, working on relaxing and releasing tense pelvic floor muscles.

USE A SEAT CUSHION

Tailbone pain is often triggered with sitting, as this puts weight directly on the bone and joint. However, sitting is a hard activity to completely avoid, considering we need to sit to drive, work, and many other activities. Using a seat cushion in the tailbone or back portion *every time you sit* can minimize irritation to the area. I recommend a dense foam cushion instead of a blow-up cushion, which can often require activation of core muscles to keep yourself upright. Using a seat cushion will not eliminate the pain by itself, but it will prolong how long you can sit comfortably before it starts.

SIT WITH AN UPRIGHT POSTURE

When you sit down, avoid what we call sacral sitting, which is essentially slouching with a rounded back and a tucked pelvis. This tightens the muscles around your tailbone and can lead to additional muscle tension and pain. Sit upright so your body weight is distributed directly on your sit bones instead of your sacrum and tailbone. Imagine a string lifting you up by the head so your torso is upright. You can use a pillow behind your back or a stool underneath your feet to help keep you in an upright position instead of sinking.

MASSAGE YOUR GLUTE MUSCLES

Your glute or buttock muscles attach to a portion of your tailbone, and tension in these outer muscles can contribute to pelvic floor tension and tailbone pain. Following the instructions in the Chapter 2 relaxation protocol, use a ball to massage the middle and outside of your buttock muscles.

STRETCH IT OUT

The best position to release tense pelvic floor muscles that attach to your tailbone is a squatting position. Focus on stretches like a deep squat stretch, child's pose, and happy baby pose, holding each for five to ten deep breaths. These should be repeated when symptoms arise after sitting or workouts and additionally throughout the day. These stretches can help release tension around the tailbone:

- Single knee to chest stretch
- Happy baby pose or modified happy baby
- Child's pose
- Deep squat stretch

RECTAL PAIN: YOUR BUTTHOLE HURTS

A literal pain in your ass, rectal pain can feel like a sharp shooting sensation in the anus, a golf ball feeling in your rectum, or a cramping ache in your butthole. In most cases, pooping problems also exist because of the tension of your pelvic floor muscles making it difficult to relax and coordinate emptying. Pelvic floor muscle spasm, particularly in the anal area, needs to be addressed to achieve relief.

RELEASE PELVIC FLOOR MUSCLE TENSION

Follow the pelvic floor relaxation protocol in Chapter 2. Start with the simple guidelines of taking deep breaths throughout the day to release tension and quiet your sympathetic nervous system. Follow the optimal posture guidelines above to avoid overclenching your buttock muscles, and use the proper pooping protocol (Chapter 4) to optimize pelvic floor muscle relaxation during bowel movements.

STRETCH IT OUT

Squatting is the best position to lengthen your pelvic floor and ease tension on your puborectalis muscle, which is often the culprit for challenges with emptying. Perform the following stretches daily and when symptoms are increased:

- Deep squat stretch
- Child's pose
- Happy baby
- Shin box stretch

RELEASE INTERNAL TRIGGER POINTS

Muscle spasm and trigger points in your pelvic floor are found in almost every person who has rectal pain with pelvic floor muscle overactivity. In order to relieve those trigger points, using a trigger point wand as described in the Chapter 2 relaxation protocol is key. But this is most effective when done in your butt. To release these internal rectal spasms, you will use the wand through the anal opening.

The best position to perform this is lying on your side or lying on your back with knees bent. Use a lot of lubricant on the wand prior to inserting. If you are using a silicone wand, avoid using a silicone lubricant, as that can break down the silicone on the wand. Insert the tip of the wand up to the first curve and gently apply pressure to the left or right side, searching for a tender spot or one that recreates the symptoms or pain you experience. Hold pressure until the pain decreases, but no longer than sixty seconds. You can do this throughout the pelvic floor muscles every other day until the tender spots are no longer present.

If inserting the trigger point wand rectally is challenging, start with anal dilators first, or use the wand vaginally to release muscle tension. Once you use the wand through the anus, do not insert that side into the vagina. Use a separate wand or the opposite side of the wand if it has two sides appropriate for internal use.

USE HEAT

Taking a warm bath or sitz bath can provide global relaxation to your pelvic area. This practice can be done daily or when pain is present to help ease symptoms. Spend fifteen to twenty minutes taking big, deep breaths to help promote muscle relaxation. When a warm bath isn't available, even lying or sitting on a heating pad or turning on your car seat warmers can be an effective way to get some warmth to the area for relaxation.

I sometimes have a sharp shooting pain in my butthole that wakes me in the middle of the night. It lasts for less than a minute and goes away quickly. What is going on back there?

A condition called proctalgia fugax is characterized by sharp, shooting, stabbing rectal pain that lasts anywhere between thirty seconds and thirty minutes, caused by a severe muscle spasm in your pelvic floor. More common in women, this spasm can wake you in the middle of the night or precede or follow a bowel movement. But rectal pain does not exist between these episodes, making it hard to diagnose and therefore treat. Treatment includes the same protocol above for rectal pain focused on pelvic floor muscle relaxation. However, many women with endometriosis also experience rectal pain, particularly with bowel movements. Check in with your gynecologist if additional symptoms of endometriosis exist. We cover endometriosis in Chapter 5, on menstruation.

Relief for Your Downstairs

Pelvic pain is a pain. Talk to any woman who has experienced it, and she'll tell you how challenging her journey has been. But also talk to any medical provider who has patients with pelvic pain. These patients are some of the hardest to manage because there is no pill or single treatment to cure it.

If you are dealing with pelvic pain, your first and most important step is to trust yourself. Don't let any doctor or healing professional dismiss your pain. If they won't partner with you to help you find relief, keep searching. Follow the managing pain protocol early in this chapter to track your pain and get to know it. Next, address your pelvic floor. Work on releasing your muscles and tissues in the area, because whether these tense muscles are the source of the pain or are a result of it, they need to be released. Last, pull in tools or providers to support the mental and emotional aspects of pain. Physical pain causes mental and emotional distress, so a mind–body approach is essential for long-term and effective management.

My patient Nancy, whom I mentioned earlier, continued to see me for treatment for nine months. We worked in physical therapy on her muscles and tissues, and she simultaneously worked with a mental health therapist who educated her on chronic pain and relaxation strategies. She started medication to help with anxiety and did daily exercises to promote gentle movement and circulation. When Nancy finished therapy with me, she was 90% better. She was not pain-free, as that was not her goal, but her quality of life was improved. She had a toolbox of exercises and strategies to manage her pain at home. She started wearing underwear again. She sat through a full movie using a seat cushion. She could pee without her vulva burning. But Nancy should have never gotten to the point she did. She deserved better care, as we all do.

CHAPTER 12

Vaginas in the Spotlight

Yesterday is history. Tomorrow is a mystery. But today is a gift. That's why it's called the present.
—KUNG FU PANDA

If you feel like you just read a lifetime's worth of pelvic floor knowledge, you're not wrong. My intention is to provide you with everything I know regarding pelvic floor therapy for women, and then you can dip in, as needed, for the rest of your lifetime. And share it—with your friends, mothers, daughters, and even complete strangers (when it isn't overly awkward). Heck, talk to your partners and sons and grandparents too.

As women, we will undoubtedly go through life transitions that affect our pelvic health, from menstruation to menopause and beyond. Many women live with pelvic floor issues, believing it's just a normal part of being a woman or are too embarrassed to talk about them. So they suffer, but *they do not have to.* Yes, we are on hormonal roller coasters monthly and have seasons of life that can make pelvic floor dysfunction seem inevitable. But we are also sending people into outerspace. More needs to be done in the healthcare system to help women prevent and overcome pelvic floor challenges and not make diapers our destiny. Until then, you have to be the driver in your care to make progress.

The education, tips, and tricks I've shared in this book are for all women—and it is meant to be used from potty-training all the way through our postmenopausal years. Teach your little girls, so that as soon as they learn to walk and talk as toddlers, they also know how to properly pee and poop. Teach the teenagers you know about their pelvic floor muscles and the impact of their periods on their pelvic health. Sex education should include conversations about pelvic health, not just discussing *how* our bodies work but also *what* to do if they aren't working optimally.

In the ideal world, I would like to see proactive pelvic health education and exercise for pregnant women that is integrated into their healthcare just as routine ultrasounds and diabetes screening are. During postpartum, you should get as much care, if not more, as the baby you just birthed. When entering menopause, your pelvic floor health should be top of mind, as much as heart health and bone health.

Incorporating the skills and ideas in this book is a lifelong journey, and it starts with making simple changes and taking one step at a time forward. I want this book to empower you to have conversations with your medical providers. Although these can feel hard and awkward, you must take control of your pelvic health and be proactive in its care. If your medical provider shuts you down, find a new one. If the next one brushes off your problems as normal, keep asking questions or keep looking. Keep going until you get the answers you need.

Struggling with pelvic floor problems can feel defeating, and relief can feel unattainable. But it's important to carry the conviction that you can get better, and you have to seek guidance and care to get there. Even if your test says no infection. Even if your medical provider says nothing is wrong. You know your body best, and if you feel in your gut that something is wrong and your pelvic floor may be involved or need attention, push for the care you deserve.

As I write this, I am currently between postpartum and menopause, raising two school-aged boys, running a business, married to a great man, and struggling to do the recommended thirty minutes of exercise five times a week (including my pelvic floor exercises). Taking care of our lives, our bodies, and our pelvic floors can feel like full-time jobs. But you don't need to overhaul your life (or your bathroom) to do this pelvic floor work. You can start with simple steps that go a really long way. Cherry-pick the few takeaways to start right now. And return to the chapters of this book at any time to manage new symptoms or navigate a new season of life. It is all here for you.

These are the actual habits that I, The Vagina Whisperer, do day in and day out to take care of my pelvic floor:

> **I don't push when I pee.** Ever. I sit down (even on public toilets unless they are really too gross) and take deep breaths when I pee. I don't push or strain. I just let it flow.
>
> **I drink a lot of water and take magnesium citrate gummies at night.** The water prevents me from getting dehydrated and, along with my mag gummies, keeps my poops regular.
>
> **I use a stool under my feet during bowel movements.** Every bathroom in my house has a pooping stool. I travel with one or use a garbage can turned on its side if one isn't available. Elevate your feet to relax the pelvic floor.
>
> **I support my perineum when I have hard poops.** Even I get constipated on occasion. To avoid straining my pelvic floor, I take a piece of toilet paper and press up firmly on my perineum and exhale as I push out to poop.
>
> **I breathe out and exhale when lifting.** Whether it's picking up one of my kids, grabbing a box of Costco groceries from my trunk, or lifting weights during my workout, I always exhale with exertion.
>
> **I use lube during sex.** After having kids, my vag is just drier. I transitioned from postpartum and breastfeeding to perimenopause without a beat and have used lube (water-soluble), which I did not require pre-pregnancy, ever since.

I use an internal trigger point wand for pelvic floor tension. I occasionally have deeper pain with sex, and I know it's linked to pelvic floor tension, often from the stress of workouts. I keep a trigger point wand in my nightstand to help release muscle tension if I experience pain with sex.

I wear an internal support (even a tampon will suffice) when coughing a lot or doing anything with high-intensity running or jumping. This is a proactive move, but I know that repetitive coughing when I am sick or lots of jumping inevitably fatigues my pelvic floor, and this keeps everything positioned where it needs to be.

I work out my pelvic floor. When exercising, I consistently contract my pelvic floor and deep abs with each repetition and exhale on the exertion part of each repetition. This is such an easy and effective way to strengthen my pelvic floor and incorporate pelvic floor strengthening into workouts that I already do.

I do not *and will not* accept that pelvic floor problems are just a normal part of being a woman.

I am a physical therapist whose practice is based on optimizing movement, improving posture, and utilizing exercise to give our bodies long-term relief and function. The tips and protocols provided in this book are not magic pills and likely won't give you immediate relief. They take time, patience, and consistency. But they are effective. And once implemented, you will see incremental improvements that will benefit your pelvic floor throughout your entire life.

If you feel you need more than what the pages of this book can offer, pelvic health therapists are located throughout the United States and the world. However, there are simply not enough of us. The United States alone has over 250 million adult women and fewer than 10,000 pelvic floor therapists nationwide. You won't find therapists in every town or city, and they are even more rare in rural areas. Although the number of us is increasing, we need more to provide all women a good standard of care. Not to mention in-person medical care can be costly, distant, or simply unavailable. The good news is that with this book, you now have a menu of options to address your pelvic floor needs, and the language for reaching out for pelvic floor care in the medical system. You can do a telehealth session, an online exercise program (like mine!), or a group workshop. You have options.

Often symptoms of pelvic floor issues persist for years before women seek care, so one therapy session or one week of exercise is not going to give you the immediate relief you desire. But as I always say, you have to learn to walk a mile before you run a marathon. Stay consistent with the small habits and simple exercises provided in this guide or by a qualified pelvic healthcare professional, and progress is possible.

And one last note worth mentioning: your pelvic floor deserves healthcare, not just the hot new wellness trend you heard about from a friend or saw on social media. Not every pelvic floor trend helps or even works—from a jade egg that promises magical pelvic floor powers to a laser wand that assures a rejuvenated vagina to a fitness professional who offers a weekend course and claims expert status on how to tighten your vagina. These options promise quick fixes, are not backed by science, and are often not coming from qualified practitioners. I'll say it again: pelvic floor care is *healthcare*, not wellness and not even fitness.

More women experience urinary leakage than diabetes, hypertension, or osteoporosis, yet women are less likely to receive treatment for pelvic floor disorders. Seventy-five percent of pregnant and postpartum women and 68% of postmenopausal women do not feel adequately educated about their pelvic floors. Women know more about erectile dysfunction than pelvic organ prolapse. It's time to bring pelvic floor education and awareness out into the open and keep it there. Start and continue the dialogue around the issues raised in this book to normalize pelvic floor *conversations* instead of normalizing pelvic floor *problems.*

If you are a medical provider, ask your patients about their pelvic health. Inquire about leakage, bowel movements, menstruation, menopause, and sexual health. Research clearly shows if we don't ask patients about their pelvic health, they are likely not to tell us. So it's on us, as their providers, to ask the questions and refer them to pelvic floor therapy if they are experiencing, or simply want to prevent, an issue.

I hope this guide not only *floors* you with the magic of your body, but also empowers you to take fabulous care of yourself. You get one pelvic floor, and you need to love it. Claim it. Reclaim it. Talk about it. Ask questions about it. And keep it in the spotlight. Reading this book may be your first step or your fiftieth in your pelvic health journey, but I hope it's certainly not your last. You deserve a healthy pelvic floor throughout your lifetime. And the power to achieve that is not just within the pages of this book. *It is within you.*

★ ★ ★ ★ ★

Your Pelvic Floor Toolkit

This list includes the tools, books, and other resources that I recommend to my patients and to my very best of friends. By no means do you need to purchase or utilize everything on this list, but I want you to have a place to get started and start exploring.

HELPFUL LINKS

- All of my recommended products can be found below or on my recommended products webpage, *https://thevagwhisperer.com/recommended-products.*
- All of the videos for stretches, strengthening exercises, and how to assess for DRA can be found on my YouTube channel, *https://www.youtube.com/@thevaginawhisperer.*
- At-home pelvic floor exercise programs for every age and stage can be found in my V-Hive pelvic floor membership at *https://thevagwhisperer.com.*

PRODUCTS AND RESOURCES

- Vaginal dilators: *https://www.intimaterose.com*
- Trigger point wand: *https://www.intimaterose.com*
- Pooping step stool: *https://www.squattypotty.com*
- Peri bottle: *https://www.fridamom.com*
- Bidet: *https://www.hellotushy.com*
- Compression socks: *https://www.sockwell.com*
- Compression garments: *https://www.lovesteady.com*
- Vaginal moisturizer: *https://www.medicinemama.com*
- Prolapse internal support: *https://www.userevive.com*
- Seat cushions for pain: *https://www.theraseat.com*

- Books on pelvic pain: *Heal Pelvic Pain* by Amy Stein, *Pelvic Pain Explained* by Stephanie Prendergast and Elizabeth Akincilar, *When Sex Hurts* by Andrew Goldstein, Caroline Pukall, Irwin Goldstein, and Jill Krapf
- Apps for tracking menstrual cycle: Flo, Ovia, Clue

MATERNAL HEALTH, PELVIC HEALTH, AND RACIAL JUSTICE ORGANIZATIONS

- Every Mother Counts: *https://everymothercounts.org*
- Chamber of Mothers: *https://chamberofmothers.com*
- Mother's Outreach Network: *https://mothersoutreachnetwork.org*
- National Black Doulas Association: *https://www.blackdoulas.org*
- TightLipped: *https://www.tightlipped.org*
- Planned Parenthood: *https://www.plannedparenthood.org*

About the Author

Since 2007, Dr. Sara Reardon has been caring for people's pelvic floors as a doctor of physical therapy and board-certified pelvic floor physical therapist. Sara was born and raised in New Orleans, Louisiana, and attended Washington University in St. Louis, graduating in 2004 with a bachelor's of science and in 2007 with a doctorate of physical therapy. She started her career as a pelvic floor therapist in Austin, Texas, eventually moving to Dallas, Texas, where she met her husband, Neil, and gave birth to her two sons, Dylan and Shaan. While pregnant, Sara started sharing pelvic health tips to navigate the physical demands of pregnancy and preparing for birth on an Instagram account, aptly called the nickname her friends had given her, The Vagina Whisperer. The account's rapid growth of followers was a testament to how much women wanted and needed more pelvic health information.

Sara and her family eventually moved back to New Orleans, where she opened the city's first pelvic health physical therapy clinic, NOLA Pelvic Health. Due to the necessity of at-home workouts following the pandemic, Sara went on to launch the V-Hive Membership, providing online, on-demand pelvic floor and core workouts for pregnancy, postpartum, menopause, painful sex, and pelvic floor weakness. Although The Vagina Whisperer started as a dancing vulva on social media educating women about their bodies, it has become a business and brand offering modern pelvic healthcare for women worldwide.

Sara has been featured in *Time* magazine, *Harper's Bazaar*, *InStyle*, *HuffPost*, the *Today* show, and numerous other podcasts, publications, and professional conferences for her advocacy and educational work as a pelvic health physical therapist. She is also a TED presenter on Rethinking Postpartum Care. When not helping people with their pelvic floors, Sara loves to travel to the mountains, play tennis, eat Asian food, read for hours on her couch, and spend time with her family and friends. *Floored: A Woman's Guide to Pelvic Floor Health at Every Age and Stage* is her first book.

Acknowledgments

Thank you to Erika Imranyi and the entire team at Park Row Books and HarperCollins Publishers, who took a chance on a dancing vulva on social media to share this much-needed information with women. Thanks to my agents, Wendy Sherman and Callie Deitrick, at Wendy Sherman Associates, who saw me as an author well before I saw myself as one. You all crafted unprecedented deals to get this book to publication and led me to my invaluable collaborator, Haven Iverson of Wordhaven. Haven, you are the best writing collaborator, cheerleader, and coach I could have asked for. With your guidance, I was able to finesse my words, capture my voice, and pour my heart onto these pages. To Richelle Friedson, thank you for helping me first put together a proposal and encouraging me to let my personality shine through. From the first word to the last, I couldn't have written *Floored* without the trust, support, and encouragement from all of you.

Thank you to Sydnei Lewis, my research assistant, who was crucial in tracking down the necessary publications and research articles for this book. You were a gift to work with. Thank you for seeing this through until the end. To my medical illustrator, Anna Bessmertnaya, thank you for being collaborative and communicative, and for creating illustrations that help readers visualize their bodies. And a huge thank-you to the small but mighty Vagina Whisperer team. You all keep my business going behind the scenes—Tova, Carly, Kelley, Robin, Rachel, and Jeremy. The ripples of your work go far in helping women and pelvic floors everywhere. Thank you for being on this journey with me.

My interest in pelvic health was sparked at Washington University in St. Louis Program in Physical Therapy. Tracy Spitznagle, you drove me across Missouri to present at a conference and help set me on this incredibly rewarding path. Thank you for being my forever mentor. To Ms. Mary Noetzel, you took me in during my last semester of PT school and gave me a home when I needed one. To the late Dr. Mike Noetzel, you gave me solid advice to follow my passion in pelvic health. That casual chat had a profound effect on me, and the ripples of your guidance have gone far. To my first boss, Kimberlee Sullivan, you taught me how to listen, deliver excellent care, and pound the pavement to let others know the importance of this work. To my former colleagues at Baylor Hospital, the University of Texas Southwestern, and currently at NOLA Pelvic Health, thank you for being great colleagues and making work a place I love to be.

To my family, the Chanimals, I couldn't ask for a better family, and to be back home with all of you is a gift. Cheers to more cousin dinners and Chan karaoke. Angela, Mike, and Ju—we have been through so much, and I am thankful every day we were put on this earth together as siblings. I can't imagine going through life without you all. I love you and your families and am eternally grateful for your support and encouragement. JAMS forever. To Ju and Evan, you both have generously helped me with The Vagina Whisperer from the very beginning. Evan, your literary genius led me to *Floored*, and Ju, your branding and marketing genius have been the backbone of TVW since day one. Thanks to you both for being my sounding boards and best friends. To Dad and Christy, thank you for being my biggest cheerleaders and always jumping at the chance to help out and cheer me and the kids on. To Dean, you're the best stepdad I could have ever asked for. From driving me to track practices and eventually off to college, I am grateful. To the Parekh family, thanks for supporting our family in so many ways. I appreciate you all cheering me on during the writing process and for being wonderful grandparents and Mamu to our boys. Last, but certainly not least, to my dear mom, Sue. When I think about the person who has been most impactful on my life, there is no question it is you. You worked hard, sent me to great schools, supported my move away for college, gave me the much-needed nudge to go to PT school, and provided me the safe haven of a home as I drifted to find my passion and myself. You demonstrated what grit, determination, and hard work can do. A thank-you doesn't do justice to how grateful I am to have you as my mom. I love you.

To my dear friends, who cheered me on while writing this book and since the start of The Vagina Whisperer. To my WashU friends who coined my nickname The Vagina Whisperer; my PT school friends (Back Right '07) who made graduate school unforgettable; to my Austin, Dallas, and Houston girls who gave me some of the most fun years; and to my NOLA girls who are the most supportive, encouraging, and funny women to have in my life. Special shout-out to Erica Noel for being my incredible attorney, guide, and student council president.

Floored was written during early mornings with a cup of coffee, over weekends while peering through my office window watching my boys play, and during late evenings after bedtime routines. Although the words and stories of *Floored* are mine, they would not have made their way onto the pages without the support of my dear husband. Neil, thank you for your endless support, encouragement, pep talks, warm cups of coffee, and more than anything, being an incredibly loving and present father to our boys so I could carve out time to write. People often ask me how I do it all, and the fact of the matter is that I simply do not. You and I do it together. You are an incredible partner and work hard to provide an amazing life for us. I would not be where I am in my career or my life without you. I am incredibly grateful for you. I love you and our life together.

To the absolute loves of my life, Dylan and Shaan: Being your mom is the greatest gift of my lifetime. I work hard to give you an incredibly loving and safe home and to make this wild world a better place for you both. Dylan, your quiet observation of the world and ability to follow what fills your heart teaches me to slow down, be present, and lean into my intuition. Shaan, your zest for life (and board games) sparks fun and excitement in our home, and your affection fills my cup. I want both of you to hold on to your spirits, your creativity, and your love of reading. I love you bigger than the multiverse and want you to always remember: You are strong. You are brave. And today is going to be a good day.

To every woman: This book is for you. For the generations of women before us who deserved access to this information, and for the generations after us who will no longer live in the dark when it pertains to their pelvic health. For my patients, who over seventeen years of practicing have trusted me with their care. For every person who follows me on social media, shares my posts, reads my blogs, or tells me their pelvic floor problem while waiting in a bathroom line. For every medical provider who refers their patients to pelvic floor therapy instead of dismissing their problems. And for every pelvic health provider who walks this lesser-known path, takes the leap to follow their passion, and works to normalize pelvic floor conversations instead of pelvic floor problems. Let's keep saving the world, one vagina at a time.

References

INTRODUCTION

Beck Cheryl T, Sue Watson, Robert K Gable. "Traumatic Childbirth and Its Aftermath: Is There Anything Positive?" Journal of Perinatal Education 27 (3) (June) *https://doi.org/10.1891/1058-1243.27.3.175*.

Jundt, Katharina, Ursula Peschers, Heribert Kentenich. 2015. "Vaginal Jade Eggs: Ancient Chinese Practice or Modern Marketing Myth?" *Female Pelvic Medicine & Reconstructive Surgery* 25 (1): 1–2. *https://doi.org/10.1097/SPV.0000000000000643*.

Jundt K, Peschers U, Kentenich H. 2015. "The investigation and treatment of female pelvic floor dysfunction." *Deutches Arzteblatt International* 112 (33–34): 564–74. *doi:10.3238/arztebl.2015.0564*.

Kenton, Kimberly, and Elizabeth R. Mueller. 2006. "The Global Burden of Female Pelvic Floor Disorders." *BJU International* 98 (s1): 1–5. *https://doi.org/10.1111/j.1464-410X.2006.06299.x*.

Subak LL, et al. 2008. "High costs of urinary incontinence among women electing surgery to treat stress incontinence." *Obstetrics and Gynecology* 111 (4): 899–907. *https://doi.org/10.1097/AOG.0b013e31816a1e12*.

CHAPTER 1: PULLING BACK THE CURTAINS

Aschkenazi, Sarit O, and Roger P Goldberg. 2009. "Female Sexual Function and the Pelvic Floor." *Expert Review of Obstetrics & Gynecology* 4 (2): 165–78. *https://doi.org/10.1586/17474108.4.2.165*.

Basnyat, Iccha. 2011. "Beyond Biomedicine: Health through Social and Cultural Understanding." *Nursing Inquiry* 18 (2): 123–34. *https://doi.org/10.1111/j.1440-1800.2011.00518.x*.

Fante, Júlia Ferreira, Thais Daniel Silva, Elaine Cristine Lemes Mateus-Vasconcelos, Cristine Homsi Jorge Ferreira, and Luiz Gustavo Oliveira Brito. 2019. "Do Women Have Adequate Knowledge about Pelvic Floor Dysfunctions? A Systematic Review." *Revista Brasileira de Ginecologia e Obstetrícia* 41 (September): 508–19. *https://doi.org/10.1055/s-0039-1695002*.

François, Isabelle, Brigitte Bagnol, Matthew Chersich, Francisco Mbofana, Esmeralda Mariano, Hipolito Nzwalo, Elise Kenter, Nazarius Mbona Tumwesigye, Terry Hull, and Adriane Martin Hilber. 2012. "Prevalence and Motivations of Vaginal Practices in Tete Province, Mozambique." *International Journal of Sexual Health* 24 (3): 205–17. *https://doi.org/10.1080/19317611.2012.691443*.

Gowda, Supreeth N., and Bruno Bordoni. 2024. "Anatomy, Abdomen and Pelvis: Levator Ani Muscle." In *StatPearls*. Treasure Island (FL): StatPearls Publishing. *http://www.ncbi.nlm.nih.gov/books/NBK556078/*.

Mwakawanga, Dorkasi L., Beatrice Mwilike, Morie Kaneko, and Yoko Shimpuku. 2022. "Local Knowledge and Derived Practices of Safety during Pregnancy, Childbirth and Postpartum: A Qualitative Study among Nurse-Midwives in Urban Eastern Tanzania." *BMJ Open* 12 (12): e068216. *https://doi.org/10.1136/bmjopen-2022-068216*.

Neels, Hedwig, Jean-Jacques Wyndaele, Wiebren A. A. Tjalma, Stefan De Wachter, Michel Wyndaele, and Alexandra Vermandel. 2016. "Knowledge of the Pelvic Floor in Nulliparous Women." *Journal of Physical Therapy Science* 28 (5): 1524–33. *https://doi.org/10.1589/jpts.28.1524*.

Pauls, Rachel N. 2015. "Anatomy of the Clitoris and the Female Sexual Response." *Clinical Anatomy* 28 (3): 376–84. *https://doi.org/10.1002/ca.22524*.

Quaghebeur, Jörgen, Peter Petros, Jean-Jacques Wyndaele, and Stefan De Wachter. 2021. "Pelvic-Floor Function, Dysfunction, and Treatment." *European Journal of Obstetrics & Gynecology and Reproductive Biology* 265 (October): 143–49. *https://doi.org/10.1016/j.ejogrb.2021.08.026*.

Rossetti, Salvatore Rocca. 2016. "Functional Anatomy of Pelvic Floor." *Archivio Italiano Di Urologia e Andrologia* 88 (1): 28–37. *https://doi.org/10.4081/aiua.2016.1.28*.

Snyder, Kailey, Elizabeth Mollard, Kari Bargstadt-Wilson, and Julie Peterson. 2022. "'We Don't Talk about It Enough': Perceptions of Pelvic Health among Postpartum Women in Rural Communities." *Women's Health* 18 (September): 17455057221122584. *https://doi.org/10.1177/17455057221122584*.

CHAPTER 2: PELVIC FLOOR HEALTH 101

Berzuk, Kelli, and Barbara Shay. 2015. "Effect of Increasing Awareness of Pelvic Floor Muscle Function on Pelvic Floor Dysfunction: A Randomized Controlled Trial." *International Urogynecology Journal* 26 (6): 837–44. *https://doi.org/10.1007/s00192-014-2599-z*.

Bø, Kari, Bary Berghmans, Siv Mørkved, and Marijke Van Kampen. 2023. *Evidence-Based Physical Therapy for the Pelvic Floor - E-Book*. Elsevier Health Sciences.

Díaz-Álvarez, Lara, Laura Lorenzo-Gallego, Helena Romay-Barrero, Virginia Prieto-Gómez, María Torres-Lacomba, and Beatriz Navarro-Brazález. 2022. "Does the Contractile Capability of Pelvic Floor Muscles Improve with Knowledge Acquisition and Verbal Instructions in Healthy Women? A Systematic Review." *International Journal of Environmental Research and Public Health* 19 (15): 9308. *https://doi.org/10.3390/ijerph19159308*.

Joseph, Christine, Kosha Srivastava, Olive Ochuba, Sheila W Ruo, Tasnim Alkayyali, Jasmine K Sandhu, Ahsan Waqar, Ashish Jain, and Sujan Poudel. n.d. "Stress Urinary Incontinence Among Young Nulliparous Female Athletes." *Cureus* 13 (9): e17986. *https://doi.org/10.7759/cureus.17986*.

Khodarahmi, S., N. Kariman, A. Ebadi, and G. Ozgoli. 2018. "Effect of Exercise on Stress Urinary Incontinence in Women: A Review Study." *Iranian Journal of Obstetrics, Gynecology and Infertility* 21 (3): 78–89.

Kim, So Young, and Jeong Sook Park. 2000. "The Effect of Pelvic Muscle Exercise Program on Women with Stress Urinary Incontinence in the Degree and Amount of Urinary Incontinence and Maximum Vaginal Contraction Pressure." *Korean Journal of Adult Nursing* 12 (2): 267–77.

Moen, Michael D., Michael B. Noone, Brett J. Vassallo, Denise M. Elser. 2009. "Pelvic
    Floor Muscle Function in Women Presenting with Pelvic Floor Disorders."
    International Urogynecology Journal 20 (7): 843–46. *https://doi.org/10.1007/s00192-
    009-0853-6.*
Nygaard, Ingrid E., and Janet M. Shaw. 2016. "Physical Activity and the Pelvic
    Floor." *American Journal of Obstetrics and Gynecology* 214 (2): 164–71. *https://doi.
    org/10.1016/j.ajog.2015.08.067.*
Sartori, Dulcegleika Vilas Boas, Paulo Roberto Kawano, Hamilton Akihissa Yamamoto,
    Rodrigo Guerra, Pedro Rochetti Pajolli, and João Luiz Amaro. 2021. "Pelvic Floor
    Muscle Strength Is Correlated with Sexual Function." *Investigative and Clinical Urology*
    62 (1): 79–84. *https://doi.org/10.4111/icu.20190248.*
The American Society of Colon and Rectal Surgeons. n.d. "Pelvic Floor Dysfunction
    Expanded Version | ASCRS." Accessed September 5, 2024. *https://fascrs.org/patients/
    diseases-and-conditions/a-z/pelvic-floor-dysfunction-expanded-version.*

CHAPTER 3: TAMING THE TINKLER
Adams, Sonia R., Sybil G. Dessie, Laura E. Dodge, Jessica L. Mckinney, Michele R.
    Hacker, and Eman A. Elkadry. 2015. "Pelvic Floor Physical Therapy as Primary
    Treatment of Pelvic Floor Disorders With Urinary Urgency and Frequency-
    Predominant Symptoms." *Urogynecology* 21 (5): 252. *https://doi.org/10.1097/
    SPV.0000000000000195.*
Berghmans, L.c.m., H.j.m. Hendriks, R.a. De Bie, E.s.c. Van Waalwijk, Van Doorn,
    K. Bø, and Ph.e.v. Van Kerrebroeck. 2000. "Conservative Treatment of Urge
    Urinary Incontinence in Women: A Systematic Review of Randomized Clinical
    Trials." *BJU International* 85 (3): 254–63. *https://doi.org/10.1046/j.1464-
    410x.2000.00434.x.*
Bø, K. 1995. "Pelvic Floor Muscle Exercise for the Treatment of Stress Urinary
    Incontinence: An Exercise Physiology Perspective." *International Urogynecology Journal*
    6(5):282–91. *https://doi.org/10.1007/BF01901527.*
Bø, K., A. C. N. L. Fernandes, T. B. Duarte, L. G. O. Brito, and C. H. J. Ferreira. 2020.
    "Is Pelvic Floor Muscle Training Effective for Symptoms of Overactive Bladder
    in Women? A Systematic Review." *Physiotherapy* 106 (March): 65–76. *https://doi.
    org/10.1016/j.physio.2019.08.011.*
Burgio, Kathryn L. 2004. "Behavioral Treatment Options for Urinary Incontinence."
    Gastroenterology 126 (January): S82–89. *https://doi.org/10.1053/j.gastro.2003.10.042.*
Cervigni, Mauro, and Franca Natale. 2014. "Gynecological
    Disorders in Bladder Pain Syndrome/Interstitial Cystitis Patients." *International Journal
    of Urology* 21 (S1): 85–88. *https://doi.org/10.1111/iju.12379.*
Chermansky, Christopher J., and Pamela A. Moalli. 2016. "Role of Pelvic Floor in Lower
    Urinary Tract Function." *Autonomic Neuroscience*, 200 (October): 43–48. *https://doi.
    org/10.1016/j.autneu.2015.06.003.*
Chisholm, Leah, Sophia Delpe, Tiffany Priest, and W. Stuart Reynolds. 2019. "Physical
    Activity and Stress Incontinence in Women." *Current Bladder Dysfunction Reports* 14
    (3): 174–79. *https://doi.org/10.1007/s11884-019-00519-6.*
FitzGerald, M. P., C. K. Payne, E. S. Lukacz, C. C. Yang, K. M. Peters,
    T. C. Chai, J. C. Nickel, et al. 2012. "Randomized Multicenter
    Clinical Trial of Myofascial Physical Therapy in Women With Interstitial Cystitis/
    Painful Bladder Syndrome and Pelvic Floor Tenderness." *Journal of Urology* June.
    https://doi.org/10.1016/j.juro.2012.01.123.

Gram, Marte Charlotte Dobbertin, and Kari Bø. 2020. "High Level Rhythmic Gymnasts and Urinary Incontinence: Prevalence, Risk Factors, and Influence on Performance." *Scandinavian Journal of Medicine & Science in Sports* 30 (1): 159–65. *https://doi.org/10.1111/sms.13548.*

Greer, Joy A., Ariana L. Smith, and Lily A. Arya. 2012. "Pelvic Floor Muscle Training for Urgency Urinary Incontinence in Women: A Systematic Review." *International Urogynecology Journal* 23 (6): 687–97.*https://doi.org/10.1007/s00192-011-1651-5.*

Lukban, James Chivian, and Kristene E. Whitmore. 2002. "Pelvic Floor Muscle Re-Education Treatment of the Overactive Bladder and Painful Bladder Syndrome." *Clinical Obstetrics and Gynecology* 45 (1): 273.

Nygaard, Ingrid E., Karl J. Kreder, Mary M. Lepic, Kathleen A. Fountain, and Ann T. Rhomberg. 1996. "Efficacy of Pelvic Floor Muscle Exercises in Women with Stress, Urge, and Mixed Urinary Incontinence." *American Journal of Obstetrics and Gynecology* 174 (1, Part 1): 120–25. *https://doi.org/10.1016/S0002-9378(96)70383-6.*

Price, Natalia, Rehana Dawood, and Simon R. Jackson. 2010. "Pelvic Floor Exercise for Urinary Incontinence: A Systematic Literature Review." *Maturitas* 67 (4): 309–15. *https://doi.org/10.1016/j.maturitas.2010.08.004.*

Rebullido, Tamara Rial, Cinta Gómez-Tomás, Avery D. Faigenbaum, and Iván Chulvi-Medrano. 2021. "The Prevalence of Urinary Incontinence among Adolescent Female Athletes: A Systematic Review." *Journal of Functional Morphology and Kinesiology* 6 (1): 12. *https://doi.org/10.3390/jfmk6010012.*

Sar, Dilek, and Leyla Khorshid. 2009. "The Effects of Pelvic Floor Muscle Training on Stress and Mixed Urinary Incontinence and Quality Of Life." *Journal of Wound Ostomy & Continence Nursing* 36 (4): 429. *https://doi.org/10.1097/WON.0b013e3181aaf539.*

Schelbert, Vasco, Lena Kriwanek, S. Ramesh Sakthivel, Lotte Kristoferitsch, Harald Gründl, and Christoph Lüthi. 2024. "How Women and Men Pee: Assessing Gender-Specific Urination Practices for a Comfortable Toilet Experience." *Ergonomics in Design* 32 (1): 5–12. *https://doi.org/10.1177/10648046211044008.*

Sung, Vivian W., Diane Borello-France, Diane K. Newman, Holly E. Richter, Emily S. Lukacz, Pamela Moalli, Alison C. Weidner, et al. 2019. "Effect of Behavioral and Pelvic Floor Muscle Therapy Combined With Surgery vs Surgery Alone on Incontinence Symptoms Among Women With Mixed Urinary Incontinence: The ESTEEM Randomized Clinical Trial." *JAMA* 322 (11): 1066–76. *https://doi.org/10.1001/jama.2019.12467.*

Thom, David H., and Guri Rortveit. 2010. "Prevalence of Postpartum Urinary Incontinence: A Systematic Review." *Acta Obstetricia et Gynecologica Scandinavica* 89 (12): 1511–22. *https://doi.org/10.3109/00016349.2010.526188.*

CHAPTER 4: THE SCOOP ON POOP

Asnong, Anne, André D'Hoore, Marijke Van Kampen, Nele Devoogdt, An De Groef, Kim Sterckx, Hilde Lemkens, et al. 2021. "Randomised Controlled Trial to Assess Efficacy of Pelvic Floor Muscle Training on Bowel Symptoms after Low Anterior Resection for Rectal Cancer: Study Protocol." *BMJ Open* 11 (1): e041797. *https://doi.org/10.1136/bmjopen-2020-041797.*

Bharucha, Adil E., and Sidney F. Phillips. 2001. "SLOW TRANSIT CONSTIPATION." *Gastroenterology Clinics of North America* 30 (1): 77–96. *https://doi.org/10.1016/S0889-8553(05)70168-0.*

Ditah, Ivo, Pardha Devaki, Henry N. Luma, Chobufo Ditah, Basile Njei, Charles Jaiyeoba, Augustine Salami, Calistus Ditah, Oforbuike Ewelukwa, and Lawrence Szarka. 2014. "Prevalence, Trends, and Risk Factors for Fecal Incontinence in United States Adults, 2005–2010." *Clinical Gastroenterology and Hepatology* 12 (4): 636–643.e2. *https://doi.org/10.1016/j.cgh.2013.07.020*.

Freeman, Alison, and Stacy Menees. 2016. "Fecal Incontinence and Pelvic Floor Dysfunction in Women: A Review." *Gastroenterology Clinics of North America* 45 (2): 217–37. *https://doi.org/10.1016/j.gtc.2016.02.002*.

Gonenne, J., T. Esfandyari, M. Camilleri, D. D. Burton, D. A. Stephens, K. L. Baxter, A. R. Zinsmeister, and A. E. Bharucha. 2006. "Effect of Female Sex Hormone Supplementation and Withdrawal on Gastrointestinal and Colonic Transit in Postmenopausal Women." *Neurogastroenterology & Motility* 18 (10): 911–18. *https://doi. org/10.1111/j.1365-2982.2006.00808.x*.

Harrington, Kendra L, and Esther M Haskvitz. 2006. "Managing a Patient's Constipation With Physical Therapy." *Physical Therapy* 86 (11): 1511–19. *https://doi.org/10.2522/ ptj.20050347*.

Jorge, J. M., and S. D. Wexner. 1993. "Etiology and Management of Fecal Incontinence." *Diseases of the Colon and Rectum* 36 (1): 77–97. *https://doi.org/10.1007/BF02050307*.

Lämås, Kristina, Lars Lindholm, Hans Stenlund, Birgitta Engström, and Catrine Jacobsson. 2009. "Effects of Abdominal Massage in Management of Constipation—A Randomized Controlled Trial." *International Journal of Nursing Studies* 46 (6): 759–67. *https://doi.org/10.1016/j.ijnurstu.2009.01.007*.

Lewicky-Gaupp, Christina, Cynthia Brincat, Aisha Yousuf, Divya A. Patel, John O. L. Delancey, and Dee E. Fenner. 2010. "Fecal Incontinence in Older Women: Are Levator Ani Defects a Factor?" *American Journal of Obstetrics and Gynecology* 202 (5): 491.e1–491.e6. *https://doi.org/10.1016/j.ajog.2010.01.020*.

Lewicky-Gaupp, Christina, Quinn Hamilton, James Ashton-Miller, Markus Huebner, John O. L. DeLancey, and Dee E. Fenner. 2009. "Anal Sphincter Structure and Function Relationships in Aging and Fecal Incontinence." *American Journal of Obstetrics and Gynecology* 200 (5): 559.e1–559.e5. *https://doi.org/10.1016/j. ajog.2008.11.009*.

Lewis, S. J., and K. W. Heaton. 1997. "Stool Form Scale as a Useful Guide to Intestinal Transit Time." *Scandinavian Journal of Gastroenterology* 32 (9): 920–24. *https://doi. org/10.3109/00365529709011203*.

Lunsford, Tisha N., Mary A. Atia, Suaka Kagbo-Kue, and Lucinda A. Harris. 2022. "A Pain in the Butt: Hemorrhoids, Fissures, Fistulas, and Other Anorectal Syndromes." *Gastroenterology Clinics of North America*, Pelvic Floor Disorders, 51 (1): 123–44. *https://doi.org/10.1016/j.gtc.2021.10.008*.

Malone, Jordan C., and Aravind Thavamani. 2024. "Physiology, Gastrocolic Reflex." In *StatPearls*. Treasure Island (FL): StatPearls Publishing. *http://www.ncbi.nlm.nih.gov/ books/NBK549888*.

Maria, Giorgio, Gerardo Anastasio, Giuseppe Brisinda, and Ignazio Massimo Civello. 1997. "Treatment of Puborectalis Syndrome with Progressive Anal Dilation." *Diseases of the Colon & Rectum* 40 (1): 89–92. *https://doi.org/10.1007/BF02055688*.

Modi, Rohan M., Alice Hinton, Daniel Pinkhas, Royce Groce, Marty M. Meyer, Gokulakrishnan Balasubramanian, Edward Levine, and Peter P. Stanich. 2019a. "Implementation of a Defecation Posture Modification Device." *Journal of Clinical Gastroenterology* 53 (3): 216–19. *https://doi.org/10.1097/ MCG.0000000000001143*.

————. 2019b. "Implementation of a Defecation Posture Modification Device: Impact on Bowel Movement Patterns in Healthy Subjects." *Journal of Clinical Gastroenterology* 53 (3): 216. *https://doi.org/10.1097/MCG.0000000000001143.*

National Institutes of Health. n.d. "Treatment for Constipation-NIDDK." National Institute of Diabetes and Digestive and Kidney Diseases. Accessed September 5, 2024. *https://www.niddk.nih.gov/health-information/digestive-diseases/constipation/treatment.*

Norton, Christine, Louise Thomas, and Jennifer Hill. 2007. "Management of Faecal Incontinence in Adults: Summary of NICE Guidance." *BMJ: British Medical Journal* 334 (7608): 1370–71. *https://doi.org/10.1136/bmj.39231.633275.AD.*

Pucciani, F., and M. Trafeli. 2021. "Sampling Reflex: Pathogenic Role in Functional Defecation Disorder." *Techniques in Coloproctology* 25 (5): 521–30. *https://doi.org/10.1007/s10151-020-02393-5.*

Rao, Satish S. C., Ashok K. Tuteja, Tony Vellema, Joan Kempf, and Mary Stessman. 2004. "Dyssynergic Defecation: Demographics, Symptoms, Stool Patterns, and Quality of Life." *Journal of Clinical Gastroenterology* 38 (8): 680. *https://doi.org/10.1097/01.mcg.0000135929.78074.8c.*

Sadeghi, Anahita, Elham Akbarpour, Fatemeh Majidirad, Serhat Bor, Mojgan Forootan, Mohammad-Reza Hadian, and Peyman Adibi. 2023. "Dyssynergic Defecation: A Comprehensive Review on Diagnosis and Management." *The Turkish Journal of Gastroenterology* 34 (3): 182–95. *https://doi.org/10.5152/tjg.2023.22148.*

Sakakibara, Ryuji, Kuniko Tsunoyama, Hiroyasu Hosoi, Osamu Takahashi, Megumi Sugiyama, Masahiko Kishi, Emina Ogawa, Hitoshi Terada, Tomoyuki Uchiyama, and Tomonori Yamanishi. 2010. "Influence of Body Position on Defecation in Humans." *LUTS* 2 (April): 16–21. *https://doi.org/10.1111/j.1757-5672.2009.00057.x.*

Srinivasan, Sushmitha Grama, Mayank Sharma, Kelly Feuerhak, Kent R. Bailey, and Adil E. Bharucha. 2021. "A Comparison of Rectoanal Pressures during Valsalva Maneuver and Evacuation Uncovers Rectoanal Discoordination in Defecatory Disorders." *Neurogastroenterology & Motility* 33 (10): e14126. *https://doi.org/10.1111/nmo.14126.*

The Rome Foundation. n.d. "Rome IV Criteria." Rome Foundation. Accessed September 5, 2024. *https://theromefoundation.org/rome-iv/rome-iv-criteria.*

Tillou, John, and Vitaliy Poylin. 2016. "Functional Disorders: Slow-Transit Constipation." *Clinics in Colon and Rectal Surgery* 30 (December): 76–86. *https://doi.org/10.1055/s-0036-1593436.*

Whitehead, William E., and Adil E. Bharucha. 2010. "Diagnosis and Treatment of Pelvic Floor Disorders: What's New and What to Do." *Gastroenterology* 138 (4): 1231–1235. e4. *https://doi.org/10.1053/j.gastro.2010.02.036.*

CHAPTER 5: THE POWER OF YOUR PERIOD

Arbuckle, Janeen L., Alison M. Parden, Kimberly Hoover, Russell L. Griffin, and Holly E. Richter. 2019. "Prevalence and Awareness of Pelvic Floor Disorders in Female Adolescents Seeking Gynecologic Care." *Journal of Pediatric and Adolescent Gynecology* 32 (3): 288–92. *https://doi.org/10.1016/j.jpag.2018.11.010.*

Bhatia, Narender N., and Mat H. Ho. 2006. "Role of Hormones in the Pathophysiology of Pelvic Floor Disorders in Women." *Current Opinion in Obstetrics and Gynecology* 18 (5): 525. *https://doi.org/10.1097/01.gco.0000242955.40491.c5.*

Blanco-Diaz, Maria, Ana Vielva-Gomez, Marina Legasa-Susperregui, Borja Perez-Dominguez, Esther M. Medrano-Sánchez, and Esther Diaz-Mohedo. 2024. "Exploring Pelvic Symptom Dynamics in Relation to the Menstrual Cycle: Implications for Clinical Assessment and Management." *Journal of Personalized Medicine* 14 (3): 239. *https://doi.org/10.3390/jpm14030239.*

Bø, Kari, and Ingrid Elisabeth Nygaard. 2020. "Is Physical Activity Good or Bad for the Female Pelvic Floor? A Narrative Review." *Sports Medicine* 50 (3): 471–84. *https://doi. org/10.1007/s40279-019-01243-1.*

Davila, G. Willy. 2009. "Hormonal Influences on the Pelvic Floor." In *Pelvic Floor Dysfunction: A Multidisciplinary Approach*, edited by G. Willy Davila, Gamal M. Ghoniem, and Steven D. Wexner, 295–99. London: Springer. *https://doi. org/10.1007/978-1-84800-348-4_50.*

Delgado, Benjamin J., and Wilfredo Lopez-Ojeda. 2024. "Estrogen." In *StatPearls*. Treasure Island (FL): StatPearls Publishing. *http://www.ncbi.nlm.nih.gov/books/ NBK538260.*

Farage, Miranda A, Kenneth W Miller, and Ann Davis. 2011. "Cultural Aspects of Menstruation and Menstrual Hygiene in Adolescents." *Expert Review of Obstetrics & Gynecology* 6 (2): 127–39. *https://doi.org/10.1586/eog.11.1.*

Fennie, Thelma, Mokgadi Moletsane, and Anita Padmanabhanunni. 2022. "Adolescent Girls' Perceptions and Cultural Beliefs about Menstruation and Menstrual Practices: A Scoping Review." *African Journal of Reproductive Health* 26 (2): 88–105. *https://doi. org/10.29063/ajrh2022/v26i2.9.*

Ferrero, Simone, Francesca Esposito, Luiza Helena Abbamonte, Paola Anserini, Valentino Remorgida, and Nicola Ragni. 2005. "Quality of Sex Life in Women with Endometriosis and Deep Dyspareunia." *Fertility and Sterility* 83 (3): 573–79. *https:// doi.org/10.1016/j.fertnstert.2004.07.973.*

Fritzer, N., D. Haas, P. Oppelt, St Renner, D. Hornung, M. Wölfler, U. Ulrich, G. Fischerlehner, M. Sillem, and G. Hudelist. 2013. "More than Just Bad Sex: Sexual Dysfunction and Distress in Patients with Endometriosis." *European Journal of Obstetrics, Gynecology, and Reproductive Biology* 169 (2): 392–96. *https://doi. org/10.1016/j.ejogrb.2013.04.001.*

Guarneri, Alissa M., and Manmohan K. Kamboj. 2019. "Physiology of Pubertal Development in Females." *Pediatric Medicine* 2 (2019). *https://doi.org/10.21037/ pm.2019.07.03.*

Hamal, M., and Susma Kc. 2014. "Hygiene, Health Problems and Socio-Cultural Practices: What School Girls Do During Menstruation?" *International Journal of Health Sciences and Research. https://www.semanticscholar.org/paper/ Hygiene%2C-Health-Problems-and-Socio-Cultural-What-Do-Hamal-Kc/ d68d740de1f0198e34282676696d647da8d3da74.*

Hebert-Beirne, Jennifer M., Rachel O'Conor, Jeni Donatelli Ihm, Molly Kirk Parlier, Missy D. Lavender, and Linda Brubaker. 2017. "A Pelvic Health Curriculum in School Settings: The Effect on Adolescent Females' Knowledge." *Journal of Pediatric and Adolescent Gynecology* 30 (2): 188–92. *https://doi.org/10.1016/j. jpag.2015.09.006.*

Hennegan, Julie, Deborah Jordan Brooks, Kellogg J. Schwab, and G. J. Melendez-Torres. 2020. "Measurement in the Study of Menstrual Health and Hygiene: A Systematic Review and Audit." *PLoS ONE* 15 (6): e0232935. *https://doi.org/10.1371/journal. pone.0232935.*

Leena, Sequira, and Soumya. 2020. "A Descriptive Study on Cultural Practices about Menarche and Menstruation." *Journal of Health and Allied Sciences NU* 06 (April): 10–13. *https://doi.org/10.1055/s-0040-1708631.*

Liu, H.-L., K.-H. Chen, and N.-H. Peng. 2012. "Cultural Practices Relating to Menarche and Menstruation among Adolescent Girls in Taiwan—Qualitative Investigation." *Journal of Pediatric and Adolescent Gynecology* 25 (1): 43–47. *https://doi. org/10.1016/j.jpag.2011.08.006.*

López-Liria, Remedios, Lucía Torres-Álamo, Francisco A. Vega-Ramírez, Amelia V. García-Luengo, José M. Aguilar-Parra, Rubén Trigueros-Ramos, and Patricia Rocamora-Pérez. 2021. "Efficacy of Physiotherapy Treatment in Primary Dysmenorrhea: A Systematic Review and Meta-Analysis." *International Journal of Environmental Research and Public Health* 18 (15): 7832. *https://doi.org/10.3390/ijerph18157832.*

Micussi, Maria Thereza, Rodrigo Pegado Freitas, Priscylla Helouyse Angelo, Elvira Maria Soares, Telma Maria Lemos, and Técia Maria Maranhão. 2015. "Is There a Difference in the Electromyographic Activity of the Pelvic Floor Muscles across the Phases of the Menstrual Cycle?" *Journal of Physical Therapy Science* 27 (7): 2233–37. *https://doi.org/10.1589/jpts.27.2233.*

Micussi, Maria Thereza, Rodrigo Pegado Freitas, Larissa Varella, Elvira Maria Soares, Telma Maria Lemos, and Técia Maria Maranhão. 2016. "Relationship between Pelvic Floor Muscle and Hormone Levels in Polycystic Ovary Syndrome." *Neurourology and Urodynamics* 35 (7): 780–85. *https://doi.org/10.1002/nau.22817.*

Monis, Carol N., and Maggie Tetrokalashvili. 2024. "Menstrual Cycle Proliferative And Follicular Phase." In *StatPearls.* Treasure Island (FL): StatPearls Publishing. *http://www.ncbi.nlm.nih.gov/books/NBK542229.*

Parden, Alison M., Russell L. Griffin, Kimberly Hoover, David R. Ellington, Jonathan L. Gleason, Kathryn L. Burgio, and Holly E. Richter. 2016. "Prevalence, Awareness, and Understanding of Pelvic Floor Disorders in Adolescent and Young Women." *Urogynecology* 22 (5): 346. *https://doi.org/10.1097/SPV.0000000000000287.*

Reed, Beverly G., and Bruce R. Carr. 2000. "The Normal Menstrual Cycle and the Control of Ovulation." In *Endotext,* edited by Kenneth R. Feingold, Bradley Anawalt, Marc R. Blackman, Alison Boyce, George Chrousos, Emiliano Corpas, Wouter W. de Herder, et al. South Dartmouth (MA): MDText.com, Inc. *http://www.ncbi.nlm.nih.gov/books/NBK279054.*

Sandhiya, Dr M., Dr Priya Kumari, A. Arulya, Dr P. Senthil Selvam, Dr M. Manoj Abraham, and Dr Tushar J. Palekar. 2021. "The Effect of Pelvic Floor Muscle Exercise on Quality of Life in Females with Primary Dysmenorrhea." *Annals of the Romanian Society for Cell Biology* 25 (6): 3111–17.

Silva, Joyce Pereira da, Bianca Maciel de Almeida, Renata Santos Ferreira, Claudia Regina de Paiva Oliveira Lima, Leila Maria Álvares Barbosa, and Caroline Wanderley Souto Ferreira. 2023. "Sensory and Muscular Functions of the Pelvic Floor in Women with Endometriosis—Cross-Sectional Study." *Archives of Gynecology and Obstetrics* 308 (1): 163–70. *https://doi.org/10.1007/s00404-023-07037-1.*

Smorgick, Noam, and Sawsan As-Sanie. 2018. "Pelvic Pain in Adolescents." *Seminars in Reproductive Medicine* 36 (December): 116–22. *https://doi.org/10.1055/s-0038-1676088.*

Stubbs, Margaret L. 2008. "Cultural Perceptions and Practices around Menarche and Adolescent Menstruation in the United States." *Annals of the New York Academy of Sciences* 1135 (1): 58–66. *https://doi.org/10.1196/annals.1429.008.*

Ten, Tjon. 2007. "Menstrual Hygiene: A Neglected Condition for the Achievement of Several Millennium Development Goals." Brussels, Belgium: Europe External Policy Advisors.

Thiyagarajan, Dhanalakshmi K., Hajira Basit, and Rebecca Jeanmonod. 2024. "Physiology, Menstrual Cycle." In *StatPearls.* Treasure Island (FL): StatPearls Publishing. *http://www.ncbi.nlm.nih.gov/books/NBK500020.*

Trant, Amelia A., Alla Vash-Margita, Deepa Camenga, Paula Braverman, Denise Wagner, Mariana Espinal, Edwina P. Kisanga, Lisbeth Lundsberg, Sangini S. Sheth, and Linda

Fan. 2022. "Menstrual Health and Hygiene among Adolescents in the United States." *Journal of Pediatric and Adolescent Gynecology* 35 (3): 277–87. *https://doi.org/10.1016/j. jpag.2021.12.014.*

CHAPTER 6: LET'S TALK ABOUT SEX

Aslan, Melike, Şeyda Yavuzkır, and Sema Baykara. 2020. "Is 'Dilator Use' More Effective Than 'Finger Use' in Exposure Therapy in Vaginismus Treatment?" *Journal of Sex & Marital Therapy* 46 (4): 354–60. *https://doi.org/10.1080/009262 3X.2020.1716907.*

Both, Stephanie, and Ellen Laan. 2007. "Simultaneous Measurement of Pelvic Floor Muscle Activity and Vaginal Blood Flow: A Pilot Study." *The Journal of Sexual Medicine* 4 (3): 690–701. *https://doi.org/10.1111/j.1743-6109.2007.00457.x.*

Darling, Carol Anderson, J. Kenneth Davidson, and Colleen Conway-Welch. 1990. "Female Ejaculation: Perceived Origins, the Grafenberg Spot/Area, and Sexual Responsiveness." *Archives of Sexual Behavior* 19 (1): 29–47. *https://doi.org/10.1007/BF01541824.*

Dias-Amaral, Ana, and André Marques-Pinto. 2018. "Female Genito-Pelvic Pain/ Penetration Disorder: Review of the Related Factors and Overall Approach." *Revista Brasileira De Ginecologia E Obstetricia: Revista Da Federacao Brasileira Das Sociedades De Ginecologia E Obstetricia* 40 (12): 787–93. *https://doi. org/10.1055/s-0038-1675805.*

Eserdag, Süleyman, Merve Ezberci Akgün, and Filiz Şükrü Gürbüz. 2023. "Outcomes of Vaginismus Therapy Assessed by Penetrative Intercourse, Psychiatric Symptoms, and Marital Satisfaction." *Journal of Sex & Marital Therapy* 49 (4): 412–19. *https://doi.org/1 0.1080/0092623X.2022.2127384.*

Fernández-Pérez, Paula, Raquel Leirós-Rodríguez, Mª Pilar Marqués-Sánchez, María Cristina Martínez-Fernández, Fernanda Oliveira de Carvalho, and Leonardo Y. S. Maciel. 2023. "Effectiveness of Physical Therapy Interventions in Women with Dyspareunia: A Systematic Review and Meta-Analysis." *BMC Women's Health* 23 (1): 387. *https://doi.org/10.1186/s12905-023-02532-8.*

Hill, D. Ashley, and Chantel A. Taylor. 2021. "Dyspareunia in Women." *American Family Physician* 103 (10): 597–604.

Korda, Joanna B., Sue W. Goldstein, and Frank Sommer. 2010. "SEXUAL MEDICINE HISTORY: The History of Female Ejaculation." *The Journal of Sexual Medicine* 7 (5): 1965–75. *https://doi.org/10.1111/j.1743-6109.2010.01720.x.*

Maldonado, Mariana, Antonio Egidio Nardi, and Aline Sardinha. 2023. "The Role of Vaginal Penetration Skills and Vaginal Penetration Behavior in Genito-Pelvic Pain/ Penetration Disorder." *Journal of Sex & Marital Therapy* 49 (7): 816–28. *https://doi.org/ 10.1080/0092623X.2023.2193587.*

Marchand, Erica. 2021. "Psychological and Behavioral Treatment of Female Orgasmic Disorder." *Sexual Medicine Reviews* 9 (2): 194–211. *https://doi.org/10.1016/j. sxmr.2020.07.007.*

Martin Hilber, Adriane, Terence H. Hull, Eleanor Preston-Whyte, Brigitte Bagnol, Jenni Smit, Chintana Wacharasin, and Ninuk Widyantoro. 2010. "A Cross Cultural Study of Vaginal Practices and Sexuality: Implications for Sexual Health." *Social Science & Medicine* 70 (3): 392–400. *https://doi.org/10.1016/j.socscimed.2009.10.023.*

Martínez-Galiano, Juan Miguel, Rocío Adriana Peinado-Molina, Sergio Martínez-Vazquez, Fidel Hita-Contreras, Miguel Delgado-Rodríguez, and Antonio Hernández-Martínez. 2024. "Influence of Pelvic Floor Disorders on Sexuality in Women." *International Journal of Gynecology & Obstetrics* 164 (3): 1141–50. *https://doi. org/10.1002/ijgo.15189.*

Pastor, Zlatko. 2013. "Female Ejaculation Orgasm vs. Coital Incontinence: A Systematic Review." *The Journal of Sexual Medicine* 10 (7): 1682–91. *https://doi.org/10.1111/ jsm.12166.*

Pastor, Zlatko, and Roman Chmel. 2018. "Differential Diagnostics of Female 'Sexual' Fluids: A Narrative Review." *International Urogynecology Journal* 29 (5): 621–29. *https:// doi.org/10.1007/s00192-017-3527-9.*

Perez, Samara, and Yitzchak M. Binik. 2016. "Vaginismus: 'Gone' But Not Forgotten," 33 (7). *https://www.psychiatrictimes.com/view/vaginismus-gone-not-forgotten.*

Raveendran, Arkiath Veettil, and Peedikakkal Rajini. 2024. "Vaginismus: Diagnostic Challenges and Proposed Diagnostic Criteria." *Balkan Medical Journal* 41 (1): 80–82. *https://doi.org/10.4274/balkanmedj.galenos.2023.2022-9-62.*

Reissing, Elke D., Heather L. Armstrong, and Caroline Allen. 2013. "Pelvic Floor Physical Therapy for Lifelong Vaginismus: A Retrospective Chart Review and Interview Study." *Journal of Sex & Marital Therapy* 39 (4): 306–20. *https://doi.org/10.1 080/0092623X.2012.697535.*

Rosenbaum, Talli Yehuda. 2005. "Physiotherapy Treatment of Sexual Pain Disorders." *Journal of Sex & Marital Therapy* 31 (4): 329–40. *https://doi. org/10.1080/00926230590950235.*

Salama, Samuel, Florence Boitrelle, Amélie Gauquelin, Lydia Malagrida, Nicolas Thiounn, and Pierre Desvaux. 2015. "Nature and Origin of 'Squirting' in Female Sexuality." *The Journal of Sexual Medicine* 12 (3): 661–66. *https://doi.org/10.1111/ jsm.12799.*

Seehusen, Dean A, Eisenhower Army Medical Center, and Fort Gordon. 2014. "Dyspareunia in Women" 90 (7).

Trahan, Jennifer, Erin Leger, Marlena Allen, Rachel Koebele, Mary Brian Yoffe, Corey Simon, Meryl Alappattu, and Carol Figuers. 2019. "The Efficacy of Manual Therapy for Treatment of Dyspareunia in Females: A Systematic Review." *Journal of Women's Health Physical Therapy* 43 (1): 28–35. *https://doi.org/10.1097/ jwh.0000000000000117.*

Wallen, Kim, and Elisabeth A. Lloyd. 2011. "Female Sexual Arousal: Genital Anatomy and Orgasm in Intercourse." *Hormones and Behavior*, Special Issue on Research on Sexual Arousal, 59 (5): 780–92. *https://doi.org/10.1016/j.yhbeh.2010.12.004.*

Wurn, Lawrence J, Belinda F Wurn, Amanda S Roscow, C Richard King, Eugenia S Scharf, and Jonathan J Shuster. 2004. "Increasing Orgasm and Decreasing Dyspareunia by a Manual Physical Therapy Technique." *Medscape General Medicine* 6 (4): 47.

CHAPTER 7: WHAT TO EXPECT FROM YOUR EXPECTING PELVIC FLOOR

Bartling, Samantha J., and Patrick M. Zito. 2016. "Overview of Pelvic Floor Dysfunction Associated with Pregnancy." *International Journal of Childbirth Education* 31 (1): 18–21.

Baruch, Yoav, Stefano Manodoro, Marta Barba, Alice Cola, Ilaria Re, and Matteo Frigerio. 2023. "Prevalence and Severity of Pelvic Floor Disorders during Pregnancy: Does the Trimester Make a Difference?" *Healthcare* 11 (8): 1096. *https://doi. org/10.3390/healthcare11081096.*

Bø, Kari, Raul Artal, Ruben Barakat, Wendy J. Brown, Gregory A. L. Davies, Michael Dooley, Kelly R. Evenson, et al. 2018. "Exercise and Pregnancy in Recreational and Elite Athletes: 2016/2017 Evidence Summary from the IOC Expert Group Meeting, Lausanne. Part 5. Recommendations for Health Professionals and Active Women." *British Journal of Sports Medicine* 52 (17): 1080–85. *https://doi.org/10.1136/ bjsports-2018-099351.*

Bø, Kari, Marie Ellstrøm Engh, and Gunvor Hilde. 2018. "Regular Exercisers Have Stronger Pelvic Floor Muscles than Nonregular Exercisers at Midpregnancy." *American Journal of Obstetrics and Gynecology* 218 (4): 427.e1–427.e5. *https://doi.org/10.1016/j.ajog.2017.12.220.*

Bø, Kari, and Ingrid Elisabeth Nygaard. 2020. "Is Physical Activity Good or Bad for the Female Pelvic Floor? A Narrative Review." *Sports Medicine* 50 (3): 471–84. *https://doi.org/10.1007/s40279-019-01243-1.*

Bozkurt, Murat, Ayşe Ender Yumru, and Levent Şahin. 2014. "Pelvic Floor Dysfunction, and Effects of Pregnancy and Mode of Delivery on Pelvic Floor." *Taiwanese Journal of Obstetrics and Gynecology* 53 (4): 452–58. *https://doi.org/10.1016/j.tjog.2014.08.001.*

Casagrande, Danielle, Zbigniew Gugala, Shannon M. Clark, and Ronald W. Lindsey. 2015. "Low Back Pain and Pelvic Girdle Pain in Pregnancy." *JAAOS-Journal of the American Academy of Orthopaedic Surgeons* 23 (9): 539. *https://doi.org/10.5435/JAAOS-D-14-00248.*

Casey, Brian M., Joseph I. Schaffer, Steven L. Bloom, Stephen F. Heartwell, Donald D. McIntire, and Kenneth J. Leveno. 2005. "Obstetric Antecedents for Postpartum Pelvic Floor Dysfunction." *American Journal of Obstetrics and Gynecology* 192 (5): 1655–62. *https://doi.org/10.1016/j.ajog.2004.11.031.*

Cattani, Laura, Judit Decoene, Ann-Sophie Page, Natalie Weeg, Jan Deprest, and Hans Peter Dietz. 2021. "Pregnancy, Labour and Delivery as Risk Factors for Pelvic Organ Prolapse: A Systematic Review." *International Urogynecology Journal* 32 (7): 1623–31. *https://doi.org/10.1007/s00192-021-04724-y.*

Daly, Deirdre, Cinny Cusack, and Cecily Begley. 2019. "Learning about Pelvic Floor Muscle Exercises before and during Pregnancy: A Cross-Sectional Study." *International Urogynecology Journal* 30 (6): 965–75. *https://doi.org/10.1007/s00192-018-3848-3.*

Davenport, Margie H., Andree-Anne Marchand, Michelle F. Mottola, Veronica J. Poitras, Casey E. Gray, Alejandra Jaramillo Garcia, Nick Barrowman, et al. 2019. "Exercise for the Prevention and Treatment of Low Back, Pelvic Girdle and Lumbopelvic Pain during Pregnancy: A Systematic Review and Meta-Analysis." *British Journal of Sports Medicine* 53 (2): 90–98. *https://doi.org/10.1136/bjsports-2018-099400.*

Davenport, Margie H., Taniya S. Nagpal, Michelle F. Mottola, Rachel J. Skow, Laurel Riske, Veronica J. Poitras, Alejandra Jaramillo Garcia, et al. 2018. "Prenatal Exercise (Including but Not Limited to Pelvic Floor Muscle Training) and Urinary Incontinence during and Following Pregnancy: A Systematic Review and Meta-Analysis." *British Journal of Sports Medicine* 52 (21): 1397–1404. *https://doi.org/10.1136/bjsports-2018-099780.*

Dufour, Sinéad, Stéphanie Bernard, Beth Murray-Davis, and Nadine Graham. 2019. "Establishing Expert-Based Recommendations for the Conservative Management of Pregnancy-Related Diastasis Rectus Abdominis: A Delphi Consensus Study." *The Journal of Women's & Pelvic Health Physical Therapy* 43 (2): 73. *https://doi.org/10.1097/JWH.0000000000000130.*

Elenskaia, Ksena, Ranee Thakar, Abdul Hameed Sultan, Inka Scheer, and Andrew Beggs. 2011. "The Effect of Pregnancy and Childbirth on Pelvic Floor Muscle Function." *International Urogynecology Journal* 22 (11): 1421–27. *https://doi.org/10.1007/s00192-011-1501-5.*

Fiat, Felicia, Petru Eugen Merghes, Alexandra Denisa Scurtu, Bogdan Almajan Guta, Cristina Adriana Dehelean, Narcis Varan, and Elena Bernad. 2022. "The Main Changes in Pregnancy—Therapeutic Approach to Musculoskeletal Pain." *Medicina* 58 (8): 1115. *https://doi.org/10.3390/medicina58081115.*

Frigerio, Matteo, Giuseppe Marino, Marta Barba, Stefania Palmieri, Alessandro
Ferdinando Ruffolo, Rebecca Degliuomini, Pasquale Gallo, et al. 2023. "Prevalence
and Severity of Bowel Disorders in the Third Trimester of Pregnancy." *AJOG Global
Reports* 3 (3): 100218. *https://doi.org/10.1016/j.xagr.2023.100218.*

Gruszczyńska, Dominika, and Aleksandra Truszczyńska-Baszak. 2018. "Exercises for
Pregnant and Postpartum Women with Diastasis Recti Abdominis—Literature
Review." *Advances in Rehabilitation* 32 (3): 27–35. *https://doi.org/10.5114/
areh.2018.80967.*

Hezel, John-Paul D. 2017. "Musculoskeletal Pain in Pregnancy." In *Medical Problems
During Pregnancy: A Comprehensive Clinical Guide*, edited by Carolyn Bernstein and
Tamara C. Takoudes, 139–53. Cham: Springer International Publishing. *https://doi.
org/10.1007/978-3-319-39328-5_8.*

Hilde, Gunvor, and Kari Bo. 2015. "The Pelvic Floor During Pregnancy and
after Childbirth, and the Effect of Pelvic Floor Muscle Training on Urinary
Incontinence-A Literature Review." *Current Women's Health Reviews* 11 (1): 19–30.

Kamisan Atan, Ixora, Wenyu Zhang, Ka Lai Shek, and Hans Peter Dietz. 2021. "Does
Pregnancy Affect Pelvic Floor Functional Anatomy? A Retrospective Study."
European Journal of Obstetrics & Gynecology and Reproductive Biology 259 (April): 26–31.
https://doi.org/10.1016/j.ejogrb.2021.01.047.

Karahan, Nazan, Hediye Arslan, and Çetin Çam. 2018. "The Behaviour of Pelvic Floor
Muscles during Uterine Contractions in Spontaneous and Oxytocin-Induced
Labour." *Journal of Obstetrics and Gynaecology: The Journal of the Institute of Obstetrics and
Gynaecology* 38 (5): 629–34. *https://doi.org/10.1080/01443615.2017.1399111.*

Kristiansson, Per, Eva Samuelsson, Bo Von Schoultz, and Kurt Svärdsudd. 2001.
"Reproductive Hormones and Stress Urinary Incontinence in Pregnancy." *Acta
Obstetricia et Gynecologica Scandinavica* 80 (12): 1125–30. *https://doi.org/10.1080/
j.1600-0412.2001.801209.x.*

Larsudd-Kåverud, Jennie, Julia Gyhagen, Sigvard Åkervall, Mattias Molin, Ian Milsom,
Adrian Wagg, and Maria Gyhagen. 2023. "The Influence of Pregnancy, Parity, and
Mode of Delivery on Urinary Incontinence and Prolapse Surgery—a National
Register Study." *American Journal of Obstetrics and Gynecology* 228 (1): 61.e1–61.e13.
https://doi.org/10.1016/j.ajog.2022.07.035.

Liu, Jiayi, Shu Qi Tan, and How Chuan Han. 2019. "Knowledge of Pelvic Floor
Disorder in Pregnancy." *International Urogynecology Journal* 30 (6): 991–1001. *https://
doi.org/10.1007/s00192-019-03891-3.*

Mckay, Elishia R., Lisbet S. Lundsberg, Devin T. Miller, Ashley Draper, Jamie Chao,
Judy Yeh, Sabrina Rangi, Priscilla Torres, Michelle Stoltzman, and Marsha K.
Guess. 2019. "Knowledge of Pelvic Floor Disorders in Obstetrics." *Female
Pelvic Medicine & Reconstructive Surgery* 25 (6): 419–25. *https://doi.org/10.1097/
SPV.0000000000000604.*

Michalska, Agata, Wojciech Rokita, Daniel Wolder, Justyna Pogorzelska, and Krzysztof
Kaczmarczyk. 2018. "Diastasis Recti Abdominis—a Review of Treatment Methods."
Ginekologia Polska 89 (2): 97–101. *https://doi.org/10.5603/GP.a2018.0016.*

"Physiotherapy in Diastasis of the Rectus Abdominis Muscle for Women during
Pregnancy and Postpartum—a Review Paper." n.d. Accessed September 10, 2024.
https://rehmed.pl/article/135015/en.

Rogers, Rebecca G., Cara Ninivaggio, Kelly Gallagher, A. Noelle Borders, Clifford
Qualls, and Lawrence M. Leeman. 2017. "Pelvic Floor Symptoms and Quality of
Life Changes during First Pregnancy: A Prospective Cohort Study." *International
Urogynecology Journal* 28 (11): 1701–7. *https://doi.org/10.1007/s00192-017-3330-7.*

Sangsawang, Bussara, and Nucharee Sangsawang. 2013. "Stress Urinary Incontinence in Pregnant Women: A Review of Prevalence, Pathophysiology, and Treatment." *International Urogynecology Journal* 24 (6): 901–12. *https://doi.org/10.1007/s00192-013-2061-7.*

Sangsawang, Bussara. 2014. "Risk Factors for the Development of Stress Urinary Incontinence during Pregnancy in Primigravidae: A Review of the Literature." *European Journal of Obstetrics & Gynecology and Reproductive Biology* 178 (July): 27–34. *https://doi.org/10.1016/j.ejogrb.2014.04.010.*

Shiri, R., D. Coggon, and K. Falah-Hassani. 2018a. "Exercise for the Prevention of Low Back and Pelvic Girdle Pain in Pregnancy: A Meta-Analysis of Randomized Controlled Trials." *European Journal of Pain* 22 (1): 19–27. *https://doi.org/10.1002/ejp.1096.*

Sperstad, Jorun Bakken, Merete Kolberg Tennfjord, Gunvor Hilde, Marie Ellström-Engh, and Kari Bø. 2016. "Diastasis Recti Abdominis during Pregnancy and 12 Months after Childbirth: Prevalence, Risk Factors and Report of Lumbopelvic Pain." *British Journal of Sports Medicine* 50 (17): 1092–96. *https://doi.org/10.1136/bjsports-2016-096065.*

Thabah, Molly, and Vinod Ravindran. 2015. "Musculoskeletal Problems in Pregnancy." *Rheumatology International* 35 (4): 581–87. *https://doi.org/10.1007/s00296-014-3135-7.*

V, Mahalakshmi, Sumathi G, Chitra Tv, and Ramamoorthy V. 2016. "Effect of Exercise on Diastasis Recti Abdominis among the Primiparous Women: A Quasi-Experimental Study." *International Journal of Reproduction, Contraception, Obstetrics and Gynecology* 5 (12): 4441–46. *https://doi.org/10.18203/2320-1770.ijrcog20164360.*

Viktrup, L, G Lose, M Rolff, and K Barfoed. 1992. "The Symptom of Stress Incontinence Caused by Pregnancy or Delivery in Primiparas." *Obstetrics and Gynecology* 79 (6): 945–49.

Wesnes, Stian Langeland, Guri Rortveit, Kari Bø, and Steinar Hunskaar. 2007. "Urinary Incontinence During Pregnancy." *Obstetrics & Gynecology* 109 (4): 922. *https://doi.org/10.1097/01.AOG.0000257120.23260.00.*

CHAPTER 8: KEEP CALM AND BIRTH ON

Abdelhakim, Ahmed Mohamed, Elsayed Eldesouky, Ibrahim Abo Elmagd, Attia Mohammed, Elsayed Aly Farag, Abd Elhalim Mohammed, Khaled M. Hamam, et al. 2020. "Antenatal Perineal Massage Benefits in Reducing Perineal Trauma and Postpartum Morbidities: A Systematic Review and Meta-Analysis of Randomized Controlled Trials." *International Urogynecology Journal* 31 (9): 1735–45. *https://doi.org/10.1007/s00192-020-04302-8.*

Araujo, Camila Carvalho de, Suelene A. Coelho, Paulo Stahlschmidt, and Cassia R. T. Juliato. 2018. "Does Vaginal Delivery Cause More Damage to the Pelvic Floor than Cesarean Section as Determined by 3D Ultrasound Evaluation? A Systematic Review." *International Urogynecology Journal* 29 (5): 639–45. *https://doi.org/10.1007/s00192-018-3609-3.*

Barasinski, Chloé, and Françoise Vendittelli. 2016. "Effect of the Type of Maternal Pushing during the Second Stage of Labour on Obstetric and Neonatal Outcome: A Multicentre Randomised Trial—the EOLE Study Protocol." *BMJ Open* 6 (12): e012290. *https://doi.org/10.1136/bmjopen-2016-012290.*

Berghella, Vincenzo, Jason K. Baxter, and Suneet P. Chauhan. 2008. "Evidence-Based Labor and Delivery Management." *American Journal of Obstetrics & Gynecology* 199 (5): 445–54. *https://doi.org/10.1016/j.ajog.2008.06.093.*

Blomquist, Joan L., Alvaro Muñoz, Megan Carroll, and Victoria L. Handa. 2018. "Association of Delivery Mode With Pelvic Floor Disorders After Childbirth." *JAMA* 320 (23): 2438–47. *https://doi.org/10.1001/jama.2018.18315.*

Bloom, Steven L., Brian M. Casey, Joseph I. Schaffer, Donald D. McIntire, and Kenneth J. Leveno. 2006. "A Randomized Trial of Coached versus Uncoached Maternal Pushing during the Second Stage of Labor." *American Journal of Obstetrics and Gynecology* 194 (1): 10–13. *https://doi.org/10.1016/j.ajog.2005.06.022.*

Bø, Kari, Gunvor Hilde, Jette Stær Jensen, Franziska Siafarikas, and Marie Ellstrøm Engh. 2013. "Too Tight to Give Birth? Assessment of Pelvic Floor Muscle Function in 277 Nulliparous Pregnant Women." *International Urogynecology Journal* 24 (12): 2065–70. *https://doi.org/10.1007/s00192-013-2133-8.*

Bø, Kari, Gunvor Hilde, Jette Stær-Jensen, Franziska Siafarikas, Merete Kolberg Tennfjord, and Marie Ellstrøm Engh. 2015. "Does General Exercise Training before and during Pregnancy Influence the Pelvic Floor 'Opening' and Delivery Outcome? A 3D/4D Ultrasound Study Following Nulliparous Pregnant Women from Mid-Pregnancy to Childbirth." *British Journal of Sports Medicine* 49 (3): 196–99. *https://doi.org/10.1136/bjsports-2014-093548.*

Boyle, Annelee, Uma M. Reddy, Helain J. Landy, Chun-Chih Huang, Rita W. Driggers, and S. Katherine Laughon. 2013. "Primary Cesarean Delivery in the United States." *Obstetrics & Gynecology* 122 (1): 33. *https://doi.org/10.1097/AOG.0b013e3182952242.*

Bozkurt, Murat, Ayşe Ender Yumru, and Levent Şahin. 2014. "Pelvic Floor Dysfunction, and Effects of Pregnancy and Mode of Delivery on Pelvic Floor." *Taiwanese Journal of Obstetrics and Gynecology* 53 (4): 452–58. *https://doi.org/10.1016/j.tjog.2014.08.001.*

Caughey, Aaron B., Alison G. Cahill, Jeanne-Marie Guise, and Dwight J. Rouse. 2014. "Safe Prevention of the Primary Cesarean Delivery." *American Journal of Obstetrics and Gynecology* 210 (3): 179–93. *https://doi.org/10.1016/j.ajog.2014.01.026.*

Chang, Su-Chuan, Min-Min Chou, Kuan-Chia Lin, Lie-Chu Lin, Yu-Lan Lin, and Su-Chen Kuo. 2011. "Effects of a Pushing Intervention on Pain, Fatigue and Birthing Experiences among Taiwanese Women during the Second Stage of Labour." *Midwifery* 27 (6): 825–31. *https://doi.org/10.1016/j.midw.2010.08.009.*

Diorgu, Faith C., Mary P. Steen, June J. Keeling, and Elizabeth Mason-Whitehead. 2016. "Mothers and Midwives Perceptions of Birthing Position and Perineal Trauma: An Exploratory Study." *Women and Birth: Journal of the Australian College of Midwives* 29 (6): 518–23. *https://doi.org/10.1016/j.wombi.2016.05.002.*

Estrada, Pamela, Laura Tipton, Rylan Chong, Dena Towner, and Kelly Yamasato. 2023. "Associations between the Safe Prevention of Primary Cesarean Delivery Care Consensus and Maternal/Neonatal Outcomes." *American Journal of Perinatology* 41 (January): e1084–89. *https://doi.org/10.1055/s-0042-1760387.*

Kadour-Peero, Einav, Shlomi Sagi, Janan Awad, Inna Bleicher, Ron Gonen, and Dana Vitner. 2022. "Are We Preventing the Primary Cesarean Delivery at the Second Stage of Labor Following ACOG-SMFM New Guidelines? Retrospective Cohort Study." *The Journal of Maternal-Fetal & Neonatal Medicine* 35 (25): 6708–13. *https://doi.org/10.1080/14767058.2021.1920913.*

Keag, Oonagh E., Jane E. Norman, and Sarah J. Stock. 2018. "Long-Term Risks and Benefits Associated with Cesarean Delivery for Mother, Baby, and Subsequent Pregnancies: Systematic Review and Meta-Analysis." *PLOS Medicine* 15 (1): e1002494. *https://doi.org/10.1371/journal.pmed.1002494.*

Le Ray, Camille, Patrick Rozenberg, Gilles Kayem, Thierry Harvey, Jeanne Sibiude, Muriel Doret, Olivier Parant, et al. 2022. "Alternative to Intensive Management of the Active Phase of the Second Stage of Labor: A Multicenter Randomized Trial (Phase Active Du Second STade Trial) among Nulliparous Women with an Epidural." *American Journal of Obstetrics and Gynecology* 227 (4): 639.e1–639.e15. *https://doi.org/10.1016/j.ajog.2022.07.025*.

Lee, Nigel, Meaghan Firmin, Yu Gao, and Sue Kildea. 2018. "Perineal Injury Associated with Hands on/Hands Poised and Directed/Undirected Pushing: A Retrospective Cross-Sectional Study of Non-Operative Vaginal Births, 2011–2016." *International Journal of Nursing Studies* 83 (July): 11–17. *https://doi.org/10.1016/j.ijnurstu.2018.04.002*.

Min, Caroline J., Deborah B. Ehrenthal, and Donna M. Strobino. 2015. "Investigating Racial Differences in Risk Factors for Primary Cesarean Delivery." *American Journal of Obstetrics and Gynecology* 212 (6): 814.e1–814.e14. *https://doi.org/10.1016/j.ajog.2015.01.029*.

Mishanina, Ekaterina, Ewelina Rogozinska, Tej Thatthi, Rehan Uddin-Khan, Khalid S. Khan, and Catherine Meads. 2014. "Use of Labour Induction and Risk of Cesarean Delivery: A Systematic Review and Meta-Analysis." *CMAJ* 186 (9): 665–73. *https://doi.org/10.1503/cmaj.130925*.

Moraloglu, Ozlem, Hatice Kansu-Celik, Yasemin Tasci, Burcu Kisa Karakaya, Yasar Yilmaz, Ebru Cakir, and Halil Ibrahim Yakut. 2017. "The Influence of Different Maternal Pushing Positions on Birth Outcomes at the Second Stage of Labor in Nulliparous Women." *The Journal of Maternal-Fetal & Neonatal Medicine* 30 (2): 245–49. *https://doi.org/10.3109/14767058.2016.1169525*.

Sampselle, Carolyn M, and Sandra Hines. 1999. "Spontaneous Pushing during Birth: Relationship to Perineal Outcomes." *Journal of Nurse-Midwifery* 44 (1): 36–39. *https://doi.org/10.1016/S0091-2182(98)00070-6*.

Shek, Ka Lai, and Hans Peter Dietz. 2019. "Vaginal Birth and Pelvic Floor Trauma." *Current Obstetrics and Gynecology Reports* 8 (2): 15–25. *https://doi.org/10.1007/s13669-019-0256-8*.

Simarro, María, José Angel Espinosa, Cecilia Salinas, Ricardo Ojea, Paloma Salvadores, Carolina Walker, and José Schneider. 2017. "A Prospective Randomized Trial of Postural Changes vs Passive Supine Lying during the Second Stage of Labor under Epidural Analgesia." *Medical Sciences* 5 (1): 5. *https://doi.org/10.3390/medsci5010005*.

Stark, Elisabeth L., William A. Grobman, and Emily S. Miller. 2019. "The Association between Maternal Race and Ethnicity and Risk Factors for Primary Cesarean Delivery in Nulliparous Women." *American Journal of Perinatology* 38 (September): 350–56. *https://doi.org/10.1055/s-0039-1697587*.

Tennfjord, M. K., G. Hilde, J. Stær-Jensen, M. Ellström Engh, and K. Bø. 2014. "Dyspareunia and Pelvic Floor Muscle Function before and during Pregnancy and after Childbirth." *International Urogynecology Journal* 25 (9): 1227–35. *https://doi.org/10.1007/s00192-014-2373-2*.

Thuillier, Claire, Sophie Roy, Violaine Peyronnet, Thibaud Quibel, Aurélie Nlandu, and Patrick Rozenberg. 2018. "Impact of Recommended Changes in Labor Management for Prevention of the Primary Cesarean Delivery." *American Journal of Obstetrics and Gynecology* 218 (3): 341.e1–341.e9. *https://doi.org/10.1016/j.ajog.2017.12.228*.

Weng, Min-Hsueh, Hung-Chieh Chou, and Jen-Jiuan Liaw. 2023. "Women's Sense of Control during Labour and Birth with Epidural Analgesia: A Qualitative Descriptive Study." *Midwifery* 116 (January): 103496. *https://doi.org/10.1016/j.midw.2022.103496*.

Yao, Jiasi, Heike Roth, Debra Anderson, Hong Lu, Xianying Li, and Kathleen Baird. 2022. "Benefits and Risks of Spontaneous Pushing versus Directed Pushing during the Second Stage of Labour among Women without Epidural Analgesia: A Systematic Review and Meta-Analysis." *International Journal of Nursing Studies* 134 (October): 104324. *https://doi.org/10.1016/j.ijnurstu.2022.104324.*

CHAPTER 9: THE POSTPARTUM AFTER-PARTY

Banaei, Mojdeh, Maryam Azizi, Azam Moridi, Sareh Dashti, Asiyeh Pormehr Yabandeh, and Nasibeh Roozbeh. 2019. "Sexual Dysfunction and Related Factors in Pregnancy and Postpartum: A Systematic Review and Meta-Analysis Protocol." *Systematic Reviews* 8 (1): 161. *https://doi.org/10.1186/s13643-019-1079-4.*

Bø, Kari, Karoline Næss, Jette Stær-Jensen, Franziska Siafarikas, Marie Ellström Engh, and Gunvor Hilde. 2022. "Recovery of Pelvic Floor Muscle Strength and Endurance 6 and 12 Months Postpartum in Primiparous Women—a Prospective Cohort Study." *International Urogynecology Journal* 33 (12): 3455–64. *https://doi.org/10.1007/s00192-022-05334-y.*

Chen, Yi, Benjamin Johnson, Fangyong Li, William C. King, Kathleen A. Connell, and Marsha K. Guess. 2016. "The Effect of Body Mass Index on Pelvic Floor Support 1 Year Postpartum." *Reproductive Sciences* 23 (2): 234–38. *https://doi.org/10.1177/1933719115602769.*

Christopher, Shefali Mathur, Gráinne Donnelly, Emma Brockwell, Kari Bø, Margie H. Davenport, Marlize De Vivo, Sinead Dufour, et al. 2024. "Clinical and Exercise Professional Opinion of Return-to-Running Readiness after Childbirth: An International Delphi Study and Consensus Statement." *British Journal of Sports Medicine* 58 (6): 299–312. *https://doi.org/10.1136/bjsports-2023-107489.*

Crockett, Katie L., Angela Bowen, Stéphanie J. Madill, Maha Kumaran, Christine Epp, and Anne-Marie Graham. 2019. "A Review of the Effects of Physical Therapy on Self-Esteem in Postpartum Women With Lumbopelvic Dysfunction." *Journal of Obstetrics and Gynaecology Canada* 41 (10): 1485–96. *https://doi.org/10.1016/j.jogc.2018.07.015.*

Dennis, Cindy-Lee, Kenneth Fung, Sophie Grigoriadis, Gail Erlick Robinson, Sarah Romans, and Lori Ross. 2007. "Traditional Postpartum Practices and Rituals: A Qualitative Systematic Review." *Women's Health* 3 (4): 487–502. *https://doi.org/10.2217/17455057.3.4.487.*

Eberhard-Gran, Malin, Susan Garthus-Niegel, Kristian Garthus-Niegel, and Anne Eskild. 2010. "Postnatal Care: A Cross-Cultural and Historical Perspective." *Archives of Women's Mental Health* 13 (6): 459–66. *https://doi.org/10.1007/s00737-010-0175-1.*

Gutzeit, Ola, Gali Levy, and Lior Lowenstein. 2020. "Postpartum Female Sexual Function: Risk Factors for Postpartum Sexual Dysfunction." *Sexual Medicine* 8 (1): 8–13. *https://doi.org/10.1016/j.esxm.2019.10.005.*

Kabakian-Khasholian, Tamar, Alexandra Ataya, Rawan Shayboub, and Faysal El-Kak. 2015. "Mode of Delivery and Pain during Intercourse in the Postpartum Period: Findings from a Developing Country." *Sexual & Reproductive Healthcare* 6 (1): 44–47. *https://doi.org/10.1016/j.srhc.2014.09.007.*

Leeman, Lawrence M., and Rebecca G. Rogers. 2012. "Sex After Childbirth: Postpartum Sexual Function." *Obstetrics & Gynecology* 119 (3): 647. *https://doi.org/10.1097/AOG.0b013e3182479611.*

Nikolopoulos, Kostis I., and Stergios K. Doumouchtsis. 2017. "Healing Process and Complications." In *Childbirth Trauma*, edited by Stergios K. Doumouchtsis, 195–211. London: Springer. *https://doi.org/10.1007/978-1-4471-6711-2_13.*

Okeahialam, Nicola Adanna, Ranee Thakar, and Abdul H Sultan. 2021. "Healing of Disrupted Perineal Wounds after Vaginal Delivery: A Poorly Understood Condition."

British Journal of Nursing 30 (Sup20): S8–16. *https://doi.org/10.12968/bjon.2021.30. Sup20.S8.*

Skoura, Anastasia, Evdokia Billis, Dimitra Tania Papanikolaou, Sofia Xergia, Charis Tsarbou, Maria Tsekoura, Eleni Kortianou, and Ioannis Maroulis. 2024. "Diastasis Recti Abdominis Rehabilitation in the Postpartum Period: A Scoping Review of Current Clinical Practice." *International Urogynecology Journal* 35 (3): 491–520. *https:// doi.org/10.1007/s00192-024-05727-1.*

Sodagar, Negin, Fariba Ghaderi, Tabassom Ghanavati, Fareshteh Ansari, and Mohammad Asghari Jafarabadi. 2021. "Related Risk Factors for Pelvic Floor Disorders in Postpartum Women: A Cross-Sectional Study." *International Journal of Women's Health and Reproduction Sciences* 10 (January): 51–56. *https://doi. org/10.15296/ijwhr.2022.10.*

Thabet, Ali A., and Mansour A. Alshehri. 2019. "Efficacy of Deep Core Stability Exercise Program in Postpartum Women with Diastasis Recti Abdominis: A Randomised Controlled Trial." *Journal of Musculoskeletal & Neuronal Interactions* 19 (1): 62–68.

Thom, David H., and Guri Rortveit. 2010. "Prevalence of Postpartum Urinary Incontinence: A Systematic Review." *Acta Obstetricia et Gynecologica Scandinavica* 89 (12): 1511–22. *https://doi.org/10.3109/00016349.2010.526188.*

Vandenburg, Tycho, and Virginia Braun. 2017. "'Basically, It's Sorcery for Your Vagina': Unpacking Western Representations of Vaginal Steaming." *Culture, Health & Sexuality* 19 (4): 470–85. *https://doi.org/10.1080/13691058.2016.1237674.*

Withers, Mellissa, Nina Kharazmi, and Esther Lim. 2018. "Traditional Beliefs and Practices in Pregnancy, Childbirth and Postpartum: A Review of the Evidence from Asian Countries." *Midwifery* 56 (January): 158–70. *https://doi.org/10.1016/j. midw.2017.10.019.*

CHAPTER 10: YOUR PELVIC FLOOR ON (MENO)PAUSE

Al-Azzawi, Farook, and Santiago Palacios. 2009. "Hormonal Changes during Menopause." *Maturitas*, Female sexual dysfunctions in the office, 63 (2): 135–37. *https://doi.org/10.1016/j.maturitas.2009.03.009.*

Angelou, Kyveli, Themos Grigoriadis, Michail Diakosavvas, Dimitris Zacharakis, and Stavros Athanasiou. n.d. "The Genitourinary Syndrome of Menopause: An Overview of the Recent Data." *Cureus* 12 (4): e7586. *https://doi.org/10.7759/cureus.7586.*

Bø, Kari, Sònia Anglès-Acedo, Achla Batra, Ingeborg H. Brækken, Yi Ling Chan, Cristine Homsi Jorge, Jennifer Kruger, Manisha Yadav, and Chantale Dumoulin. 2023. "Strenuous Physical Activity, Exercise, and Pelvic Organ Prolapse: A Narrative Scoping Review." *International Urogynecology Journal* 34 (6): 1153–64. *https://doi. org/10.1007/s00192-023-05450-3.*

Carcelén-Fraile, María del Carmen, Agustín Aibar-Almazán, Antonio Martínez-Amat, David Cruz-Díaz, Esther Díaz-Mohedo, María Teresa Redecillas-Peiró, and Fidel Hita-Contreras. 2020. "Effects of Physical Exercise on Sexual Function and Quality of Sexual Life Related to Menopausal Symptoms in Peri- and Postmenopausal Women: A Systematic Review." *International Journal of Environmental Research and Public Health* 17 (8): 2680. *https://doi.org/10.3390/ijerph17082680.*

Caretto, M., G. Misasi, A. Giannini, E. Russo, and T. Simoncini. 2021. "Menopause, Aging and the Failing Pelvic Floor: A Clinician's View." *Climacteric* 24 (6): 531–32. *https:// doi.org/10.1080/13697137.2021.1936484.*

Crandall, Carolyn J., Jaya M. Mehta, and JoAnn E. Manson. 2023. "Management of Menopausal Symptoms: A Review." *JAMA* 329 (5): 405–20. *https://doi.org/10.1001/ jama.2022.24140.*

Djapardy, Veronica, and Nicholas Panay. 2022. "Alternative and Non-Hormonal Treatments to Symptoms of Menopause." *Best Practice & Research Clinical Obstetrics & Gynaecology*, Menopause Management, 81 (May): 45–60. *https://doi.org/10.1016/j. bpobgyn.2021.09.012.*

Dumoulin, C., L. Pazzoto Cacciari, and J. Mercier. 2019. "Keeping the Pelvic Floor Healthy." *Climacteric* 22 (3): 257–62. *https://doi.org/10.1080/13697137.2018.1552934.*

Duralde, Erin R., Talia H. Sobel, and JoAnn E. Manson. 2023. "Management of Perimenopausal and Menopausal Symptoms." *BMJ* 382 (August): e072612. *https:// doi.org/10.1136/bmj-2022-072612.*

Erekson, Elisabeth A., Fang-Yong Li, Deanna K. Martin, and Terri R. Fried. 2016. "Vulvovaginal Symptoms Prevalence in Postmenopausal Women and Relationship to Other Menopausal Symptoms and Pelvic Floor Disorders." *Menopause* 23 (4): 368. *https://doi.org/10.1097/GME.0000000000000549.*

Franco, Maíra M., Caroline C. Pena, Leticia M. de Freitas, Flávia I. Antônio, Lucia A.S. Lara, and Cristine Homsi Jorge Ferreira. 2021. "Pelvic Floor Muscle Training Effect in Sexual Function in Postmenopausal Women: A Randomized Controlled Trial." *The Journal of Sexual Medicine* 18 (7): 1236–44. *https://doi.org/10.1016/j. jsxm.2021.05.005.*

Gandhi, Jason, Andrew Chen, Gautam Dagur, Yiji Suh, Noel Smith, Brianna Cali, and Sardar Ali Khan. 2016. "Genitourinary Syndrome of Menopause: An Overview of Clinical Manifestations, Pathophysiology, Etiology, Evaluation, and Management." *American Journal of Obstetrics and Gynecology* 215 (6): 704–11. *https://doi. org/10.1016/j.ajog.2016.07.045.*

Giannini, Andrea, Eleonora Russo, Antonio Cano, Peter Chedraui, Dimitrios G. Goulis, Irene Lambrinoudaki, Patrice Lopes, et al. 2018. "Current Management of Pelvic Organ Prolapse in Aging Women: EMAS Clinical Guide." *Maturitas* 110 (April): 118–23. *https://doi.org/10.1016/j.maturitas.2018.02.004.*

Gibson, William, and Adrian Wagg. 2017. "Incontinence in the Elderly, 'Normal' Ageing, or Unaddressed Pathology?" *Nature Reviews Urology* 14 (7): 440–48. *https://doi. org/10.1038/nrurol.2017.53.*

Ignácio Antônio, Flávia, Robert D. Herbert, Kari Bø, Ana Carolina Japur Sá Rosa-E-Silva, Lúcia Alves Silva Lara, Maira de Menezes Franco, and Cristine Homsi Jorge Ferreira. 2018. "Pelvic Floor Muscle Training Increases Pelvic Floor Muscle Strength More in Post-Menopausal Women Who Are Not Using Hormone Therapy than in Women Who Are Using Hormone Therapy: A Randomised Trial." *Journal of Physiotherapy* 64 (3): 166–71. *https://doi.org/10.1016/j.jphys.2018.05.002.*

Johnston, S. L. 2019. "Pelvic Floor Dysfunction in Midlife Women." *Climacteric* 22 (3): 270–76. *https://doi.org/10.1080/13697137.2019.1568402.*

Kagan, Risa, Susan Kellogg-Spadt, and Sharon J. Parish. 2019. "Practical Treatment Considerations in the Management of Genitourinary Syndrome of Menopause." *Drugs & Aging* 36 (10): 897–908. *https://doi.org/10.1007/s40266-019-00700-w.*

Mannella, Paolo, Giulia Palla, Massimo Bellini, and Tommaso Simoncini. 2013. "The Female Pelvic Floor through Midlife and Aging." *Maturitas*, 76 (3): 230–34. *https:// doi.org/10.1016/j.maturitas.2013.08.008.*

Menezes Franco, Maíra de, Patricia Driusso, Kari Bø, Daniela Cristina Carvalho de Abreu, Lucia Alves da Silva Lara, Ana Carolina Japur de Sá Rosa E Silva, and Cristine Homsi Jorge Ferreira. 2017. "Relationship between Pelvic Floor Muscle Strength and Sexual Dysfunction in Postmenopausal Women: A Cross-Sectional Study." *International Urogynecology Journal* 28 (6): 931–36. *https://doi.org/10.1007/s00192-016-3211-5.*

Mercier, J., C. Dumoulin, and G. Carrier-Noreau. 2023. "Pelvic Floor Muscle Rehabilitation for Genitourinary Syndrome of Menopause: Why, How and When?" *Climacteric* 26 (4): 302–8. *https://doi.org/10.1080/13697137.2023.2194527.*

Mercier, Joanie, Mélanie Morin, Dina Zaki, Barbara Reichetzer, Marie-Claude Lemieux, Samir Khalifé, and Chantale Dumoulin. 2019. "Pelvic Floor Muscle Training as a Treatment for Genitourinary Syndrome of Menopause: A Single-Arm Feasibility Study." *Maturitas* 125 (July): 57–62. *https://doi.org/10.1016/j.maturitas.2019.03.002.*

Meziou, Nadia, Clare Scholfield, Caroline A. Taylor, and Heather L. Armstrong. 2023. "Hormone Therapy for Sexual Function in Perimenopausal and Postmenopausal Women: A Systematic Review and Meta-Analysis Update." *Menopause* 30 (6): 659–71. *https://doi.org/10.1097/GME.0000000000002185.*

Neels, Hedwig, Wiebren A. A. Tjalma, Jean-Jacques Wyndaele, Stefan De Wachter, Michel Wyndaele, and Alexandra Vermandel. 2016. "Knowledge of the Pelvic Floor in Menopausal Women and in Peripartum Women." *Journal of Physical Therapy Science* 28 (11): 3020–29. *https://doi.org/10.1589/jpts.28.3020.*

Santoro, Nanette. 2016. "Perimenopause: from Research to Practice." *Journal of Women's Health* 25 (4): 332–39. *https://doi.org/10.1089/jwh.2015.5556.*

Santoro, Nanette, and John F. Randolph. 2011. "Reproductive Hormones and the Menopause Transition." *Obstetrics and Gynecology Clinics* 38 (3): 455–66. *https://doi.org/10.1016/j.ogc.2011.05.004.*

Twiss, Janice J., Jodi Wegner, Michelle Hunter, Melissa Kelsay, Mindy Rathe-Hart, and Wendy Salado. 2007. "Perimenopausal Symptoms, Quality of Life, and Health Behaviors in Users and Nonusers of Hormone Therapy." *Journal of the American Association of Nurse Practitioners* 19 (11): 602. *https://doi.org/10.1111/j.1745-7599.2007.00260.x.*

Wolfman, Wendy, Yonah Krakowsky, and Michel Fortier. 2021. "Guideline No. 422d: Menopause and Sexuality." *Journal of Obstetrics and Gynaecology Canada* 43 (11): 1334–1341.e1. *https://doi.org/10.1016/j.jogc.2021.09.005.*

Woods, Nancy Fugate, and Ellen Sullivan Mitchell. 2005. "Symptoms during the Perimenopause: Prevalence, Severity, Trajectory, and Significance in Women's Lives." *The American Journal of Medicine*, The NIH State-of-the-Science Conference on Management of Menopause-Related Symptoms March 21–23, 2005, 118 (12, Supplement 2): 14–24. *https://doi.org/10.1016/j.amjmed.2005.09.031.*

Wu, Chen, Diane Newman, Todd A. Schwartz, Baiming Zou, Janis Miller, and Mary H. Palmer. 2021. "Effects of Unsupervised Behavioral and Pelvic Floor Muscle Training Programs on Nocturia, Urinary Urgency, and Urinary Frequency in Postmenopausal Women: Secondary Analysis of a Randomized, Two-Arm, Parallel Design, Superiority Trial (TULIP Study)." *Maturitas* 146 (April): 42–48. *https://doi.org/10.1016/j.maturitas.2021.01.008.*

Zhuo, Zhihong, Chuhan Wang, Huimin Yu, and Jing Li. 2021. "The Relationship Between Pelvic Floor Function and Sexual Function in Perimenopausal Women." *Sexual Medicine* 9 (6): 100441. *https://doi.org/10.1016/j.esxm.2021.100441.*

CHAPTER 11: WHEN YOUR PELVIC FLOOR IS A PAIN

Cain, Abigail, Kimberly Carter, Christina Salazar, and Amy Young. 2022. "When and How to Utilize Pudendal Nerve Blocks for Treatment of Pudendal Neuralgia." *Clinical Obstetrics and Gynecology* 65 (4): 686. *https://doi.org/10.1097/GRF.0000000000000715.*

Calafiore, Dario, Nicola Marotta, Claudio Curci, Francesco Agostini, Rita Ilaria De Socio, Maria Teresa Inzitari, Francesco Ferraro, Andrea Bernetti, Antonio

Ammendolia, and Alessandro de Sire. 2024. "Efficacy of Rehabilitative Techniques on Pain Relief in Patients With Vulvodynia: A Systematic Review and Meta-Analysis." *Physical Therapy* 104 (7): pzae054. *https://doi.org/10.1093/ptj/pzae054.*

"Coccydynia: A Literature Review of Its Anatomy, Etiology, Presentation, Diagnosis, and Treatment." 2018. *International Journal of Musculoskeletal Disorders* 1 (1). *https://doi.org/10.29011/2690-0149.000009.*

Dharmshaktu, Ganesh Singh, Navneet Adhikari, and Binit Singh. 2019. "Coccydynia: A Lean Topical Review of Recent Updates on Physical Therapy and Surgical Treatment in the Last 15 Years." *Journal of Orthopaedic Diseases and Traumatology* 2 (3): 44. *https://doi.org/10.4103/JODP.JODP_18_19.*

Goldstein, Andrew T., Caroline F. Pukall, Candace Brown, Sophie Bergeron, Amy Stein, and Susan Kellogg-Spadt. 2016. "Vulvodynia: Assessment and Treatment." *The Journal of Sexual Medicine* 13 (4): 572–90. *https://doi.org/10.1016/j.jsxm.2016.01.020.*

Hibner, Michael, Nita Desai, Loretta J. Robertson, and May Nour. 2010. "Pudendal Neuralgia." *Journal of Minimally Invasive Gynecology* 17 (2): 148–53. *https://doi.org/10.1016/j.jmig.2009.11.003.*

Khalife, Tarek, Amy M. Hagen, and Jessica E. C. Alm. 2022. "Retroperitoneal Causes of Genitourinary Pain Syndromes: Systematic Approach to Evaluation and Management." *Sexual Medicine Reviews* 10 (4): 529–42. *https://doi.org/10.1016/j.sxmr.2022.06.009.*

Klifto, Kevin M., and A. Lee Dellon. 2020. "Persistent Genital Arousal Disorder: Review of Pertinent Peripheral Nerves." *Sexual Medicine Reviews* 8 (2): 265–73. *https://doi.org/10.1016/j.sxmr.2019.10.001.*

Lamvu, Georgine, Jorge Carrillo, Kathryn Witzeman, and Meryl Alappattu. 2018. "Musculoskeletal Considerations in Female Patients with Chronic Pelvic Pain." *Seminars in Reproductive Medicine* 36 (December): 107–15. *https://doi.org/10.1055/s-0038-1676085.*

Malcolm, Allison, and Satish S. C. Rao. 2023. "Chapter 22-Anorectal Disorders: Fecal Impaction, Structural Disorders of the Pelvic Floor and Anorectal Pain Syndromes." In *Handbook of Gastrointestinal Motility and Disorders of Gut-Brain Interactions (Second Edition)*, edited by Satish S. C. Rao, Henry P. Parkman, and Richard W. McCallum, 313–27. Academic Press. *https://doi.org/10.1016/B978-0-443-13911-6.00023-2.*

Martín-Vivar, María, Alejandro Villena-Moya, Gemma Mestre-Bach, Felipe Hurtado-Murillo, and Carlos Chiclana-Actis. 2022. "Treatments for Persistent Genital Arousal Disorder in Women: A Scoping Review." *The Journal of Sexual Medicine* 19 (6): 961–74. *https://doi.org/10.1016/j.jsxm.2022.03.220.*

Morrison, Pamela, Susan Kellogg Spadt, and Andrew Goldstein. 2015. "The Use of Specific Myofascial Release Techniques by a Physical Therapist to Treat Clitoral Phimosis and Dyspareunia." *Journal of Women's Health Physical Therapy* 39 (1): 17–28. *https://doi.org/10.1097/JWH.0000000000000023.*

Parada, Mayte, Tanya D'Amours, Rhonda Amsel, Leah Pink, Allan Gordon, and Yitzchak M. Binik. 2015. "Clitorodynia: A Descriptive Study of Clitoral Pain." *The Journal of Sexual Medicine* 12 (8): 1772–80. *https://doi.org/10.1111/jsm.12934.*

Pereira, Augusto, Lucia Fuentes, Belen Almoguera, Pilar Chaves, Gema Vaquero, and Tirso Perez-Medina. 2022. "Understanding the Female Physical Examination in Patients with Chronic Pelvic and Perineal Pain." *Journal of Clinical Medicine* 11 (24): 7490. *https://doi.org/10.3390/jcm11247490.*

Pérez-López, F. R., and F. Hita-Contreras. 2014. "Management of Pudendal Neuralgia." *Climacteric* 17 (6): 654–56. *https://doi.org/10.3109/13697137.2014.912263.*

Prendergast, Stephanie A. 2017. "Pelvic Floor Physical Therapy for Vulvodynia: A Clinician's Guide." *Obstetrics and Gynecology Clinics of North America*, Evaluation and Management of Vulvar Disease, 44 (3): 509–22. *https://doi.org/10.1016/j.ogc.2017.05.006.*

Robson, Kristen M, MD, MBA, FACG, and Barto, Amy, MD. 2022. "Proctalgia Fugax." July 21, 2022. *https://medilib.ir/uptodate/show/2590.*

Rosen, Natalie O., Samantha J. Dawson, Melissa Brooks, and Susan Kellogg-Spadt. 2019. "Treatment of Vulvodynia: Pharmacological and Non-Pharmacological Approaches." *Drugs* 79 (5): 483–93. *https://doi.org/10.1007/s40265-019-01085-1.*

Scott, Kelly M., Lauren W. Fisher, Ira H. Bernstein, and Michelle H. Bradley. 2017. "The Treatment of Chronic Coccydynia and Postcoccygectomy Pain With Pelvic Floor Physical Therapy." *PM&R* 9 (4): 367–76. *https://doi.org/10.1016/j.pmrj.2016.08.007.*

Stein, Amy, Sara K. Sauder, and Jessica Reale. 2019. "The Role of Physical Therapy in Sexual Health in Men and Women: Evaluation and Treatment." *Sexual Medicine Reviews* 7 (1): 46–56. *https://doi.org/10.1016/j.sxmr.2018.09.003.*

Temme, Kate E., and Jason Pan. 2017. "Musculoskeletal Approach to Pelvic Pain." *Physical Medicine and Rehabilitation Clinics of North America* 28 (3): 517–37. *https://doi.org/10.1016/j.pmr.2017.03.014.*

Vural, Meltem. 2018. "Pelvic Pain Rehabilitation." *Turkish Journal of Physical Medicine and Rehabilitation* 64 (4): 291–99. *https://doi.org/10.5606/tftrd.2018.3616.*

White, William D., Melinda Avery, Holly Jonely, John T. Mansfield, Puneet K. Sayal, and Mehul J. Desai. 2022. "The Interdisciplinary Management of Coccydynia: A Narrative Review." *PM&R* 14 (9): 1143–54. *https://doi.org/10.1002/pmrj.12683.*

Index